T0190279

Occupational Therapy for Adults With Intellectual Disability

Occupational Therapy for Adults With Intellectual Disability

Kimberly Bryze, PhD, OTR/L
Program Director
Professor
College of Health Sciences Occupational Therapy Program
Midwestern University
Downers Grove, Illinois

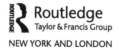

Routledge
Taylor & Francis Group

NEW YORK AND LONDON

First published in 2020 by SLACK Incorporated

Published 2024 by Routledge
605 Third Avenue, New York, NY 10158

and by Routledge
4 Park Square, Milton Park, Abingdon, Oxon OX14 4RN

Routledge is an imprint of the Taylor & Francis Group, an informa business

Cover Artist: Katherine Christie

Library of Congress Cataloging-in-Publication Data

Names: Bryze, Kimberly, editor.
Title: Occupational therapy for adults with intellectual disability /
  [edited by] Kimberly Bryze.
Description: Thorofare, NJ : SLACK Incorporated, [2020] | Includes
  bibliographical references and index.
Identifiers: LCCN 2019038275 (print) | ISBN 9781630912215 (paperback)
Subjects: MESH: Intellectual Disability--rehabilitation | Occupational
  Therapy--methods
Classification: LCC HV3004 (print) | NLM WM 308
  DDC 362.306--dc23
LC record available at https://lccn.loc.gov/2019038275

ISBN: 9781630912215 (pbk)
ISBN: 9781003525301 (ebk)

DOI: 10.4324/9781003525301

Dedication

To my husband, Ron, who always sees the good in everyone. You have made me a better person.

Contents

ACKNOWLEDGMENTS

This book is about occupational therapy and the chapters have been written by occupational therapists. This has been a labor of love and a journey shared with family, valued friends, and colleagues. Many people helped prepare me for this journey, and many have been with me along the way. My thanks go out to each and every person who has contributed to this text, discussed the ideas therein, and is living the good work of supporting persons with intellectual disability. I thank all those who have given their time and presence to individuals with intellectual disability—sitting with them, learning from them, laughing, crying, dancing, and dreaming with them, while recognizing that each of us brings our gifts and vulnerability to these relationships.

I am fortunate to have many colleagues who care about the concerns faced by persons with intellectual disability and take steps to actively make the lives of these persons better. Many of these colleagues have contributed chapters to this text, have thoughtfully challenged the established ways we treat those with intellectual disability, offered their wisdom, and celebrated the vision that we, as occupational therapists, can and should do and be better as human beings.

I would like to thank too many people to name from the various organizations in which I have worked as a teacher, occupational therapist, and educator. I have learned invaluable lessons from each person and each organization. I have seen the transformative power of occupation in the lives of persons who were never expected to be able to perform the necessary daily life tasks, and to derive meaning from doing for themselves and with others. I am most grateful for the L'Arche Chicago community with whom I have been affiliated the past 5 years. L'Arche is an intentional community comprised of individuals with and without disabilities who, through mutual relationships, celebrate the unique value of every person, make known the gifts of those with intellectual disability, and work together toward a more human society. Each chapter in this text is introduced with a photograph of some of the core members of L'Arche Chicago: Jean, Elbert, Christianne, Chris, Noah, Elisha, Dana, Anders, and Tim. Additionally, Tim Stone's original artwork provided the cover design for this book. Thank you, Tim.

I am grateful for the remarkable support of many occupational therapy students who read, reread, and suggested refinements to chapters in this text: Alexandria Barnard, Caroline Hogan, Alexa Kacerovskis, Katie Palmer, Maggie Sompolski, and Kayla Trewartha. These individuals are now practicing occupational therapists who have grown from their experiences with adults with intellectual disability.

I thank Brien Cummings and the excellent editorial team at SLACK Incorporated for their skillful and intelligent efforts to make this dream real. The quality of their work, guidance, and attention to detail has been invaluable.

I thank my good husband who has always supported my professional and personal efforts. He has willingly opened our home in welcome to friends with intellectual and developmental disabilities. I admire his patience, kindness, and creativity. I continue to be amazed at his ability to happily discuss topics of great importance to some of my friends with special interests, such as sump pumps, ceiling fans, and "bingo buns" to name a few. I am thankful for him every day.

Finally, I thank the readers of this book. I hope you learn something new and come to care more about, and for, those who need us to truly see them for who they are and to believe in a more hopeful future.

—kb

About the Editor

Kimberly Bryze, PhD, OTR/L is Program Director and Professor of Occupational Therapy at Midwestern University in Downers Grove, Illinois. In her faculty role, she teaches courses focused on occupation, intellectual disability, and professional development. She mentors students through their qualitative research studies as well as their doctoral capstone projects. She earned a baccalaureate degree in Special Education from Bradley University in Peoria Illinois, bachelor and master of science degrees in Occupational Therapy from the University of Illinois at Chicago, and a doctor of philosophy degree in Special Education from the University of Illinois at Chicago.

In addition to her academic teaching in university settings, Dr. Bryze taught children with special education needs for several years before earning a second baccalaureate degree in Occupational Therapy. As an occupational therapist since 1982, she has worked with children, adolescents, and adults who have intellectual, developmental, and social-emotional disabilities in a variety of practice arenas, including public and therapeutic day schools, outpatient pediatric clinics, early intervention, home health, and residential settings. Her 1991 master's thesis focused on functional assessment of adults with developmental disabilities, and her 2006 doctoral dissertation addressed collaboration between special educators and occupational therapists who serve students with autism.

Dr. Bryze began her service to adults with intellectual disability as a volunteer while still in high school and has never veered far from this first professional love. She now serves as a member of the Board of Directors for L'Arche Chicago. In addition to her academic life, she continues to consult to various agencies, teach workshops and seminars, and practice occupational therapy with adults with intellectual disability. In her personal life, she enjoys being a wife, mother, "cat mom," gardener, and, especially, "Grammy" to three precious grandchildren.

CONTRIBUTING AUTHORS

Meghan G. Blaskowitz, DrPH, MOT, OTR/L (Chapter 2)
Assistant Professor
Duquesne University
Pittsburgh, Pennsylvania

Susan M. Cahill, PhD, OTR/L, FAOTA (Chapter 15)
Associate Professor and Department Chair
Lewis University
Romeoville, Illinois

Ricardo C. Carrasco, PhD, OTR/L, FAOTA (Chapter 19)
Director & Professor
Nova Southeastern University, Tampa Bay Regional Campus
Entry-Level Doctor of Occupational Therapy Program
Clearwater, Florida

Katie Coakley, MOT, OTR/L (Chapter 10)
Adjunct Instructor
Midwestern University
Downers Grove, Illinois

Mariana D'Amico, EdD, OTR/L, FAOTA (Chapter 6)
Associate Professor
Nova Southeastern University, Tampa Bay Regional Campus
Clearwater, Florida

Evan E. Dean, PhD, OTR/L (Chapter 5)
Associate Director
Kansas University Center on Developmental Disabilities
University of Kansas
Lawrence, Kansas

Kelsea Rose A. Grampp, OTD, OTR/L (Chapter 19)
California Children's Services—Medical Therapy Program
Los Angeles, California

Joy Hammel, PhD, OTR/L, FAOTA (Chapter 14)
Professor & Endowed Chair
University of Illinois at Chicago
Departments of Occupational Therapy and Disability & Human Development
Joint Doctoral Program in Disability Studies
Chicago, Illinois

Jenna Heffron, PhD, OTR/L (Chapter 14)
Assistant Professor
Department of Occupational Therapy
Ithaca College
Ithaca, New York

E. Adel Herge, OTD, OTR/L, FAOTA (Chapter 17 and Foreword)
Associate Professor
Director
BSMS OT Program
Thomas Jefferson University
Philadelphia, Pennsylvania

Joy M. Hyzny, MS, OTR/L (Chapter 13)
Assistive Technology Team Collaborator
The School Association for Special Education
DuPage County, Illinois

Anne F. Kiraly-Alvarez, OTD, OTR/L, SCSS (Chapter 11)
Associate Professor
Director of Capstone Development
Occupational Therapy Program
Midwestern University
Downers Grove, Illinois

Lisa Mahaffey, PhD, OTR/L, FAOTA (Chapter 2)
Associate Professor
Midwestern University
Downers Grove, Illinois

Wanda J. Mahoney, PhD, OTR/L (Chapters 1 and 8)
Associate Professor
Program in Occupational Therapy
Washington University School of Medicine
St. Louis, Missouri

Monika Robinson, DrOT, OTR/L (Chapter 16)
Assistant Professor
College of Health Sciences
Occupational Therapy Department
Midwestern University
Downers Grove, Illinois

Alisa Jordan Sheth, PhD, OTR/L (Chapter 14)
Assistant Professor
School of Occupational Therapy
College of Health Professions
Pacific University
Hillsboro, Oregon

Daniel Stumpf, OTR/L (Chapter 16)
Occupational Therapist
Rush Copley Medical Center
Aurora, Illinois

Minetta Wallingford, DrOT, OTR/L (Chapter 13)
Adjunct Faculty
Midwestern University
Downers Grove, Illinois

PREFACE

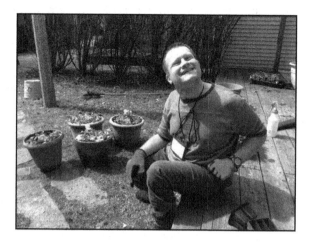

Typical of many occupational therapists, my enthusiasm for serving persons with intellectual disability was embedded in personal life experiences. I grew up on the northwest side of Chicago, and for the first 9 years of my life my parents and I lived in a small apartment in a quiet residential neighborhood. In my apartment building lived one of my playmates, a young woman named Carol, who was chronologically an adult but enjoyed hopscotch, swinging, and jumping rope as much as I did. She and I would meet every afternoon in the gangway between our building and the next and play in the backyard or at the nearby park. I never questioned the fact that Carol was an adult who chose to play with me, an elementary-aged child, or why she was bigger than me, or why she didn't work like my mother and father did. Somewhere in my mind I knew she was "a grown-up," but she was my friend. I never knew that anything was "different" about Carol until one day when I apparently said something in my impetuous way that made Carol angry. She slapped my face. Then she ran away from me, leaving me alone in the gangway. Crying from the physical sting and the emotional hurt, I ran upstairs to my mother. No one had ever slapped me before, nor did I know what I had said to Carol to deserve her expression of anger. As my mother comforted me and wiped the tears from my cheeks, she explained to me that Carol was "different," and that she did not mean to hurt me so, but that she could not always control her actions. The words, and Carol's surprising actions that day, introduced to me one experience of "difference."

Later, as a directionless 15-year-old, my mother informed me that even though I could not yet work to earn much money, I would need to stay busy and productive during the summer weeks. She provided me with a few options for volunteering from which to choose, one of which was at a park district special recreation program with children, adolescents, and adults with "mental retardation." While the term is now personally offensive, politically incorrect, and inappropriate, that was the term that defined the program and described the individuals served. The individuals' ages, abilities, and characteristics varied, as did their behavioral quirks, communication styles, and capacities for participation. The program offered swimming, crafts, sports, games, social time, lunch and snacks, and my role as a volunteer was to help those who needed extra attention or encouragement, preparing supplies and general "whatever needed doing." This first, formal exposure to persons with intellectual disability was both frightening and exciting for a quiet teenager like myself. I was attracted, yet hesitant to become too close with some of the individuals initially. It was hard to understand their speech, and even harder when they were nonverbal; I startled when someone would scream out, whether from joy, agitation, or the compulsions of Tourette syndrome. I was challenged to understand their aversion to touch or movement, and the resultant behavioral responses, when an individual was accidently bumped by another person. To this day, several individuals are held firmly in my memory.

I continued to volunteer and eventually work for pay in the park district program for years thereafter. I recognized the value and inherent good in what the program was attempting to do with individuals who otherwise had no place to spend the long days and weeks of the year. I learned several successful strategies and approaches to working with those with unique needs and characteristics. I sought opportunities to develop creative experiences and opportunities for them to make simple crafts, experiment with art media, engage with music, play games together, and just spend time with them. I sought to make a difference in their world.

I researched and decided to pursue a career in special education for my undergraduate degree in college with a focus on children with "mental handicaps" (another unfortunate term not used today). My mother, then a school psychologist and embroiled in the educational diagnostic challenges within the public school system, attempted to sway me from considering children with cognitive disorders and lean toward those with learning disabilities, who she perceived as being more likely to benefit from special education than those with "mental retardation." One of her attempts to sway me involved a visit to a nearby state "hospital," rather institution, for individuals with significant cognitive impairments. Using her influence, we were allowed into the wards that few ever experienced unless they were housed there or worked there as a caregiver, or were a family member to visit their relative or charge who had been placed.

The ward was hidden, dark, stripped bare, and offensive to one's olfactory and auditory senses. It was a large room made from stone and plaster with barred windows, yet included nothing that was soft, comforting, cheerful, or colorful. Large metal cribs were placed along the periphery of the room, and I walked across the room toward one crib placed next to a window. In the crib lay a woman who was essentially naked except for a diaper and a thin cotton gown that covered her torso. Her legs were positioned in ungainly and uncomfortable-looking angles, and her flaccid arms lay at her sides. Her head was huge, misshapen from hydrocephalus that obviously had not been prevented or corrected with ventricular shunting. Her head and face were turned toward the window, and while I stood there just looking, she slowly turned her eyes in my direction. Not knowing what else to do but, surprisingly not feeling afraid or repulsed, I said "hello." She quietly said, "hi." I asked her name, to which she replied, "Barbara." In the midst of this cold and foreign setting, I naively asked, "what are you doing?" (Alright, I was only 16 years old and my grasp of the obvious was limited in unusual social situations.) Barbara told me she was "watching sunshine"; it was indeed a sunny day outside. I remember thanking her before stepping away to return to where my mother waited outside the ward doors. I told my mother that I was sure I wanted to pursue special education—no doubts.

I did pursue special education, and amidst other life events, like falling in love and getting married, I taught elementary-aged children with mild cognitive delays in a large public school system. My life took a different path after 4 years of teaching, when I accepted a position as a teacher in a private school for children and adults with significant cognitive and other developmental disabilities. It was in this environment that I first learned that there was such a profession as occupational therapy that had to do with helping the children and adults we served learn to do what they needed and wanted to do in everyday life. The occupational therapist soon became my mentor and had answers based on neuroscience and development to the questions I had had as a teacher: Why can't some children copy words from the chalkboard? Why do some children have such aversive responses to everyday sounds? Why does he fall out of his chair when he reaches into his desk to retrieve a book? The late 1970s was also the time when sensory integration was an emerging, innovative practice theory. Although it was, and is, primarily used with children with mild learning, behavioral, and processing disorders, the occupational therapist at this private school was beginning to integrate sensory integrative principles into everyday social and leisure opportunities, designing movement, tactile, and multisensory activities and utilizing innovative pieces of equipment into play-based opportunities for children and adults alike. She had specially designed swings and movement platforms constructed; she enlisted my woodworker husband to construct a large, sturdy ramp on which to walk, slide, scoot, and roll balls up and down. She considered complex activities of daily living from a sensory perspective, exploring gardening as a tactile and heavy work activity that required digging, raking, pulling, and watering the vegetables and flowers. She lent me her books on neurology and development, and recommended to me the classic, blue, book of all books, A. Jean Ayres' *Sensory Integration and Learning Disorders*, which I read from cover to cover several times.

I decided to become an occupational therapist and return to school for another baccalaureate degree in Occupational Therapy. I have since focused my efforts on occupational performance, sensory processing, and the meaningfulness of everyday life in my practice with children and adults for 35 years. Most of these years as an occupational therapist have been spent serving adults with intellectual and developmental disabilities. I never left this, my first professional love, and firmly believe in the interconnectedness of occupational therapy's values, principles, and practices and the needs, abilities, and possibilities for persons with intellectual disability. Occupational therapy holds dear the ideal and promotes the reality of living life to the fullest, embracing the art of possibility for all individuals who seek to live their lives well regardless of cognitive, physical, psychosocial, or environmental challenges. Further, occupational therapy affirms and promotes engagement in occupation by supporting full participation in activities of daily living, education, work, play, and social participation.

With all the goodness, values, and resources within occupational therapy, we still tend to neglect certain individuals who need our strength and skilled interventions. One such population is adults with intellectual disability. These individuals are under- or poorly served in our society today, with limited funding, ineffective policies that attempt to protect, yet delimit the possibilities for, choice and independence, and an unspoken yet recognizable perspective that their worth (or lack thereof) is determined by their capacity to contribute economically to society. It is common for and notable that occupational therapists and other helping professions address the needs of infants, children, and adolescents, and their educational rights and privileges are protected and even supported by funding through 21 years of age. However, in most states, when an individual with intellectual disability achieves the age of 22 years, the policies, funding sources, possibilities for employment and productive engagement, and their perceived value and overall worth decrease. This portion of humanity appears to be largely forgotten. Those who once received expert and valued services grow up to become adults with few possibilities and limited exposure to the professionals who understand and can create occupational possibilities for enriched lives worth living.

My goal in conceptualizing this book is to inspire and encourage professionals who value and support occupation to expand their personal and professional focus to include adults with intellectual disability. There are few books available that address the unique needs of this population, and only one text, published by the American Occupational Therapy Association, is written by and for occupational therapy practitioners. Books from the fields of developmental disabilities, psychology, education, and even philosophy exist to present issues related to these persons from a historical, developmental, behavioral, or neurological perspective. However, there exists a need for a book that is dedicated to an occupational perspective, strengthening our consideration of and belief in the worth of adults with intellectual disability and their need for living meaningful lives that are enriched by engagement in occupationally relevant pursuits. Adults with intellectual disability deserve both the compassion and critical reflexivity that come from an educated and inclusive approach to understanding and believing in the possibilities for this population. This book will foster the development of an occupational perspective for their enhanced quality of life, social well-being, role competence, occupational identity, self-advocacy, and occupational justice. Occupational therapy practitioners and students alike will be challenged to serve and empower individuals with intellectual disability, their families and caregivers toward a more self-determined, authentic life in our society.

FOREWORD

Over 30 years ago, as a young therapist just entering clinical practice, I had the opportunity to work on a short-term project that examined process skills (as defined in the Model of Human Occupation). As a new therapist working with adults with intellectual disability, I was intrigued by this opportunity so I accepted the invitation. There I met an amazing occupational therapist, Kim Bryze, who shared my passion for working with this underserved population.

Fast forward 25+ years. I met up again with (now) Dr. Bryze. We instantly reconnected based on our mutual passion for clinical practice with adults with intellectual disability that never wavered. She shared her vision for creating a book that would address occupational therapy intervention for adults and aging adults with intellectual disability. The book would differ from previous works in this area in that this text would provide a resource for: practitioners who have a vision for advancing occupational justice for adults with intellectual disability; practitioners who seek new, innovative ways to enable full engagement in life and total participation in the community; and practitioners who think outside the box when designing interventions. The book would serve as an inspiration for the next group of occupational therapy leaders who will advance practice in this area.

Dr. Bryze amassed a group of accomplished experts in the field of adult intellectual disability occupational therapy practice and released them to the task of creating this incredible body of work. Through her consistent support and dedication, along with her thoughtful feedback and editing of our words, the vision has become a reality.

The timing of the creation of this book is ideal for the profession of occupational therapy. As we begin the move from volume- to value-based service, occupational therapy practice has wonderful new opportunities ahead of us. As someone who has chosen this book, you now have a valuable resource that will help you navigate through this transition. Well-composed chapters offer current information on conceptual models, philosophies, and perspectives rooted in intellectual disability literature that will help you understand the context of service delivery, which is especially critical if you are new to working in this industry. As you read this resource you will be inspired to develop innovative ways to demonstrate the unique contribution of occupational therapy in the practice area of intellectual disability in home, work, and community. The book provides information on everything from specific methodologies such as the use of technology or peer mentoring to support occupational engagement, to strategies for effective consultation, collaboration, and coaching with other members of the interprofessional team. You will be motivated to create new, evidence-informed, state-of-the art programs to meet the unique needs of this often underserved population in new practice areas such as health promotion and primary care. You will learn strategies to support individuals with intellectual disability and their caregivers as they experience the changes that come along with aging and chronic conditions such as dementia.

You have made a wise choice in selecting this book. May it serve as an inspiration to you as you ignite your passion and assume the role of leader in occupational therapy practice with adults with intellectual disability.

E. Adel Herge, OTD, OTR/L, FAOTA
Associate Professor
Director
BSMS OT Program
Thomas Jefferson University
Philadelphia, Pennsylvania

1

Intellectual Disability and Occupational Therapy

Wanda J. Mahoney, PhD, OTR/L

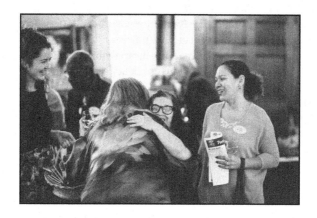

Key Words: adaptive behavior, co-occupation, developmental disability, habilitation, intellectual disability, occupational engagement, occupational justice, supportive environment

Bryze, K.
Occupational Therapy for Adults With Intellectual Disability (pp. 1-9).
© 2020 Taylor & Francis Group.

Adults with intellectual disability have lifelong disabilities that impact information processing, problem solving, and occupational performance. They require various contextual supports to successfully participate in necessary occupations, and occupational therapy can be an invaluable support for these individuals. This chapter will provide a general framework for considerations for occupational therapy practitioners who work with adults with intellectual disability in a variety of settings.

INTELLECTUAL DISABILITY

Intellectual disability is a type of developmental disability that consists of significant cognitive limitations that begin in childhood, are expected to last throughout life, and impact multiple areas of life such that supports are required for their participation (American Association on Intellectual and Developmental Disabilities [AAIDD], 2019). The cause of intellectual disability is often unknown, and individuals may also have additional diagnoses, such as Down syndrome, fragile X syndrome, fetal alcohol syndrome, seizure disorders, or brain injury that occurred before birth or during childhood (Centers for Disease Control and Prevention, 2019). Individuals with diagnoses of cerebral palsy or autism may have co-existing cognitive disabilities, but these are separate conditions and occupational therapy practitioners should not assume that individuals with other developmental disabilities have cognitive impairments.

In the *Diagnostic and Statistical Manual of Mental Disorders, Fifth Edition* (DSM-5) intellectual disability is categorized as a neurodevelopmental disorder (American Psychiatric Association [APA], 2013). Intellectual disability was formerly known as "mental retardation," and is diagnosed in the presence of significantly below average intellectual ability, identified through standardized intelligence quotient (IQ) evaluation and concurrent deficits in adaptive behavior. For the diagnosis of intellectual disability, the low intelligence and deficits in adaptive behavior must be identified in childhood (APA, 2013). Adaptive behavior consists of three major areas: conceptual or academic, social, and practical domains (APA, 2013). Although all of these areas are relevant to occupational therapy, the practical domain most closely aligns with the occupation domain of occupational therapy because it includes the basic and instrumental activities of daily living, leisure, and work (APA, 2013). The severity of intellectual disability is largely determined by the amount of support required within the areas of adaptive functioning rather than by an IQ determination alone.

Severity of intellectual disability is divided into four categories: mild, moderate, severe, and profound (APA, 2013). The AAIDD has criteria similar to the DSM-5 for the diagnosis of intellectual disability, including significantly limited intellectual functioning and adaptive behavior that originates prior to 18 years of age (Schalock et al., 2010). Profound intellectual multiple disabilities is a category to describe individuals with significant cognitive limitations, neuromotor dysfunction, and communication impairments. These individuals often experience co-existing sensory and medical conditions (Nakken & Vlaskamp, 2007). Total assistance is typically needed for self-care. It can be challenging to provide appropriate supports to foster their maximal participation in other occupations.

It is important to be aware of assumptions when working with persons with intellectual disability (Schalock et al., 2010). Limitations in persons' functioning must be considered within the context of the environments in which occupations are performed and that are typical of the individuals' same-age peers and culture. Further, while individuals possess cognitive and other limitations, such limitations coexist with individual strengths. The identification of a person's strengths and limitations is important for developing a plan for appropriate, individualized supports to enhance the person's quality of life (Schalock et al., 2010).

The prevalence of intellectual disability is approximately 1% of the population (APA, 2013). The number of individuals with intellectual and other significant developmental disabilities is approximately 4.9 million individuals in the United States (Braddock et al., 2015). The majority (71%) of adults with intellectual disability live with a family caregiver, with those remaining adults living in supported living arrangements, such as nursing homes and group homes, and a small population of adults with intellectual disability live independently, although they likely require some support to do so (Braddock et al., 2015).

OCCUPATIONAL CONCERNS FOR
ADULTS WITH INTELLECTUAL DISABILITY

Adults with intellectual disability may experience participation restrictions that limit their involvement in life activities. Although they may be physically present in a community or occupational environment, multiple research studies have shown they often have limited opportunities for them to access occupation and social interaction (Amado, Stancliffe, McCarron, & McCallion, 2013; Badia, Orgaz, Verdugo, & Ullán, 2013; Channon, 2013; Crowe, Salazar Sedillo, Kertcher, & LaSalle, 2015; Iacono, Bould, Beadle-Brown, & Bigby, 2019; Mahoney & Roberts, 2009; Mansell & Beadle-Brown, 2012). Each person with an intellectual disability requires different levels of individualized supports to access relevant occupations from childhood through adulthood. As adults with intellectual disability often require contextual and social supports to enact occupations that are meaningful and relevant, they are at risk for occupational injustice. Occupational injustice occurs when conditions beyond one's control prevent individuals from participating in occupations that are necessary for physical, spiritual, mental, economic, or social well-being (Wilcock & Townsend, 2019). Fostering occupational justice for adults with intellectual disability by enabling access to occupation is an important role for occupational therapy practitioners. This may involve environmental modification, caregiver training, establishing routines, and skill development.

Promoting Access to Occupation Through Social Support

Adults with intellectual disability spend a lot of time "doing nothing," which is an occupational justice issue (Crowe et al., 2015; Iacono et al., 2019; Mansell & Beadle-Brown, 2012; Taylor & Hodapp, 2012). These individuals require a supportive environment to access occupation and compensate for decreased abilities in information processing and potential issues with communication and physical skills (Mahoney, Roberts, Bryze, & Parker Kent, 2016). The quality of the support the individuals receive significantly impacts their access to occupation (Badia et al., 2013; Beadle-Brown et al., 2015; Iacono et al., 2019; Qian, Tichá, Larson, Stancliffe, & Wuorio, 2015). While adults with mild intellectual disability may only require changes to the physical environment and a familiar routine to enable their occupational participation, those with more significant intellectual disability often require additional assistance. As another person supports and assists an individual to engage in occupational experiences, they are engaging in co-occupation. Co-occupation is an interactive occupation that requires more than one person (Pierce, 2009). When the person providing support to the adult with intellectual disability has the skills to enable co-occupation, it benefits both the adult and the support person, as they are more likely to find the experience meaningful and reduce the risk of occupational injustice (Mahoney & Roberts, 2009).

Occupational therapy practitioners may have a role in skill development with people who provide support to adults with intellectual disability. Paid staff members often receive limited training on how to offer support, and knowing how to appropriately grade the amount of support for an individual can be challenging. Support persons may also believe that doing *for* adults with intellectual disability is the best way to help, although, doing *with* is more likely to lead to occupational participation and promote occupational justice. Family members who provide support often have long-standing, ingrained habits surrounding the ways they offer assistance. Therefore, it is important to collaborate with the adults with intellectual disability, as well as the individuals providing support to ensure that goals and outcomes are shared by all involved. For example, it is often helpful to discuss how providing appropriate supports to enable greater participation of the adults with intellectual disability often leads to less physical demands for the caregiver, as well as a more satisfying experience for both the caregiver and the individual with intellectual disability. In addition to potentially decreasing staff member frustration and increasing job satisfaction, occupational therapy practitioners can link explanations for change to the purpose and mission of the organization or program in which the staff member works. For family members, occupational therapy practitioners need to acknowledge the difficulty of changing habits and the care and experience provided over time. It is important to determine the family members' goals and link recommendations for change to those goals. This is also essential for the individual with intellectual disability, and when the occupational therapy practitioner provides clear connections between personal goals and recommended changes in an easily understandable format, such as with visual supports, it can be beneficial for everyone.

Although it is likely that providing graded assistance to enable fuller participation for adults with intellectual disability takes more time than doing the activity *for* them, there is another benefit that likely balances and outweighs this concern. Increased participation of adults with intellectual disability often decreases the incidence of challenging behaviors (Ball & Fazil, 2013; Beadle-Brown, Hutchinson, & Whelton, 2012). These challenging behaviors, such as yelling, hitting, or refusal, may lead to stress and burnout among support personnel. Providing graded support and opportunities for co-occupation can foster participation and well-being and decrease stress associated with challenging behavior (Ball & Fazil, 2013; Beadle-Brown et al., 2012).

Promoting High Occupational Engagement

Access to occupation is an important first step, but adults with intellectual disability also need positive occupational experiences. Adults with and without intellectual disability need opportunities for meaningful occupation and to experience high occupational engagement. In this context, occupational engagement is conceptualized as a range of subjective states of being involved or engrossed in meaningful activity (Mahoney & Austin, 2014). As the quality of their occupational performance may not be strong, the depth of their engagement in occupation is an important aspect for occupational therapy practitioners to consider when addressing the occupational needs of adults with intellectual disability.

An individual with severe to profound intellectual disability may find certain actions or activities meaningful, which cannot be clearly placed into a recognizable occupational category. Because what they can do on their own is limited, they may develop occupational repertoires that include actions or activities an outsider may consider to be fidgeting or self-stimulating behavior. However, these may be meaningful experiences for the individual and may serve a purpose (e.g., self-soothing, self-regulating). As long as the behaviors are not harmful to the individual or others, it is important for the occupational therapy practitioner to not attempt to remove these personally meaningful activities from the individual's repertoire.

Determining what is meaningful to adults with more severe intellectual disability can be challenging. Although individuals with mild to moderate intellectual disability may be able to verbally communicate their preferences, individuals with more severe intellectual disability often require someone to interpret their behavioral indications of interest, self-determination, or occupational engagement. In one study, adults with moderate to severe intellectual disability expressed their occupational engagement through their actual physical performance of an activity, focused attention on other people or objects for the activity, and/or expressing positive affect with an activity (Mahoney et al., 2016). Occupational therapy practitioners can help individuals who provide support to adults with intellectual disability to recognize and respond to these behavioral indicators of engagement that may be subtle or challenging to interpret in individuals with more severe disabilities.

OCCUPATIONAL THERAPY SERVICES FOR ADULTS WITH INTELLECTUAL DISABILITY

The primary concern of occupational therapy practitioners is occupation; therefore, it is essential to understand the occupations of adults with intellectual disability. The actual occupations an individual finds meaningful, necessary, and desirable will vary, and it is the occupational therapy practitioner's responsibility to determine the individual occupational needs of a client. The family, staff members, and person with intellectual disability may provide differing perspectives about the individual's occupational needs. Further, the importance of the different perspectives will be based on the setting and reason for referral, but it is always essential to understand the perspective of the person with intellectual disability. Information from significant others is important for obtaining background information and potential insights into strategies for working with the individual. However, information from others must never substitute for understanding the person's perspective. As the receptive and expressive communication abilities of people with intellectual disability span a wide range, occupational therapy practitioners need a diverse repertoire of strategies to ascertain individuals' perspectives of their own occupational needs.

Strategies to Build Occupational Profiles

Asking open-ended questions is the most common way for occupational therapy practitioners to obtain information from clients, and while it is an important place to start, many adults with intellectual disability need additional support to provide information. Adults with intellectual disability may take longer to process verbal information, so it is helpful for an occupational therapy practitioner to pause for up to 10 seconds after asking a question or giving an instruction to allow for extended processing time. Occupational therapy practitioners and others who work with adults with intellectual disability also need to be aware of potential response bias when individuals answer questions. For example, acquiescence, or saying yes to any option, and selecting/repeating the last option provided are common (Heal & Sigelman, 1995).

Visual supports are useful to compensate for difficulties processing verbal information and to address response bias. Visual supports may include drawings, photographs, or objects that relate to the question asked or to provide potential responses from which to choose. The occupational therapy practitioner must consider the physical arrangement of the options presented to the individual (i.e., vertical, horizontal, grid), whether the individual consistently selects the option from the same placement, and how the individual can indicate choices, especially if the person has a co-existing physical disability. Providing 2 to 4 options with objects or pictures is typically the most reliable method of ascertaining an individual's preferences (Heal & Sigelman, 1995; Iacono et al., 2019). Another option is having adults with intellectual disability photograph important aspects of their lives and using those photographs as discussion points (Ottmann & Crosbie, 2013; St. John, Hladik, Romaniak, & Ausderau, 2018; Zakrajsek, Hammel, & Scazzero, 2014). The prevalence of camera phones makes photography an accessible communication method for many individuals with intellectual disability. Ottmann and Crosbie (2013) found that individuals with mild to moderate intellectual disability provided the most information about their lives using a combination of interviews and photography.

Regardless of the strategies employed, occupational therapy practitioners need to use active listening techniques and repeat their understanding of the individuals' responses as the interview progresses. Not only does this verify the occupational therapy practitioners' comprehension, it reinforces how the individual communicates, especially when the individual's communication skills are limited.

Even if the occupational therapy practitioner gains limited information directly from the adult with intellectual disability, going through the process to ascertain the individual's perspective provides a valuable opportunity to build rapport and demonstrate respect for the individual, which is a key aspect of building a positive therapeutic relationship (Gjermestad, Luteberget, Midjo, & Witsø, 2017; Mahoney & Roberts, 2009).

Occupational Therapy in Community-Based Settings

In the United States, many children with intellectual disability receive occupational therapy as a related service in school under the Individuals with Disabilities Education Act. However, funding and therapeutic services are no longer readily available once the individual is 22 years of age. Accessing occupational therapy services can be especially challenging for adults with intellectual disability.

Most services for adults with intellectual disability are funded through Medicaid, and the availability of payment for occupational therapy varies throughout the United States (Braddock et al., 2015; Friedman & Vanpuymbrouck, 2018). In the United States, only 13% of adults with intellectual disability live in supervised residential settings, and only 12% access other formal support services, such as day programs, sheltered workshops, and supported employment (Braddock et al., 2015). Habilitation is a newly covered service through Medicaid and other health insurances as a provision of essential health benefits under the Affordable Care Act of 2010 (Brown, 2014). *Habilitation* refers to services provided to individuals for the purpose of acquiring or developing new skills, whereas *rehabilitation* refers to restoring or retraining skills once they have been previously acquired. Occupational therapy's focus on habilitation may be covered through the individual's health insurance, although most plans only cover a limited number of visits. Occupational therapy may also be funded through Medicaid Home and Community-Based Services waiver programs (Friedman & Vanpuymbrouck, 2018).

Beyond the work with individuals with intellectual disability, occupational therapy practitioners may work with community programs that provide services to adults with intellectual disability. As social support is a major factor in supporting participation and occupational engagement for adults with intellectual disability, occupational therapy practitioners may advocate for being involved with training staff members to set up the environment, provide graded support, and promote group interaction. Whether in a residential, employment, or day program setting, occupational therapy practitioners can work with staff members to foster increased participation and co-occupational experiences with adults with intellectual disability (Crowe et al., 2015; Johnson et al., 2019). Occupational therapy practitioners in these settings often need to advocate and explain their role to service providers (Cullen & Warren, 2013). Due to these individuals' diversity of needs, occupational therapy practitioners may find it challenging to measure specific outcomes of services, so describing anticipated and actual changes is essential (Cullen & Warren, 2013).

Occupational Therapy in Medical Settings

For the last 20 years, the population of people with intellectual disability has been growing. Adults with intellectual disability are living longer due to advances in health care, and their life spans approach those of individuals without disabilities (Coppus, 2013). Older adults with intellectual disability are a relatively new population, and occupational therapy practitioners are likely to encounter these individuals in traditional medical settings, such as hospitals, rehabilitation centers, and nursing homes (Mahoney, Ceballos, & Amir, 2019). Adults with intellectual disability undergo age-related changes at earlier ages than typically developing populations, and the combination of longer life spans and accelerated aging has led to an increasing numbers of older adults with intellectual disability experiencing issues associated with aging and health conditions, such as dementia, stroke, mental illness, and orthopedic injuries (Coppus, 2013; Kim, El Hoyek, & Chau, 2011). In addition, adults with intellectual disability have higher complication rates when they are hospitalized and experience disparities with access to appropriate health care (Ailey, Johnson, Fogg, & Friese, 2015; Kim et al., 2011; Williamson, Contreras, Rodriguez, Smith, & Perkins, 2017).

An occupational therapy practitioner in a medical setting may receive a referral for services to an adult with intellectual disability because of a co-existing health condition, and the purpose of treatment may be rehabilitative rather than habilitative. This may present challenges due to insufficient information about the individual's previous medical history and his or her routines, communication difficulties, and potential challenging behaviors. In a medical setting, it is essential for occupational therapy practitioners to learn their clients' level of functioning and necessary supports for best service provision.

Providing services to adults with intellectual disability in medical settings often involves additional considerations than those factors one faces when working with clients without intellectual disability (Villacrusis, Mahoney, & Bruneau, 2016; Williamson et al., 2017). Evaluation and intervention sessions with adults with intellectual disability often take more time than sessions with individuals without disabilities, which may impact scheduling considerations. Occupational therapy practitioners may need to implement various strategies discussed earlier in this chapter (e.g., providing multiple means of communication for the client; allowing extended processing time; utilizing gestures, modeling, short verbal phrases, and pictures). In addition to seeking information from the person with intellectual disability, the occupational therapy practitioner should attempt to obtain information about the client's communication preferences, behavioral triggers, and typical routines from family or staff members. Challenging behavior, such as aggression or self-injury, may be a way for an adult with intellectual disability to express pain or discomfort, and it is almost always a form of communication (Cronin, 2013; Villacrusis et al., 2016). Occupational therapy practitioners working with adults with intellectual disability in medical settings may need to use picture pain scales or other strategies to assess a client's' pain. Pain tools designed for individuals with dementia may be appropriate to consider and may be more helpful than tools designed for individuals with intellectual disability, which are often targeted to children.

CONCLUSION

Adults with intellectual disability have occupational needs throughout their lives. Occupational therapy practitioners may work with adults with intellectual disability to address their occupational concerns through habilitation services, community-based programs, or medical services. Occupational therapy practitioners can provide quality services by recognizing individual differences and strengths, fostering relationship building, and ensuring adults with intellectual disability have a supportive environment to enable their participation and occupational engagement.

REFERENCES

Ailey, S. H., Johnson, T. J., Fogg, L., & Friese, T. R. (2015). Factors related to complications among adult patients with intellectual disabilities hospitalized at an academic medical center. *Intellectual and Developmental Disabilities, 53*(2), 114-119. doi: 10.1352/1934-9556-53.2.114

Amado, A. N., Stancliffe, R. J., McCarron, M., & McCallion, P. (2013). Social inclusion and community participation of individuals with intellectual/developmental disabilities. *Intellectual and Developmental Disabilities, 51*(5), 360-375. doi: 10.1352/1934-9556-51.5.360

American Association on Intellectual and Developmental Disabilities. (2019). Frequently asked questions on intellectual disability. Retrieved from http://aaidd.org/intellectual-disability/definition/faqs-on-intellectual-disability#. WSboX2jyuUk

American Psychiatric Association. (2013). *Diagnostic and statistical manual of mental disorders* (5th ed.). Washington, D.C.: Author.

Badia, M., Orgaz, M. B., Verdugo, M. Á., & Ullán, A. M. (2013). Patterns and determinants of leisure participation of youth and adults with developmental disabilities. *Journal of Intellectual Disability Research, 57*(4), 319-332. doi: 10.1111/j.1365-2788.2012.01539.x

Ball, J., & Fazil, Q. (2013). Does engagement in meaningful occupation reduce challenging behaviour in people with intellectual disabilities? A systematic review of the literature. *Journal of Intellectual Disabilities, 17*(1), 64-77. doi: 10.1177/1744629512473557

Beadle-Brown, J., Hutchinson, A., & Whelton, B. (2012). Person-centred active support—increasing choice, promoting independence and reducing challenging behaviour. *Journal of Applied Research in Intellectual Disabilities, 25*(4), 291-307. doi: 10.1111/j.1468-3148.2011.00666.x

Beadle-Brown, J., Leigh, J., Whelton, B., Richardson, L., Beecham, J., Baumker, T., & Bradshaw, J. (2015). Quality of life and quality of support for people with severe intellectual disability and complex needs. *Journal of Applied Research in Intellectual Disabilities, 29*(5), 409-412. doi: 10.1111/jar.12200

Braddock, D. Hemp, R., Rizzolo, M. C., Tanis, E. S., Haffer, L., & Wu, J. (2015). *The state of the States in intellectual and developmental disabilities: Emerging from the great recession.* Washington, D.C.: American Association on Intellectual and Developmental Disabilities.

Brown, D. (2014). Habilitative services: An essential health benefit and an opportunity for occupational therapy practitioners and consumers. *American Journal of Occupational Therapy, 68*(2), 130-138. doi: 10.5014/ajot.2014.682001

Centers for Disease Control and Prevention. (2019). Facts about intellectual disability. Retrieved from www.cdc.gov/ncbddd/actearly/pdf/parents_pdfs/IntellectualDisability.pdf

Channon, A. (2013). Intellectual disability and activity engagement: Exploring the literature from an occupational perspective. *Journal of Occupational Science, 21*(4), 443-458. doi: 10.1080/14427591.2013.829398

Coppus, A. M. W. (2013). People with intellectual disability: What do we know about adulthood and life expectancy? *Developmental Disabilities Research Reviews, 18*(1), 6-16. doi: 10.1002/ddrr.1123

Cronin, A. F. (2013). Adults with developmental and intellectual disabilities in nursing home settings. *OT Practice, 18*(15), CE1-CE7.

Crowe, T. K., Salazar Sedillo, J., Kertcher, E. F., & LaSalle, J. H. (2015). Time and space use of adults with intellectual disabilities. *The Open Journal of Occupational Therapy, 3*(2), 2. doi: 10.15453/2168-6408.1124

Cullen, S., & Warren, A. (2013). Reflecting on quality in an occupational therapy intellectual disability service. *Irish Journal of Occupational Therapy, 40*(1), 3-10.

Friedman, C., & Vanpuymbrouck, L. (2018). Occupational therapy in Medicaid home and community-based services waivers. *American Journal of Occupational Therapy, 72*(2), 7202205120. doi: 10.5014/ajot.2018.024273

Gjermestad, A., Luteberget, L., Midjo, T., & Witsø, A. E. (2017). Everyday life of persons with intellectual disability living in residential settings: A systematic review of qualitative studies. *Disability and Society, 32*(2), 213–232. doi: 10.1080/09687599.2017.1284649

Heal, L. W., & Sigelman, C. K. (1995). Response biases in interviews of individuals with limited mental ability. *Journal of Intellectual Disability Research, 39*(4), 331-340. doi: 10.1111/j.1365-2788.1995.tb00525.x

Iacono, T., Bould, E., Beadle-Brown, J., & Bigby, C. (2019). An exploration of communication within active support for adults with high and low support needs. *Journal of Applied Research in Intellectual Disabilities, 32*(1), 61–70. doi: 10.1111/jar.12502

Johnson, K. R., Blaskowitz, M., & Mahoney, W. J. (2019). Occupational therapy practice with adults with intellectual disability: What more can we do? *The Open Journal of Occupational Therapy, 7*(2), 12. doi: 10.15453/2168-6408.1573

Kim, N. H., El Hoyek, G., & Chau, D. (2011). Long-term care of the aging population with intellectual and developmental disabilities. *Clinics in Geriatric Medicine, 27*(2), 291-300. doi: 10.1016/j.cger.2011.02.003

Mahoney, W. J., & Austin, S. (2014). Theoretical perspective of occupational engagement. In *Conference Proceedings: Society for the Study of Occupation 13th Annual Research Conference* (pp. 74-75). Minneapolis, MN: SSO:USA.

Mahoney, W. J., Ceballos, J., & Amir, N. (2019). Occupational therapy practitioners' perceptions about older adults with developmental disabilities in traditional health care settings. *American Journal of Occupational Therapy, 73*(3), 7303345010p1-6. doi: 10.5014/ajot.2019.029835

Mahoney, W. J., & Roberts, E. (2009). Co-occupation in a day program for adults with developmental disabilities. *Journal of Occupational Science, 16*(3), 170-179. doi: 10.1080/14427591.2009.9686659

Mahoney, W. J., Roberts, E., Bryze, K., & Parker Kent, J. A. (2016). Occupational engagement and adults with intellectual disabilities. *American Journal of Occupational Therapy, 70*, 7001350030p1-6. doi: 10.5014/ajot.2016.016576

Mansell, J., & Beadle-Brown, J. (2012). *Active support: Enabling and empowering people with intellectual disabilities.* London, United Kingdom: Jessica Kingsley Publishers.

Nakken, H., & Vlaskamp, C. (2007). A need for a taxonomy for profound intellectual and multiple disabilities. *Journal of Policy and Practice in Intellectual Disabilities, 4*(2), 83-87. doi: 10.1111/j.1741-1130.2007.00104.x

Ottmann, G., & Crosbie, J. (2013). Mixed method approaches in open-ended, qualitative, exploratory research involving people with intellectual disabilities: A comparative methods study. *Journal of Intellectual Disabilities, 17*(3), 182-197. doi: 10.1177/1744629513494927

Pierce, D. (2009). Co-occupation: The challenges of defining concepts original to occupational science. *Journal of Occupational Science, 16*(3), 203-207. doi: 10.1080/14427591.2009.9686663

Qian, X., Tichá, R., Larson, S. A., Stancliffe, R. J., & Wuorio, A. (2015). The impact of individual and organisational factors on engagement of individuals with intellectual disability living in community group homes: A multilevel model. *Journal of Intellectual Disability Research, 59*(6), 493-505. doi: 10.1111/jir.12152

Schalock, R. L., Borthwick-Duffy, S. A., Bradley, V. J., Buntinx, W. H. E., Coulter, D. L., Craig, E. M., ... Yeager, M. H. (2010). *Intellectual disability: Definition, classification, and systems of supports* (11th ed.). Washington, D.C.: American Association on Intellectual and Developmental Disabilities.

St. John, B. M., Hladik, E., Romaniak, H. C., & Ausderau, K. K. (2018). Understanding health disparities for individuals with intellectual disability using Photovoice. *Scandinavian Journal of Occupational Therapy, 25*(5), 371–381. doi: 10.1080/11038128.2018.1502349

Taylor, J. L., & Hodapp, R. M. (2012). Doing nothing: Adults with disabilities with no daily activities and their siblings. *American Journal on Intellectual and Developmental Disabilities, 117*(1), 67-69. doi: 10.1352/1944-7558-117.1.67.

Villacrusis, M., Mahoney, W., & Bruneau, L. (2016). Adults with developmental disabilities: Strategies to address a population trend. *ILOTA Communique*, (2), 12–13.

Wilcock, A. A., & Townsend, E. A. (2019). Occupational justice. In B. A. B. Schell & G. Gillen (Eds.), *Willard & Spackman's occupational therapy* (13th ed., pp. 643–660). Philadelphia, PA: Wolters Kluwer.

Williamson, H. J., Contreras, G. M., Rodriguez, E. S., Smith, J. M., & Perkins, E. A. (2017). Health care access for adults with intellectual and developmental disabilities: A scoping review. *OTJR: Occupation, Participation, and Health, 37*, 227–236. doi: 10.1177/1539449217714148

Zakrajsek, A. G., Hammel, J., & Scazzero, J. A. (2014). Supporting people with intellectual and developmental disabilities to participate in their communities through support staff pilot intervention. *Journal of Applied Research in Intellectual Disabilities, 27*(2), 154-162. doi: 10.1111/jar.12060

2

Health Policy and Funding for Adults With Intellectual Disability

Past, Present, and Future Directions

Meghan G. Blaskowitz, DrPH, MOT, OTR/L and
Lisa Mahaffey, PhD, OTR/L, FAOTA

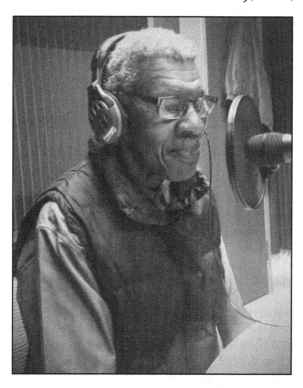

Key Words: Americans with Disabilities Act, health policy, health reform, intellectual disability, long-term supports and services, Olmstead Decision

Bryze, K.
Occupational Therapy for Adults With Intellectual Disability (pp. 11-27).
© 2020 Taylor & Francis Group.

If you have ever gotten married, applied for college, a mortgage, or a car loan, or simply driven to work, you have been impacted by policy. People mostly go about their lives, engaging in their daily occupations, unaware of the legislation or regulations that make those activities safe, possible and organized. Most people are aware that politicians in Congress are crafting, debating, and voting on bills that might become laws. For many, that process remains distant, something that resides in the hands of federal and state governments and rarely trickles down to their daily lives. However, people with intellectual disability must often arrange their lives within the confines of federal and state policies, as policy and funding streams impact almost all aspects of their lives: where they attend school, if and where they can work, how much they get paid, where they live, and the supports and services they receive to live a quality life. Services for people with intellectual disability, including occupational therapy, rely on policies that dictate funding, reimbursement rates, and where and how often therapists can provide services.

The role of public perception on health policy reform is vital, as policymakers are highly impacted by prevailing societal attitudes, beliefs, and expert opinions from medical and educational institutions. The disability rights movement affects all persons with disabilities, but persons with intellectual disability are impacted more than other disability groups due to the high level of stigma they experience, and societal views that perceive them as "less than" (American Association on Intellectual and Development Disabilities, n.d.). Societal viewpoints on integration of individuals with intellectual disability into classrooms, workplaces, and communities have been slow to change.

This chapter provides an overview of significant civil rights legislation and health policies that impact adults with intellectual disability historically, now and moving into the future. It is vital that occupational therapists understand the opportunities, as well as limitations, created by policy in order to be successful in supporting and enhancing occupational participation for adults with intellectual disability.

A History of Intellectual Disability Policy in the United States

The first policies directed toward people with disabilities emerged in the 1800s. Increases in industry, manufacturing, and migration from rural areas to larger cities left people with disabilities unable to meet the demands of manufacturing positions; many became poor and were left to beg in the streets. Societal attitudes were intolerant of the poor and stigma was rampant. People with intellectual disability were considered "feeble-minded" and "idiots," while those with mental illness were considered "mad." As a result, institutions were developed to get beggars, and people with disabilities and mental illness off the streets and out of the public eye (Minnesota Developmental Disabilities Council, n.d.).

In the 1800s, policymakers developed a growing understanding that people with "idiocy" had developmental differences that varied from mental illness and separate structures of care were created for them (Trent, n.d.; Wehmeyer, 2013). Further, the new science of eugenics influenced social policy and the care of those deemed "unproductive" to society. As this "science" gained greater acceptance, attitudinal shifts impacted legislation and institutional action. Some of the most disturbing beliefs emerged regarding who should be allowed to reproduce (and subsequent sterilization efforts), to euthanasia of "defective" infants and adults; the most dramatic period in euthanasia's history occurred between 1939 to 1945 (Hudson, 2011). The medical professionals at that time, also strongly influenced by political powers, contributed to the policies and procedures for managing individuals with intellectual disability within society. While the influences of Nazi Germany and history have been most often reconstructed and disseminated, the effects of eugenics were seen throughout the western world from the mid-1800s until the mid-1900s.

In the second half of the 20th century, humanistic thought began to dominate, with values directed toward the promotion of an individual's right to participate, the protection of human and civil rights for all, the rise of quality of life discourses, and the call for humane treatment. Models of deinstitutionalization were founded on constructs of moral treatment and normalization (Wolfensberger, 1972). Normalization attempts to replicate conditions that are normal for the society in which the person dwells, and inform the foundation of policies regarding deinstitutionalization (Burrell & Trip, 2011).

Specific institutions for people with intellectual disability, called *developmental centers*, were established in the 20th century. Budding developmental centers were initially viewed as places where residents could obtain a "cure" for intellectual deficits and acquire new adaptive skills. However, these institutions gradually shifted from places of recovery to permanent housing for people who "refused" to improve. Tremendous growth of medical-based models made institutionalization the preferred intervention for people with intellectual disability (Wehmeyer, 2013). Families of children born with intellectual disability were often advised by health professionals to place their loved ones in institutions, away from general society. By the mid-20th century, institutions in the United States had grown by 50% and institutionalized populations doubled in size. Unfortunately, this was without additional funding. Conditions in institutions became deplorable and dangerous for residents, secondary to overcrowding and poorly qualified staff.

The 20th century was also characterized by an era of science, professionalism, and classification within the field of disability. Understanding historical policies for people with intellectual disability involves recognition that "intellectual disability" was largely constructed by policy. Classifying people as having an intellectual disability began secondarily to an increase in prevalence and a limited number of available resources to support them, forcing governments to identify thresholds of "normal" vs. "below normal." People with intellectual disability were classified based on their level of intellect, cognition, and social ability. These classifications allowed government institutions to determine eligibility for state and federally-funded resources and to allocate vital services, such as welfare, entitlements, and access to long-term supports and services (LTSS).

Between 1950 and 1980, a parent-led movement demanded better services for their children and sparked the formation of a number of community-based, non-profit organizations, offering a wider range of individualized services and housing options for people with intellectual disability. Many of these organizations, such as the Association of Retarded Citizens (now referred to as The Arc), still exist today.

The 1961 election of President John F. Kennedy and his policy efforts on behalf of his sister Rosemary, who had an intellectual disability, shifted policy reform for people with intellectual disability into high gear. The Kennedy's had a strong influence on the American public's perception of disability. The President's siblings, Eunice and Robert, were credited for their influence in generating policy that opened doors to community living for people with intellectual disability. In addition to leading the President's Panel on Mental Retardation, which resulted in 72 recommendations on best practices and services for people with intellectual disability, Eunice worked toward policy changes that increased access to educational services. She was also instrumental in developing the Special Olympics, the largest sports organization promoting physical activity and social participation for people with intellectual disability, both in the United States and globally.

CIVIL RIGHTS POLICIES IMPACTING PEOPLE WITH INTELLECTUAL DISABILITY

The 1970s were an incredibly important period of reform for people with disabilities, who were demanding equal rights as U.S. citizens. The Rehabilitation Act of 1973 was the first bill to include formal language banning discrimination on the basis of disability. For people with disabilities, including those with intellectual disability, the Rehabilitation Act established requirements for vocational supports as well as protections for employees with disabilities in the workplace (U.S. Department of Justice [DOJ], 2009).

Section 504 of the Rehabilitation Act breathed new life into the disability rights movement and upended the disability landscape. Section 504 states that "no qualified individual with a disability in the United States shall be excluded from, denied the benefits of, or be subjected to discrimination under" any program or activity that receives Federal funding or is conducted by an Executive agency of the United States (U.S. DOJ, 2009). Because of its broad scope, Section 504 influenced almost every aspect of life for people with disabilities: where they could live, go to school, work, and access services to support their daily lives. It also impacted every organization in supporting those with disabilities. These regulations served as the springboard for the Americans with Disabilities Act (ADA; Kendrick, 2007).

The ADA was signed into law in 1990 and was the culmination of a legislative period that began in the 1960s. Fifty congressional acts had been passed as part of this process to improve access to services and environments for people with disabilities so they could fully participate in their daily life roles, tasks, and activities, and achieve more satisfying, quality lives. These acts redefined disability supports, making access to support a basic human right rather than a moral responsibility. This paradigm shift, from caring for people with disabilities out of moral responsibility to legislative oversight, came from grassroots activism by self-advocates with disabilities.

The intent of the ADA was to advance basic civil rights and equity for people with disabilities by improving their access to physical and societal spaces. For people with disabilities to live and work in places of their choosing, they may require accommodations and/or environmental modifications that come with a cost to community workplaces, commercial spaces, restaurants, educational and government buildings, and public transportation. By failing to provide these adaptations, which are now enforced by the ADA, people with disabilities' rights are being violated (Bazelon Center for Mental Health Law, 2014).

THE OLMSTEAD DECISION

In 1999, a landmark lawsuit led to greater access to community-based housing for people with intellectual disability. Two women with intellectual disability, residing in a Georgia institution, filed suit against the state for keeping them in a hospital after they were deemed capable of living in the community, which violated Title II of the ADA. The state failed to provide accommodations these women needed to live independently. The lawsuit went all the way to the Supreme Court and resulted in a ruling known as the Olmstead Decision. The Olmstead Decision set a nationwide precedent that unnecessary institutionalization constitutes unjustifiable discrimination against people with intellectual disability and that all community-based services must be provided to people in the "least restrictive, most integrated" setting (*Olmstead v. L.C.*, 1999).

Rapid closures of congregate settings across the country were caused by the Olmstead Decision and the concurrent Willowbrook Consent Decree, which required New York state to create community-based opportunities for "Willowbrook Class" clients (institutionalized individuals with intellectual and developmental disabilities; Dewan, 2000). Between 1997 and 2009, 36.2% of adults with intellectual disability moved from institutional settings (Centers for Disease Control and Prevention [CDC], 2010) to less restrictive group home settings and supported apartments. Since 2008, the DOJ, state and local governments, and disability rights organizations have been active in a nationwide effort to enforce the Olmstead Decision. Several states, including Oregon, South Dakota, and Illinois, are currently involved in class action litigation or have settled consent decrees with the DOJ secondary to violations of Title II of the ADA for people with intellectual disability (ADA.gov, n.d.). For example, the state of Illinois is currently under a consent decree called *Ligas v. Marem*, a class action lawsuit filed on behalf of 320 residents with intellectual disability living in institutional settings and

4000 residents living at home, all of whom expressed interest in living in more integrated community settings (American Civil Liberties of Illinois, 2011).

Understanding historical perspectives of the civil rights movement for people with intellectual disability is an integral part of providing services to this population and advocating in the fight for more inclusive policies. Although people with intellectual disability still continue to experience segregation, there is hope that, as public opinion shifts and communities demonstrate the value that people with intellectual disability bring, they will attain full integration in work, community, and social settings.

SOCIAL SERVICES FOR PEOPLE WITH INTELLECTUAL DISABILITY

People with intellectual disability are largely supported through social insurance programs, which are designed to help families and workers replace lost income due to unemployment, retirement, or disability (National Priorities Project, 2014). Social insurance programs are largely funded through taxes and premiums collected by employers. People with intellectual disability are deemed eligible for Social Security benefits, including Supplemental Security Income (SSI) or Social Security Disability Insurance (SSDI), by federal statute. A person's benefit is typically determined by how long they have worked and paid taxes; however, in the years following passage of the Social Security Act, a number of amendments have enabled coverage of medical costs for older adults, as well as monetary and medical supports for specific groups, including veterans, federal employees, those in poverty, and children and adults with disabilities.

SSI is a means-tested welfare program run by the Social Security Administration (SSA) and administered by individual states. SSI is designed to provide income to people who are over age 65, blind, disabled, and can demonstrate that their income (or "means") are below a certain threshold. SSI is provided to people who are unemployed or underemployed, and, consequently, have not paid enough social security tax to qualify for SSDI benefits. Unlike the ADA, in which *disability* is defined by a physical, intellectual, or psychiatric impairment that interferes with one or more major life activities, disability by SSI standards is determined by a person's inability to participate in paid work. In 2017, the federal SSI benefit was $735 a month for an individual and approximately $1100 for a married couple if both persons are collecting SSI (SSA, 2017). It is worth noting that disabled couples who choose to engage in the valued occupational role of spouse often lose much needed SSI. Earning income above a certain threshold or receiving support from a family member may also affect SSI wages. This loss of SSI benefits often deters people with intellectual disability from engaging in occupational roles, such as spouse or worker.

SSDI, an additional amendment to the Social Security Act, provides a safety net for workers who are disabled and unable to continue working. A person must work a minimum of a quarter of their life, or 5 of the last 10 years, to qualify for and collect SSDI. People with intellectual disability who work pay social security tax until they reach age 65 or are unable to maintain work that brings in substantial income per month (Laurence, n.d.). Their SSDI benefit amount depends on how much social security tax they have paid to the federal government throughout their work history.

People with intellectual disability fund their supports and services through private insurance, Medicare or Medicaid's Home- and Community-Based Services (HCBS) waiver. Medicaid, a government-funded health insurance program overseen by the Centers for Medicare & Medicaid Services (CMS), funds the majority of supports and services for adults with intellectual disability. Medicaid operates through combined state and federal dollars. The federal government provides 57% to 90% of a state's Medicaid funds through federal matching programs and block grants (Medicaid.gov, n.d.a.), while each state contributes the remainder of funding to their Medicaid program. Medicaid covers a broad range of services for people with disabilities, children, and their parents with low socioeconomic status, and in some states, low socioeconomic status adults without children (this last group was part of the Medicaid expansion that states can opt into under the Patient Protection and Affordable Care Act (ACA) of 2009; Kaiser Family Foundation, 2017). State Medicaid plans are mandated to provide physician, hospital, and nursing home services for people with intellectual disability; however, states can also choose to cover prescription drugs, diagnostic screenings, preventive services, and occupational, physical, and/or speech therapy services.

Medicaid HCBS waivers allow states to waive certain requirements of Medicaid in order to provide services in the community and test new and/or existing means of health care delivery (Medicaid. gov, n.d.b.). The HCBS waiver allows states to use Medicaid money to provide alternative community supports to people with intense support needs who would otherwise be institutionalized (University of Colorado, 2008). In 2014, 53% of all Medicaid spending was on HCBS waiver services for adults with intellectual disability, in the form of community-based residential, day, employment, and therapy services to help them live in community settings rather than in institutions. However, while adults with intellectual disability receive the majority of Medicaid HCBS services, only about 17% of families who support their children with intellectual disability at home are accessing and benefiting from these vital waiver supports.

Many adults with intellectual disability are eligible for dual Medicaid and Medicare benefits. Medicare, another federally-funded program, provides health insurance for people over 65 who are eligible for social security benefits and people under 65 who have disabilities. In 2012, Medicare covered approximately 49 million people (Kaiser Family Foundation, 2012), including those with intellectual disability. Medicare Parts A and B are most essential for people with intellectual disability. Medicare Part A covers hospital services, including inpatient mental health, skilled nursing, long-term care, hospice, and home health services, such as nursing, occupational, and physical therapy services. Medicare Part B covers diagnostic testing, preventive services, like cancer screens and immunizations, and durable medical equipment, adaptive equipment, and walkers (SSA, 2016).

Policies That Impact Meaningful Occupational Engagement

The following policies impact the day-to-day lives of people with intellectual disability, as they engage in daily occupations that are most meaningful to them. These are not all-encompassing; therefore, therapists are encouraged to research additional information on specific policies that may impact the lives of the clients they serve.

Employment Policy

Much debate exists around the impact of the ADA on employment for people with intellectual disability, with most data indicating only a slight increase in employment rates since its passage (Burgdorf, 2013). According to 2010 U.S. census data, the employment rate for people with severe disabilities was approximately 27%, compared to 71% in the general public (Brault, 2012). The rate of competitive employment among people with intellectual disability is even lower. The 2014 American Community Survey found that only 15% to 24% of people with a self-care or intellectual disability were employed, and rates were lowest for adolescents, with only 8% to 10% of young adults with intellectual disability employed (Cornell University, 2016).

Even with strong evidence of the positive outcomes that result from people with intellectual disability working in competitive jobs, supported employment, or customized employment, *The State of the States in Intellectual Disabilities* (Braddock, Hemp, Tanis, Wu, & Haffer, 2017) still reports that hundreds of thousands of people with intellectual disability continue to attend congregate day settings and segregated sheltered workshops. These numbers are unfortunate and do not reflect the policy efforts made to date to increase employment opportunities for adults with intellectual disability.

The disability rights movements of the 1970s resulted in the Rehabilitation Act, which established grant programs to create day habilitation and supported employment programs focused on vocational skills training. This legislation also established funding for research and training in vocational rehabilitation. Possibly the most impactful statute of the Rehabilitation Act was the banning of discrimination in the workplace on the basis of disability. Specifically, the Rehabilitation Act requires that agencies and contractors that receive federal funding, including schools, universities, and public transportation, take affirmative action to hire a diverse workforce, including people with intellectual disability (U.S. DOJ, 2009).

More recently, Congress passed the Higher Education Opportunity Act of 2008 and the Workforce Innovation and Opportunity Act (WIOA) of 2014, both of which established transition services for adolescents and adults with intellectual disability. Transition services include vocational training services and opportunities to access college courses to earn certificates and degrees that will better prepare people with intellectual disability for work. The Higher Education Opportunity Act provides monetary support for pilot projects to create and expand post-secondary educational programs for adolescents with intellectual disability through Transition and Post-Secondary Programs for People with Intellectual Disability funding. As of 2012, 250 college campus-based, post-secondary programs existed for people with intellectual disability, allowing approximately 10% of the population to access higher education. The WIOA requires states to provide person-centered job exploration, work counseling, in-school or after-school work-based learning experiences, self-advocacy training, and counseling to students with intellectual disability during their post-secondary education (U.S. Department of Labor [DOL], 2015). States are now mandated to dedicate 15% of vocational rehabilitation budgets to pre-employment services and to use person-centered planning approaches to help individuals identify their strengths, capacities, needs, and employment goals. Finally, states must include community business owners, executives with hiring power, and representatives from labor organizations on their workforce development boards to further address employment barriers for people with intellectual disability (U.S. DOL, 2015).

An additional aspect of the WIOA, Section 511, helped to shift employment supports from congregate to community-based settings by restricting sub-minimum hourly wages for people with intellectual disability, stating that "no entity which holds a 14(c) Special Wage Certificate under the Fair Labor Standards Act of 1938 may compensate at a wage which is less than the federal minimum wage." In the past, the 14(c) certificate had been the basis for continued support of the sheltered workshop model. With increasing enforcement of the WIOA, the Olmstead Decision, and more states emphasizing "Employment First" (a stance that community-based employment be the first and preferred service option for people with intellectual disability), significant restrictions are being placed on sheltered workshop funding. Many states instead emphasize exploration, discovery, and attainment of competitive employment for adults with intellectual disability over placement in a sheltered workshop (U.S. DOL, 2015).

As is the case with other civil rights and disability policies, policy does not always reflect practice. Although the WIOA and Employment First address important barriers for people with intellectual disability, there are still disincentives built into social systems that impact their ability to achieve competitive employment. One example is income restrictions placed on people who receive SSI. As SSI is tied to Medicaid services, there are limits on the amount of income a person with intellectual disability can earn if they want to retain their SSI and Medicaid. If someone earns above these limits, they are at risk of losing their Social Security benefits and health services through Medicaid. This is a huge barrier for people with intellectual disability as they attempt to obtain jobs and do meaningful work of their choosing. Some recent efforts, such as the Ticket to Work program and Work Incentive Improvement Act, are designed to mitigate these limitations and help individuals' retain their Medicaid supports by increasing the amount of income permitted by SSI/Medicaid and offering buy-in programs for Medicaid services.

Housing Policy

Despite widespread institutional closures, the U.S. General Accounting Office estimates that more than 100,000 people with intellectual disability still live in institutional and congregate settings (Hayden & Kim, 2002), with an additional 60,000 currently waiting for housing opportunities (Stancliffe & Lakin, 2004). The Fair Housing Act, amended most recently in 1988, was meant to make accessible housing options more available to people with disabilities. Most community housing for people with intellectual disability is supported by Medicaid, Social Security, and through low-income housing vouchers. However, this law specifically addresses physical accessibility and requires communities to increase accessible housing stock. In many states, people with intellectual disability access low-income housing options. The U.S. Department of Housing and Urban Development and Section 8 housing vouchers allow renters to pay as little as 30% or less of their income toward rent (U.S. Department of Housing and Urban Development, n.d.). The 2015 National Housing Trust Fund (Aurand et al., 2016) also provides subsidies to building owners who agree to maintain units in their buildings for people with disabilities, with the hope of increasing housing stock for people with all types of disabilities.

With the Olmstead Decision mandating that states provide services in the least restrictive setting, supported housing options have expanded. *Supported housing* is defined as permanent, integrated housing offering multi-disciplinary services, including independent living skills training, employment skills training, coordination of medical needs, and more (Dohler, Bailey, Rice, & Katch, 2016; Bazelon Center for Mental Health Law, 2014). Supported housing is largely funded through federal/state rental subsidies and Medicaid start-up funds, and exists along a continuum from institutional, highly supportive settings (e.g., intermediate care facilities) to community-based, independent living arrangements (e.g., individualized residential alternatives, supported apartments). Many states are working to create an even wider menu of community housing options for people with intellectual disability, including apartments with smart home technologies, rural housing, specialized housing for older adults with intellectual disability, shared living, and live-in caregiver models (Office for People With Developmental Disabilities, 2013).

CMS is also helping states establish more community housing options for people with intellectual disability through a demonstration project called Money Follows the Person (MFP; Medicaid.gov, n.d.c.). Demonstration projects provide federal funds to states to implement innovative programs and then measure the impact of these programs on the intended populations. The goal of the MFP Demonstration Grant is to help states rebalance funding streams, so that a larger share of state budgets are funneled into community-based services and directed away from congregate living/work settings. MFP has already demonstrated a lower per-person service delivery cost with provision of services in community contexts rather than congregate settings. As of December 2015, more than 63,000 people with intellectual and developmental disabilities had moved into the community because of MFP programs.

Social Welfare Policy

Adults with intellectual disability are more likely to have lower socioeconomic status than those in the general public (Emerson, 2013). Adults with severe disabilities, in particular, experience persistent poverty (10.8%) more often than adults with mild disabilities (4.9%) or those without disability (3.8%; Brault, 2012). In addition to low-income housing policies, there are a number of social policies, such as transportation, meal assistance, and telecommunication programs, that help people with disabilities live independently. The Food and Nutrition Act of 2008 demonstrated the federal government's commitment to food assistance for people living in poverty. These policies are not unique to people with intellectual disability, but support people living in poverty with disabilities and mitigate food accessibility challenges.

Supplemental Nutrition Assistance Program (SNAP), also known as food stamps, was implemented to fight stigma surrounding food assistance. SNAP dispenses food and meets the nutritional needs of individuals and families with low socioeconomic status through education (U.S. Department of Agriculture, n.d.). Income eligibility for SNAP is determined annually and based on cost of living. Generally, if a person receives Social Security benefits (SSI or SSDI), they will meet SNAP eligibility requirements.

Finally, telecommunication policies provide basic cell phones and a set number of monthly minutes to people who qualify for Medicaid. Unfortunately, these policies do not include access to personal computers or the internet (The Arc, n.d.).

Family Support Services

The United States relies heavily on family caregivers as the primary providers of LTSS for people with intellectual disability. Over 75% of adults with intellectual disability live at home with family (Heller, 2010). More than 3.5 million families are caring for their loved ones with intellectual disability, far exceeding the number of people supported by state and governmental agencies (Braddock & Rizzolo, 2013). Despite the country's reliance on family caregivers, minimal supports are in place for them. The Arc Family and Individual Needs for Disability Supports Survey (FINDS, 2010) found that most family members of people with intellectual disability spend between 40 and 80 hours per week doing caregiving activities and incur approximately $6000 to $16,000 in out-of-pocket caregiving costs annually (Anderson, Larson & Wuorio, 2011; The Arc, 2013).

The FINDS survey also highlights that caregivers receive little support for their own needs, with most caregivers reporting physical, emotional, and/or financial strain (Anderson et al., 2018). Many find it necessary to give up their employment due to caregiving responsibilities. Adding to the caregiver crisis, more and more caregivers are retiring, creating subsequently less income for the family unit, and many are aging, leaving uncertainty about who will care for the family member with intellectual disability once the caregiver is gone. Despite these concerns, many families continue to provide caregiving services to their loved ones with intellectual disability, motivated by fear of placing them in a congregate setting and dissatisfaction with government-funded employment, housing, transportation, personal care, and therapy services (Anderson et al., 2018).

One HCBS waiver provision, the Community First Choice (CFC) option, provides support to families in the form of additional funding for community-based services, such as home attendant services for people with intellectual disability living in the community who need assistance with activities of daily living and instrumental activities of daily living like shopping, household management, and money management. The National Family Caregiver Support Program also provides families with monetary support for respite care, training, and counseling. However, families are not eligible to receive these supports until their family member with intellectual disability is over the age of 18. Despite recent efforts to increase family support services and funding, parents and policymakers are increasingly concerned about where many adults with intellectual disability will live and receive supports and services once family members are no longer in a position to care for them.

Long-Term Supports and Services

Most individuals with intellectual disability have complex medical, psychosocial, and behavioral health needs, requiring specialty health care and LTSS over the course of their lives. With advances in technology and preventative health care, individuals with intellectual disability are living longer, with life spans almost equivalent to the general public (Heller, 2010; Office of the Surgeon General, National Institute of Child Health and Human Development, CDC, & U.S. Department of Health and Human Services, 2002; Janicki et al., 2002). At the same time, incidence of specific developmental disabilities is on the rise, with autism prevalence alone skyrocketing to 1 in 68 children, a 289% increase from 1996 to 2010 (Boyle et al., 2011; CDC, 2016). Furthermore, diagnosis of parent-reported intellectual disability has increased 17% from 1997 to 2008 (CDC, 2016). This growth combined with increasing life spans has led to an increased need for LTSS among those with intellectual disability.

Transition of individuals with intellectual disability out of institutional settings and into community-based living has also contributed to a growing need for community-based LTSS. Over the last 40 years, deinstitutionalization trends and *Olmstead v. L.C.* brought about rapid closures of congregate settings. This further compounds a demand for LTSS (Medicaid.gov, 2013). From 1991 to 2002, community-based LTSS utilization increased by 19.3% (Stancliffe & Lakin, 2004). Extremely high wait lists for community-based LTSS still exist in many regions of the United States, with over 300,000 people with intellectual disability currently waiting to receive much-needed LTSS (The Arc, 2013; Hayden & Kim, 2002; Stancliffe & Lakin, 2004).

High rates of chronic health conditions among people with intellectual disability also lead them to use health care services to a greater degree than the general population (Walsh, Kastner, & Criscione, 1997). For instance, people with intellectual disability seek emergency department services and are admitted to hospitals more frequently than people without disabilities. A 2006 to 2008 U.S. Medical Expenditure Panel Survey of community-based residents (N = 53,586) found that people with disabilities accounted for up to 40% of annual visits to the emergency department. Other studies of emergency department and hospital utilization among adults with intellectual disability in New York State found that 30% to 38% of adults with intellectual disability used the emergency department in the year prior, a rate 10% higher than utilization in the general public (Blaskowitz, 2014; Janicki et al., 2002).

Each of the aforementioned factors have substantially increased utilization of LTSS and U.S. spending on services for people with intellectual disability (Stancliffe & Lakin, 2004). As a result, U.S. policymakers have identified a critical need for Medicaid reform, which primarily funds services for people with intellectual disability and other populations with chronic health needs requiring lifelong supports and services.

RECENT HEALTH CARE REFORMS

In 2008, public spending on programs for people with disabilities reached more than $619 billion, representing 12% of all federal, state, and local budgets (University of Colorado, 2008). As of 2017, spending on supports and services specifically for people with intellectual and developmental disabilities totaled more than $65 billion (Braddock et al., 2017). With Medicaid spending increasing by 2% to 3% a year (Kaiser Family Foundation, 2015), President Obama's administration and CMS recognized a critical need to reform Medicaid and the health systems that support high-need populations, including older adults, individuals with mental health and substance abuse issues, children with medical complexities, and individuals with intellectual disability (New York State Department of Health, n.d.).

As a result, the Obama administration proposed new health reforms and a series of grants to support innovative pilot programs that would improve the quality of care for people with intellectual disability, but also contain health care costs. The ACA was a comprehensive health care reform that jumpstarted new initiatives for people with intellectual disability and expanded Medicaid coverage to a greater number of people with disabilities and low income (U.S. Department of Health and Human Services, 2010).

The Patient Protection and Affordable Care Act

The ACA was signed into law in 2010 to increase health care access and enrollment for more Americans, improve the quality of care provided, and contain growing health care costs. The ACA has made significant improvements to the lives of people with intellectual disability, particularly in their ability to access health services and receive quality care. The ACA draws from a health care framework called the *Triple Aim*. The Triple Aim strives to (1) improve the personal experience of

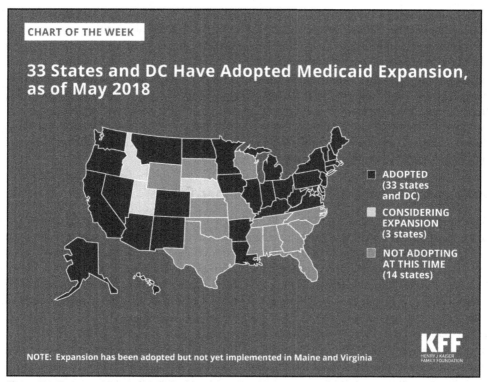

Figure 2-1. States participating in Medicaid expansion under the ACA as of 2018. (Reprinted from Kaiser Family Foundation: Charts and Slides, 2018, Retrieved from www.kff.org/medicaid/slide/33-states-and-dc-have-adopted-medicaid-expansion-as-of-may-2018. Copyright [2018] by the Henry J. Kaiser Family Foundation. Reprinted with permission.)

health care services; (2) improve the health of the population; and (3) reduce the per capita expense of health care (Institute for Health Care Improvement, 2015). The ACA was implemented to improve health care experiences and better address the needs of all citizens of the United States, but a number of provisions have specifically impacted people with intellectual disability.

Many people with intellectual disability are not in the labor pool, have low socioeconomic status, have a high prevalence of health disparities, and lack access to health care coverage and specialty health services. Even people with intellectual disability who have employer-sponsored insurance still lack access to specialty services, as many are not covered by private insurance. ACA provisions allowed more people with intellectual disability to gain access to health insurance by expanding Medicaid coverage. For states who opted in, people with intellectual disability who work and are paid minimum-wage can now qualify for Medicaid. Figure 2-1 demonstrates the states that opted for Medicaid Expansion as of 2018. This allows states to offer additional home- and community-based services for people with intellectual disability through expanded Waiver options such as the CFC program. While approximately 40% of Medicaid funds went toward institutional care in 2015 (Paradise, 2015), the CFC incentivizes states to create comprehensive, community-based services for adults with intellectual disability (Mathews Burwell, 2015). CFC offers states a 6% increase in federal Medicaid matching funds to provide community-based services to people who would otherwise be institutionalized. CFC was designed to help states rebalance their Medicaid monies in favor of person-centered, community-based services, which demonstrate better outcomes at a lower cost (McDaid, 2005). However, as of July, 2015 only five states had implemented CFC programs as part of their state Medicaid plans (Mathews Burwell, 2015).

Under the ACA, the quality of insurance plans also improved for people with intellectual disability due to the removal of the pre-existing conditions clause. Insurance plans offered through the

Health Insurance Marketplace are no longer permitted to turn people away, charge more, or refuse to pay for essential health benefits if someone has a diagnosed medical condition prior to the start of their coverage (Healthcare.gov, n.d.). Thus far, 33 states chose to expand their Medicaid programs under the ACA (Kaiser Family Foundation, 2017).

In addition to these provisions, the ACA ensures that minimum-covered benefits in each state includes access to habilitation and rehabilitation services, as well as adaptive devices that help people with intellectual disability live and function independently in the community. With increased focus on quality care, the ACA also ensures coverage for prevention services and training for direct support staff on how to treat people with disabilities with dignity and respect so that they can encourage people to live quality lives of their choosing (The Arc, 2016).

From Fee-for-Service to Medicaid Managed Care

In order to continue providing valuable LTSS to people with intellectual disability amidst rising Medicaid costs, many states are actively moving intellectual disability service systems from a traditional fee-for-service model to Medicaid Managed Care. While managed care is not a new concept, it has not been widely used in serving people with intellectual disability. Fee-for-service payment systems used by health providers are, in part, to blame for rising health care costs. Under a fee-for-service model, payers reimburse for all services provided. Clinicians can order as many assessments and tests as they deem necessary (even if not always essential) to diagnose a client, with little or no oversight built into the system to deter them (Barnes, 2012).

One key component of Medicaid Managed Care is that each managed care organization would instead receive a per member, per month capitated payment; a fixed amount of money provided by federal and state governments to manage health care costs for a managed care organization's entire pool of clients. These per member, per month payments are determined by each managed care organization's population of clients served, their health needs, and combined health risks. This payment plan aims to rid the health care system of wasteful spending and disincentivize organizations from providing unnecessary, high-cost services to people within their networks, including people with intellectual disability. Agencies that provide services to people with intellectual disability within a managed care network are mandated to collect and track health and quality of life outcomes data on the clients they serve. Using an incentive-based model, agencies found to provide high-quality services to people with intellectual disability and decrease unnecessary service utilization will be rewarded with additional monies and/or higher reimbursement rates (CMS, 2016). A number of states with Medicaid Managed Care options have already demonstrated cost savings (The Lewin Group, 2004), while others have inconclusive results. One certainty is that redesigning Medicaid will require major reform to multiple, intertwined health systems, and will likely take years to effectively implement.

Innovative Affordable Care Act Approaches for People With Intellectual Disability

The ACA made available additional grant funds to states and non-profit provider agencies to pilot innovative, cost-saving demonstration projects for people with intellectual disability in preparation for the transition to managed care. Some interventions have shown preliminary positive outcomes including use of the patient-centered medical home (PCMH) and accountable care organization (ACO) models, care coordination, population health standardized assessments, behavioral health programs, and chronic disease prevention and health management programs for people with intellectual disability (The Lewin Group, 2004; Peter et al., 2011). Some of these programs are highlighted in the following section.

PCMHs and ACOs are two program-level interventions that foster community partnerships between hospitals, non-profit agencies, rehabilitation professionals, and mental/behavioral health organizations through use of special liaisons called *care coordinators*. Care coordinators perform individualized assessments of people with intellectual disability and develop comprehensive, integrated care plans, liaise between community primary care physicians, specialists, hospitals, the patient, and his or her family, and ensure that all necessary services and medications are provided. PCMHs and ACOs using care coordination have begun to demonstrate improved quality and continuity of care, as well as cost savings through improved health management and reduction of emergency department visits and hospital admissions (Academy Health Panel, 2012; Counsell et al., 2007). If PCMH and ACO programs meet quality benchmarks and save on health expenditures, they receive incentives that can be distributed to all partners and reinvested in program operations (CMS, 2011). The first ACO for people with intellectual disability who have dual Medicare/Medicaid eligibility was launched in New York State in 2014. If this pilot increases the quality of intellectual disability services while saving money, it may be a highly effective solution to sustaining LTSS for people with intellectual disability (Karon et al., 2019).

New behavioral health programs, such as the Systemic Therapeutic Assessment, Respite, and Treatment (START) model, are also being piloted for prevention of mental health crises among people with intellectual disability who have co-occuring mental illnesses (Center for START Services, 2013). With up to 40% of persons with intellectual disability having a mental illness, behavioral health models are especially vital and gaining recognition (Razzano et al., 2015). They provide individualized prevention plans, regular mental health supports, cross-systems communication between mental health providers, short-term and emergency respite, and round-the-clock telephone and in-person response systems to people and their families during crisis events. Tennessee, North Carolina, Virginia, and New York have all begun using START behavioral health programs for people with intellectual disability and have seen cost savings and decreased psychiatric hospitalizations (Center for START Services, 2013). North Carolina found that, when utilizing START, 66% of people with intellectual disability remained in their homes rather than utilizing the emergency department or emergency respite (North Carolina START, 2010).

Person-directed services, or self-direction models, are also gaining popularity across many states. Self-direction offers people with intellectual disability maximum flexibility and control over their lives by providing them budget authority control over how they spend their Medicaid funds on supports and services and employer authority control over choosing, hiring, and firing staff who support them in habilitation, life skills training, and employment (In the Driver's Seat, n.d.). Research on self-directed services has already begun to demonstrate a positive impact of people with intellectual disability, including greater flexibility in their daily schedules, greater satisfaction with their supports, services, and staff, and a higher overall quality of life (Alakeson, 2007).

The Future of Intellectual Disability Health Reform

The U.S. health care system is a complex, ever-changing landscape. Health policies change rapidly and are heavily dependent on sociopolitical forces, advocacy, and the ideology of the current political administration. With an administration change in early 2017, and the threat to "repeal or replace" the ACA, some estimates predict that 12.9 million people could lose their Medicaid coverage (Blumberg, Buettgens & Holahan, 2016). Replacement options propose that the federal government provide states with Medicaid block grants or per capita lump sums to manage all of the needs of their Medicaid recipients. However, if these lump sums fail to provide adequate funding for the needs of a state's constituents with intellectual disability, due to increases in enrollment, increases in enrollee health needs, or an aging population, the state will need to make up the difference and make tough choices about who should be eligible to receive much-needed coverage. These changes could greatly impact insurance access and the health and quality of life of people with intellectual disability.

It is critical that self-advocates, the intellectual disability community, and support professionals, including occupational therapists, remain vigilant in their advocacy and outreach efforts, especially on behalf of those who struggle with self advocacy. Eliminating the ACA, without simultaneously replacing it with a coordinated, functional alternative, jeopardizes the civil rights of people with intellectual disability and puts equal access to comprehensive, affordable health care at grave risk.

Policy Matters to Occupational Therapists

Occupational therapists' role in supporting adults with intellectual disability in daily life skills, and their hopes and dreams for the future, is influenced by health policy and demands that occupational therapists understand the power these policies have on a person's ability to engage in meaningful occupations of their choosing. Reflection on policy issues and an understanding of how they impact clients' school, work, community, health, and social lives is critical to occupational therapy practice.

Many resources people use every day are regulated at the state level, and each state has its own legislative processes surrounding policy and funding for people with intellectual disability. Therapists are encouraged to research and understand their own state intellectual disability policies and use the resources available to them including the Arc, the American Occupational Therapy Association, the American Occupational Therapy Association Legislative Action Center (American Occupational Therapy Association, n.d.), and their state occupational therapy associations. Occupational therapy practitioners can benefit from forming advocacy networks with each other, and with other self-advocates, family caregivers, non-profit providers, and state agencies who serve people with intellectual disability, in order to protect reimbursement of their occupational therapy services, the livelihood of the people they serve, and to navigate the ever-changing policy landscape.

CONCLUSION

The history of disability rights legislation, including the passage of the ADA, Olmstead Decision and ACA, have all greatly impacted equal rights, inclusion, access to health care, and quality of life for people with intellectual disability. However, many disparities still exist for this community in the areas of employment, health, housing, and social inclusion. Self-advocates and a system of health care agencies and professionals who support people with intellectual disability are working to make positive strides in health policy, funding, and improved access to innovative programs designed to improve quality outcomes for this population.

While this chapter focuses heavily on health policy and funding, occupational therapists are encouraged to always think of the person at the heart of these issues—an individual with unique talents and a voice that deserves our constant consideration and advocacy as we provide occupational therapy services and design future health systems with and for people with intellectual disability.

REFERENCES

Academy Health Panel. (2012). What works in care coordination? Activities to reduce spending in Medicare fee-for-service. Retrieved from www.academyhealth.org/sites/default/files/publications/files/RICareCoordination.pdf

ADA.gov. (n.d.). Olmstead Enforcement: Olmstead Litigation in the 12 U.S. Circuit Courts of Appeals. Retrieved from www.ada.gov/olmstead/olmstead_enforcement.htm

Alakeson, V. (2007). The contribution of self-direction to improving the quality of mental health services. Office of the Assistant Secretary for Planning and Evaluation. Retrieved from https://aspe.hhs.gov/basic-report/contribution-self-direction-improving-quality-mental-health-services#satisfy

American Association on Intellectual and Development Disabilities. (n.d.). Definition of intellectual disability. Retrieved from http://aaidd.org/intellectual-disability/definition#.V3VUvuswhD8

American Civil Liberties Union of Illinois. (2011). Williams v. Quinn fact sheet. Retrieved from http://www.aclu-il.org/wp-content/uploads/2011/02/Fact-Sheet-on-Williams-v-Quinn-10-1-10.pdf

Americans with Disabilities Act. (2010). Retrieved from www.ada.gov/pubs/adastatute08.pdf

American Occupational Therapy Association. (n.d.) AOTA legislative action center. Retrieved from www.aota.org/takeaction

Anderson, L., Hewitt, A., Pettingell, S., Lulinski, A., Taylor, M., & Reagan, J. (2018) *Family and individual needs for disability supports (V. 2) community report 2017.* Research and Training Center on Community Living, Institute on Community Integration, University of Minnesota. Retrieved from https://ici.umn.edu/products/docs/FINDS_survey_2018.pdf

The Arc. (n.d.a.). The Affordable Care Act: What disability advocates need to know. Retrieved from http://www.thearcppr.org/wp-content/uploads/2015/03/The-Affordable-Care-Act.pdf

The Arc. (n.d.b.). Long term services and supports. Retrieved from http://www.thearc.org/what-we-do/public-policy/policy-issues/long-term

The Arc. (2013). Long term services and supports (LTSS) issues for people with disabilities. Retrieved from http://www.thearc.org/page.aspx?pid=2640

The Arc. (2016). How people with intellectual and/or developmental disabilities (I/DD) benefit from the Affordable Care Act (ACA). Retrieved from www.thearc.org/document.doc?id=5647

Aurand, A., Emmanuel, D., Crowley Errico, E., Leong, G. M., & Rodrigues, K. (2016). *The affordable housing GAP analysis 2016.* Washington, D.C.: The National Low Income Housing Coalition.

Barnes, J. (2012). Moving away from fee-for-service. *The Atlantic.* Retrieved from www.theatlantic.com/health/archive/2012/05/moving-away-from-fee-for-service/256755

Bazelon Center for Mental Health Law. (2014). A place of my own: How the ADA is creating integrated housing opportunities for people with mental illness. Retrieved from www.bazelon.org/portals/0/Where We Stand/CommunityIntegration/Olmstead/A Place of My Own. Bazelon Center for Mental HealthLaw.pdf.

Blaskowitz, M. G. (2014). Predictors of emergency room and hospital utilization among adults with intellectual disabilities (ID) in New York City. Retrieved from http://www.manhattanddcouncil.org/wp-content/uploads/Presentation-DD-Council-12.11.14.pdf

Blumberg, L., Buettgens, M., & Holahan, J. (2016). Implications of partial repeal of the ACA through reconciliation. The Urban Institute. Retrieved from http://www.urban.org/research/publication/implications-partial-repeal-aca-through-reconciliation

Boyle, C. A., Boulet, S., Schieve, L. A., Cohen, R. A., Blumberg, S. J., Yeargin-Allsopp, M., … Kogan, M. D. (2011). Trends in the prevalence of developmental disabilities in U.S. children, 1997-2008. *Pediatrics, 127*(6), 1034-1042. doi: 10.1542/peds.2010-2989

Braddock, D. L., Hemp, R. E., Tanis, E. S., Wu, J., & Haffer, L. (2017). *The state of the States in intellectual and developmental disabilities: 2017.* Boulder, CO: University of Colorado, Coleman Institute for Cognitive Disabilities, Department of Psychiatry.

Braddock, D., & Rizzolo, M. K. (2013). Intellectual disabilities services in the U.S.: 2013. [PowerPoint Slides]. Retrieved from www.researchgate.net/publication/309493631_Intellectual_and_Developmental_Disabilities_Services_in_the_United_States_2013

Brault, M. W. (2012). Americans with disabilities: Household economic studies. United States Census Bureau. Retrieved from http://www.census.gov/prod/2012pubs/p70-131.pdf

Burgdorf, R. L. (2013). A promising start: Preliminary analysis of court decisions under the ADA amendments act. National Council on Disability. Retrieved from http://www.ncd.gov/publications/2013/07232013/

Centers for Disease Control and Prevention. (2010). Healthy People 2010: Disability and secondary conditions. Retrieved from www.cdc.gov/nchs/data/hpdata2010/hp2010_final_review_focus_area_06.pdf

Centers for Disease Control and Prevention. (2016). Key findings: Trends in the prevalence of developmental disabilities in U. S. children, 1997–2008. Retrieved from https://www.cdc.gov/ncbddd/developmentaldisabilities/features/birth-defects-dd-keyfindings.html.

Centers for Medicare & Medicaid Services. (n.d.a.). Community First Choice 1915 (k). Retrieved from http://www.medicaid.gov/medicaid-chip-program-information/by-topics/long-term-services-and-supports/home-and-community-based-services/community-first-choice-1915-k.html

Centers for Medicare & Medicaid Services. (n.d.b.). Your Medicare coverage choices. Retrieved from https://www.medicare.gov/sign-up-change-plans/decide-how-to-get-medicare/your-medicare-coverage-choices.html#collapse-313

Centers for Medicare & Medicaid Services. (2011). What providers need to know: Accountable Care Organizations. Retrieved from www.cms.gov/newsroom/fact-sheets/what-providers-need-know-accountable-care-organizations

Centers for Medicare & Medicaid Services. (2016). Quality payment program. Retrieved from https://qpp.cms.gov

Center for START Services. (2013). A systems linkage approach: START. Retrieved from http://www.centerforstartservices.com/Files/NewsEvents/START_Presentation_Indiana_2013jbb%20edit3.pdf

Cornell University. (2016). Disability statistics. Retrieved from https://www.disabilitystatistics.org

Counsell, S. R., Callahan, C. M., Clark, D. O., Tu, W., Buttar, A. B., Stump, T. E., & Ricketts, G. D. (2007). Geriatric care management for low-income seniors: A randomized controlled trial. *Journal of the American Medical Association, 298*(22), 2623-2633.

Dewan, S. K. (2000). Recalling a victory for the disabled. *The New York Times.* Retrieved from www.nytimes.com/2000/05/03/nyregion/recalling-a-victory-for-the-disabled.html

Dohler, E., Bailey, P., Rice, D., & Katch, H. (2016). Supportive housing helps vulnerable live and thrive in the community. Center on Budget and Policy Priorities. Retrieved from http://www.cbpp.org/research/housing/supportive-housing-helps-vulnerable-people-live-and-thrive-in-the-community

Emerson, E. (2013). Commentary: Childhood exposure to environmental adversity and the well-being of people with intellectual disabilities. *Journal of Intellectual Disability Research, 57*(7), 589-600.

Hayden, M. F., & Kim, S. H. (2002). Health status, health care utilization patterns, and health care outcomes of persons with intellectual disabilities: A review of the literature. *Policy Research Brief (University of Minnesota: Minneapolis, Institute on Community Integration).* Retrieved from https://ici.umn.edu/products/view/81

HealthCare.gov. (n.d.). Coverage for pre-existing conditions. Retrieved from https://www.healthcare.gov/coverage/pre-existing-conditions

Heller, T. (2010). People with intellectual disabilities growing old: An overview. *Impact, 23*(1), 1-36.

Hudson, L. (2011). From small beginnings: The euthanasia of children with disabilities in Nazi Germany. *Journal of Paediatrics and Child Health, 47,* 508-511.

Institute for Healthcare Improvement. (2015). The IHI Triple Aim initiative. Retrieved from www.ihi.org/Engage/Initiatives/TripleAim/pages/default.aspx

In the Driver's Seat. (n.d.). What is self-direction? Retrieved from http://inthedriversseat.org/what-is-self-direction/

Janicki, M. P., Davidson, P. W., Henderson, C. M., McCallion, P., Taets, J. D., Force, L. T., … Ladrigan, P. M. (2002). Health characteristics and health services utilization in older adults with intellectual disability living in community residences. *Journal of Intellectual Disability Research, 46*(4), 287-298.

Kaiser Family Foundation. (2012). *Total number of Medicare beneficiaries.* Retrieved from http://kff.org/medicare/state-indicator/total-medicare-beneficiaries

Kaiser Family Foundation. (2015). Medicaid enrollment and spending growth: FY 2015 & 2016. Retrieved from http://kff.org/medicaid/issue-brief/medicaid-enrollment-spending-growth-fy-2015-2016/.

Kaiser Family Foundation. (2017). Status of state action on the medicaid expansion decision. Retrieved from https://www.kff.org/health-reform/state-indicator/state-activity-around-expanding-medicaid-under-the-affordable-care-act/?currentTimeframe=0&sortModel=%7B%22colId%22:%22Location%22,%22sort%22:%22asc%22%7D

Karon, S. L., Knowles, M., Lyda-McDonald, B., Thach, N., Wiener, J. M., Justice, D., … Sowers, M. (2019). Final outcome evaluation of the balancing incentive program. Retrieved from https://aspe.hhs.gov/basic-report/final-outcome-evaluation-balancing-incentive-program.

Kendrick, D. (2007). The sit-in that ended segregation of the disabled. *Cincinnati City Beat.* Retrieved from http://citybeat.com/cincinnati/print-article-2503-print.html#

Laurence, B. (n.d.). What is substantial gainful activity (SGA) for social security disability purposes. *Disability Secrets.* Retrieved from http://www.disabilitysecrets.com/sga.html

The Lewin Group. (2004). *Medicaid managed care cost savings—A synthesis of fourteen studies: Final report.* Falls Church, VA: Lewin Group for America's Health Insurance Plans

Mathews Burwell, S. (2015). *Community first choice: Final report to Congress as required by the Patient Protection and Affordable Care Act of 2010 (P.L. 111-148) from the Department of Health and Human Services Office of the Secretary.* Retrieved from ww.advancingstates.org/sites/nasuad/files/Community%20First%20Choice.pdf

McDaid, D. (2005). Mental health II: Balancing institutional and community-based care. World Health Organization. Retrieved from http://www.euro.who.int/__data/assets/pdf_file/0007/108952/E85488.pdf

Medicaid.gov (n.d.a.). Financing and reimbursement. Retrieved from http://www.medicaid.gov/medicaid-chip-program-information/by-topics/financing-and-reimbursement/financing-and-reimbursement.html

Medicaid.gov (n.d.b.). Home and community-based services 1915(C). Retrieved from https://www.medicaid.gov/medicaid/hcbs/authorities/1915-c/index.html

Medicaid.gov (n.d.c.). Money follows the person (MFP). Retrieved from http://www.medicaid.gov/Medicaid-CHIP-Program-Information/By-Topics/Long-Term-Services-and-Supports/Balancing/Money-Follows-the-Person.html

Medicaid.gov (2013). Long-term services & supports. Retrieved from http://www.medicaid.gov/Medicaid-CHIP-Program-Information/By-Topics/Long-Term Services-and-Support/Long-Term-Services-and-Support.html

Minnesota Developmental Disabilities Council. (n.d.). Parallels in time: A history of developmental disabilities (Part one: The ancient era to the 1950s). Retrieved from http://mn.gov/mnddc/parallels/index.html

National Priorities Project. (2014). Federal budget tip sheet: Social insurance and earned benefits. Retrieved from https://media.nationalpriorities.org/uploads/publications/social insurance.tipsheet.9_23_14.pdf

New York State Department of Health. (n.d.). A plan to transform the empire state's medicaid program. Retrieved from https://www.health.ny.gov/health_care/medicaid/redesign/docs/mrtfinalreport.pdf

North Carolina START. (2010). North Carolina Systemic, Therapeutic, Assessment, Respite, and Treatment program (NC START) annual report. Retrieved from http://www.iod.unh.edu/pdf/START/Annual_report_NC_START_final.pdf

Office for People with Developmental Disabilities. (2013). Services & supports. Retrieved from www.opwdd.ny.gov/opwdd_services_supports/home

Office of the Surgeon General, National Institute of Child Health and Human Development, Centers for Disease Control and Prevention, & U.S. Department of Health and Human Services. (2002). Closing the gap: A national blueprint to improve the health of persons with mental retardation: Report of the Surgeon General's conference on health disparities and mental retardation. Retrieved from www.ncbi.nlm.nih.gov/books/NBK44354

Olmstead V. L. C. (98-536). 527 U.S. 581. (1999).138 F.3d 893.

Paradise, J. (2015). Medicaid moving forward. *Kaiser Family Foundation.* Retrieved from http://kff.org/health-reform/issue-brief/medicaid-moving-forward

Peter, S., Chaney, G., Zappia, T., van Veldhuisen, C., Pereira, S., & Santamaria, N. (2011). Care coordination for children with complex care needs significantly reduces hospital utilization. *Journal for Specialists in Pediatric Nursing, 16,* 305-312.

Razzano, L. A., Cook, J. A., Yost, C., Jonikas, J. A., Swarbrick, M. A., Carter, T. M., & Santos, A. (2015). Factors associated with co-occurring medical conditions among adults with serious mental disorders. *Schizophrenia Research, 161*(2-3), 458-464. doi:10.1016/j.schres.2014.11.021

Social Security Administration. (2016). Medicare. Retrieved from https://www.ssa.gov/pubs/EN-05-10043.pdf

Social Security Administration. (2017). SSI federal payment amounts. Retrieved from https://www.ssa.gov/oact/cola/SSIamts.html.

Stancliffe, R. J., & Lakin, C. (2004). Costs and outcomes of community services for persons with intellectual disabilities. *Policy Research Brief, 15*(1), 1-12.

Trent, J. W. (n.d.). Moral treatment. Disability History Museum. Retrieved from http://www.disabilitymuseum.org/dhm/edu/essay.html?id=19

University of Colorado. (2008). State of the states in developmental disabilities: Disability spending in the states (1997-2008). Retrieved from http://www.stateofthestates.org/index.php/all-disabilities/overview

U.S. Department of Agriculture. (n.d.). Supplemental nutrition assistance program (SNAP). Retrieved from http://www.fns.usda.gov/snap/

U.S. Department of Health and Human Services. (2010). The Affordable Care Act. Retrieved from http://www.hhs.gov/healthcare/rights/laws

U.S. Department of Housing and Urban Development. (n.d.a.). HUD history. Retrieved from http://portal.hud.gov/hudportal/HUD?src=/about/hud_historyhttp://portal.hud.gov/hudportal/HUD?src=/about/hud_history

U.S. Department of Justice. (n.d.b.). Olmstead: Community integration for everyone. Retrieved from http://www.ada.gov/olmstead/index.htm

U.S. Department of Justice. (n.d.c.). Information and technical assistance on the American with Disabilities Act. Retrieved from https://www.ada.gov/index.html

U.S. Department of Justice. (2009). A guide to disability rights laws. Retrieved from http://www.ada.gov/cguide.htm#anchor65610

U.S. Department of Labor. (2015). WIOA overview. Retrieved from https://www.doleta.gov/WIOA/Overview.cfm

Walsh, K., Kastner, T., & Criscione, T. (1997). Characteristics of hospitalizations for people with developmental disabilities: Utilization, costs, and impact of care coordination. *American Journal on Mental Retardation, 101*(5), 505-520.

Wehmeyer, M. L. (2013). *The story of intellectual disability: An evolution of meaning, understanding and public perception.* Baltimore MD: Paul H. Brookes Publishing.

Wolfensberger, Wolf P. (1972). *The principle of normalization in human services.* Toronto, ON, Canada: National Institute on Mental Retardation.

3

Neurobehavior

Kimberly Bryze, PhD, OTR/L

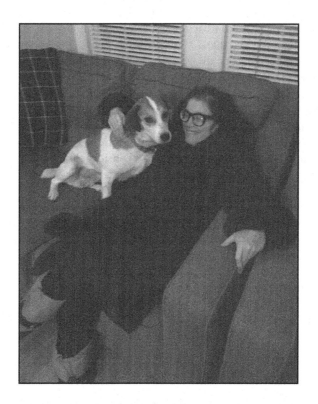

Key Words: arousal, autonomic nervous system, diagnostic overshadowing, emotion and behavior, limbic system, sensory modulation, sensory processing, stress

Bryze, K.
Occupational Therapy for Adults With Intellectual Disability (pp. 29-39).
© 2020 Taylor & Francis Group.

Human beings are remarkably complicated in the ways they think, move, feel, act, and interact with each other. Many disciplines exist to help make sense of why we humans do what we do, and often the diverse disciplinary arguments counter each other, compelling therapists to make decisions regarding evaluation and intervention that are the most understandable—or the clearest, or loudest—and which best make sense of the client's behavior. Programmatic or therapeutic decisions are often made based on the logic or reasoning specific to a particular discipline's explanation, and as new knowledge and research emerges from the neuroscience arena, beliefs and assumptions are slowly challenged; however, the brain remains the most intriguing organ.

Persons with intellectual disability, by diagnostic definition, experience significant cognitive challenges that impact many areas of daily life. Cognitive functions originate and are controlled by the brain, yet the central nervous system, as a whole, manages other essential functions, such as the motor, sensory, autonomic, and social-emotional dimensions that afford one's capacity to enact those occupations that he or she needs and wants to perform. In addition to cognitive challenges, approximately 60% of individuals with intellectual disability present with additional mental health concerns, such as anxiety, depression, and psychotic disorders (Turygin, Matson, & Adams, 2014). The prevalence of dual diagnoses (i.e., concurrent intellectual and psychiatric disorders) ranges up to more than 50%, depending on the methodologies utilized in the various studies (Cooper, Smiley, Morrison, Williamson, & Allan, 2007; Cooper et al., 2015). Psychiatric disorders are frequently under-reported for adults with intellectual disability because of *diagnostic overshadowing* (Reiss, Levitan, & Szyszko, 1982), which refers to the tendency on the part of professionals to attribute psychological and behavioral symptoms symptomatic of mental illness to the primary diagnosis of intellectual disability (Jopp & Keys, 2001; Mason & Scior, 2004). The attribution of what may be a psychiatric disorder to the intellectual disability creates barriers to receiving appropriate diagnoses and implementation of the most effective interventions for the individual.

Occupational therapists have typically directed their focus toward serving individuals with intellectual disability through restorative or acquisitional interventions using cognitive supports, neuromotor, and sensorimotor approaches, as well as therapeutic and behavioral techniques. However, many intervention approaches are typically directed toward a specific aspect of neurobehavioral concern or functioning. Practitioners may neglect to consider the interdependence and interplay between different neurofunctional components as they affect behavior, occupational engagement, and interactions with the social and physical environment.

This chapter will present the reader with an overarching perspective of the ways in which various neurological functions interrelate and contribute to behavior and occupational engagement. An exhaustive explanation of the many detailed facets of nervous system functioning will not be provided here, and the reader who desires such specificity is referred to other, more scholarly sources (Kandel, Schwartz, Jessell, Sieglbaum, & Hudspeth, 2013). The intent of this chapter is to provide practitioners with a foundational understanding of the interaction between autonomic, limbic, and sensory processing functions, and inform strategies for designing thoughtful interventions to positively influence emotional safety, behavioral control, and to enhance occupational engagement.

NEURAL NETWORKS

Human brains are comprised of an incredible number of interconnected neurons and neuronal systems. While there are many different types of neurons (i.e., motor, sensory, and interneurons), each neuron is then connected to between 5000 to 200,000 other neurons through synapses that transmit chemical and electrical information throughout the entire nervous system (Kandel et al., 2013; Zull, 2002). These neuronal networks are established and influenced by our genetic make-up, as well as every experience encountered in our lives—each sensory, motor, emotional, and learning experience—and interlink the many components of the nervous system. However, the complexity of the nervous system can be organized into five overarching, interrelated functions:

1. Autonomic and automatic functions that support life and state
2. Sensory processing and perception
3. Motor control, including gross, fine, oral, and ocular motor abilities
4. Emotional and behavioral control
5. Cognitive functions, specifically the ways in which one learns, thinks, and remembers

Higher cognitive functions, such as the executive functions of judgment, problem solving, and decision making, are also included in this cognitive category. These five categories are interdependent; deficits or dysfunction in one area will influence and impact the others.

Autonomic Functions and Responsibilities

The autonomic nervous system (ANS) is the primary control system for regulating bodily functions and internal organs (e.g., heart, lungs, digestive system), and controlling vasomotor activity and certain reflexive actions (e.g., coughing, sneezing, vomiting). The ANS is comprised of two primary branches that work together in concert: the sympathetic nervous system (SNS) and the parasympathetic nervous system (PSNS).

The SNS is responsible for quickly mobilizing an individual to enable the fight or flight response. It provides the basis for the body's mobilizing responses by increasing heart rate and cardiac contractility, constricting visceral vasculature, sweating to dissipate heat, etc. The SNS quickly exerts its influences over widespread regions of the body for quick action on the person's part; however, the effects of the SNS are slow to dissipate and return to baseline. The systemic distribution of the neurochemicals released by the SNS initiation (e.g., norepinephrine, epinephrine) are slow to metabolize (Black, 2002). Many of us have experienced the SNS effects while driving, when suddenly, a child's ball bounces in front of our car. We react by forcefully braking to stop, seemingly an inch away from the child, who runs into the street after the ball. We see the child, surprised, grab his or her ball and scamper back to his or her lawn. While we are grateful that nothing unfortunate happened, we are left with the knee-shaking, heart-pounding, sweaty-palm effects of the SNS, which activated the reflexive motoric responses. We proceed slowly and carefully, trying to drive calmly while our body slowly returns to normal breathing and heart rate.

Conversely, the PSNS is responsible for the conservation and restoration of body resources. It responds slower to specific stimuli and for short durations of time. It serves to decrease heart rate, increase peristaltic activity in the gut, slow breathing, etc. The overall effects of the PSNS include a calming, organizing, and restorative sense of well-being. Parasympathetic influences also facilitate the readiness for learning and cognitive capacity. As an example, consider the outdated belief that cramming for exams or pulling all-nighters is a good thing to do. Scholars have recognized that a more effective way of preparing for high-stakes examinations is to maintain a disciplined approach to integrating and reviewing the material a bit every day rather than memorizing and attempting to digest the material just for the examination (Levine, 1999; Zull, 2002). It is now believed that maintaining good nutrition, hydration, and sleep cycles will contribute to a more organized state when interacting with the learned material and utilizing cognitive functions more effectively during the examination. Moreover, in this PSNS biased state, one can retain new material, and efficiently assimilate new material into existing cognitive schemas (Zull, 2002). While adults with intellectual disability may not need to study for high-stakes examinations, there are opportunities for substantive learning to take place in their daily lives, as when mastering new tasks on a job, acquiring the routines of a new home, or discovering a community center for new leisure pursuits. If the individual is biased toward the PSNS state, such new learning will be enhanced.

Regarding the ANS and its effect on health and stress, SNS responses promote widespread inflammation (Janig, 2014), whereas the calming effects of the PSNS promote anti-inflammatory responses throughout the body. Inflammation is the body's attempt to protect itself from harm, irritation, or pathogens while attempting to heal. The inflammatory response results in pain, swelling, and cellular action where arteries dilate, blood flow increases, and capillaries become permeable to allow white blood cells, hormones, and nutrients to move into interstitial spaces. Chronic inflammation, caused by environmental factors, poor diet, or prolonged stress, has been linked to a variety of health risks, ailments, and inflammation within joints, arteries, and organs. For example, an imbalanced ANS, with reduced PSNS and increased SNS influences, has been a consistent finding in persons with autoimmune disorders (Black, 2002; Koopman et al., 2011). Attaining and maintaining PSNS tone is important for promoting the organized state that is conducive to homeostasis, cognitive functioning, and restoration of the body and mind (Schaaf et al., 2010).

Limbic System

The limbic system is a complex system of neural networks and structures in the brain that are primarily responsible for one's emotional life, the formation of memories, and the integration of all sensory systems with autonomic functions. The limbic system controls our basic emotions (e.g., fear, pleasure, anger) and basic drives. Each of the limbic system structures contributes to the functions of the whole system yet interconnect with each other to also interact with the autonomic and sensory systems for neurobehavior.

For example, the hypothalamus is a limbic system structure that helps regulate the functioning of the ANS. It works to monitor and control one's hunger, thirst, response to pain, and to regulate one's level of pleasure and sexual satisfaction, anger, aggression, etc. This structure is affected by intense stress and releases hormones and neurochemicals in response to the stressors, including pain. The hippocampus, another of the limbic structures, serves to integrate all sensory inputs. Various types of sensory information are processed as they are derived from specific situations and events in order to create images, patterns, faces, sounds, and locations, which build explicit, long-term memories. The hippocampus is responsible for converting things "in your mind" now into things that you will remember long term. Hence, explicit memories are built in the hippocampus and then stored at the cortical level. Without the ability to build new memories, each new experience or bit of knowledge does not convert to acquired knowledge for use, although older or emotional memories may remain. An individual who is highly motivated to learn a new task may acquire the knowledge and skill more easily and faster than a task he or she may not be motivated to perform. Similarly, individuals with intellectual disability may require specific, step-wise training with repetition to learn new tasks, which may not be highly motivating or that are complex. The repetition and specificity of learning the task will help form the explicit memories for habit formation.

The formation and long-term storage of emotional (implicit) memories, however, have been attributed to the work of the amygdala, another limbic structure. Sensory inputs and emotionally-laden experiences are transmitted directly to the amygdala, and automatic processing and resultant action responses are initiated before cognitive awareness occurs (Schroeder & Shinnick-Gallagher, 2005). The amygdala is considered a fear/danger center that receives information directly from concrete experiences. It constantly monitors our experience and screens for possible negative emotional content. With its primary role in forming and storing long-term, emotional memories, the effect of chronic stress and trauma should be considered. Individuals who have experienced significant life challenges (e.g., abuse, military battle, chronic maltreatment) may have a neurophysiological inability to recover fully from such toxic stress and may carry residual memories or response patterns beyond the acute stress phase. Adults with intellectual disability who have experienced institutionalization or abuse may have emotional memories that are well-ingrained; their lives require the supports of consistency, physical, and emotional safety within natural, less restrictive contexts (Reynolds, Lane & Richards, 2010). The amygdala can relax its vigilance and become less active when the person perceives no threats or fearful situations (Willner, 2015) and when the brain is actively engaged in meaningful cognitive tasks. This is likened to the total engagement and absorption when one is in "the flow", as when one feels energized and fully involved in an enjoyable activity, losing "all track of time"(Csikszentmihályi, 1990).

Along with the hippocampus, the amygdala also receives information from all sensory modalities and helps modulate sensory processing in the association areas of the brain (Davidson, 2003). It assists with processing dual sensations as seen when one type of input triggers the perception of a second sensory input. For example, seeing a lovely, red, crispy apple can generate the sensation that one can almost hear the crunch as it is bitten, or feel the weight of the apple in one's hand. The responsibilities for processing sensory information extend to a parallel responsibility to establish connections between those sensory inputs and resultant affective states (e.g., aversive touch can trigger aggression).

Sensory Processing

The coordination and integration of the various sensory systems influence the responsiveness and actions of the ANS and the limbic system functions. One's autonomic state and emotional-behavioral stability is dependent on the efficient coordination of the sensory systems, especially the more primal, body-centered senses of tactile proprioception and vestibular proprioception. Many occupational therapists are knowledgeable and trained in sensory integration theory, assessment, and intervention, especially in practice with children. However, the neurobehavioral constructs are important considerations for one's practice with adults with intellectual disability, although little has been studied or written in this area (Roley, Blanche, & Schaaf, 2001). While *sensory integration* is a term that refers to the specific practice theory developed by Ayres (1972) and expanded by others (Bundy, Murray, & Lane, 2001; Roley, Blanche & Schaaf, 2001), the term sensory processing is more inclusive and consistent with neurobehavioral constructs founded on research.

Sensory processing is the dynamic, neurological process of taking in, processing, and organizing sensation from one's own body and from the environment for use (Bundy et al., 2001). Sensory information that has been processed and integrated affords the ability to plan and organize one's movements, emotions, and behavior effectively. There are more senses than the commonly known five senses (i.e., touch, hearing, vision, taste, smell). Four sensory systems serve some of the most pervasive and essential functions within the nervous system: vestibular, proprioception, interoception, and tactile. The *vestibular* (response to gravity and movement), *proprioceptive* (information from muscles, joints, tendons, ligaments), *interoceptive* (response to internal sensations related to digestion, elimination, hunger, etc.) and *tactile* (fine and deep touch) systems provide the capacity for experiencing our internal and external worlds. The literature related to sensory integration and sensory processing has accorded the tactile, proprioceptive, and vestibular proprioceptive sensory systems greater focus and study, in that these systems develop early in gestation and have a pervasive effect on an individual's overall state and development.

Tactile and proprioception are the first sensory systems to develop in the embryonic stage, in as early as the 7th week in utero. The vestibular nerve begins to develop simultaneously but vestibular system maturity does not culminate until long after birth, at approximately 10 years of age (Moore & Persaud, 2015). Because the touch, vestibular, and proprioceptive sensory systems are the first to develop, they have an influential and pervasive interrelationship with other sensory systems. Disorders in these primary sensory systems often create greater challenges for behavior, emotional regulation, and, ultimately, occupational performance.

Sensory modulation refers to the ability to derive affective or emotional meaning from incoming sensory inputs. An individual who experiences dysmodulation of touch or movement may demonstrate hyperresponsive or fluctuating emotional responses that are out of proportion to the incoming input. For example, an individual who is overresponsive to tactile inputs may perceive common touch to be aversive. He or she may overreact and pull away from being touched, misinterpret a comforting hug, or perceive socks with seams to be unbearably uncomfortable. An individual who is overresponsive to movement may react with fear when his or her feet leave the ground to step up onto the bus and may react with resultant fight or flight responses. Given the affective emotional responses to sensory inputs, a caregiver may notice the behavioral problems or emotional outbursts but may not attribute the behavior to the sensory dysmodulation that causes the behavior. Sensory dysmodulation or overresponsivity may take such forms as tactile defensiveness, gravitational insecurity, intolerance to movement, visual or auditory defensiveness, and hypersensitivity to smells, tastes, or food textures. Apart from proprioception, dysmodulation may involve any sensory system, and it is common for individuals to be oversensitive to more than one sensation at a time (e.g., tactile and auditory hypersensitivities, visual and vestibular modulation disorders, taste and smell sensitivities).

Moreover, individuals who are hypersensitive, or who demonstrate fluctuation in their modulation ability, also do not habituate effectively to sensory stimuli; they do not easily "get used to" recurring stimuli like other individuals (Brett-Green, Miller, Schoen, & Nielsen, 2010). While we engage in sensory experiences in our daily occupations, the inability to habituate impacts the ease of completing certain tasks. Individuals may resist certain self-care tasks due to, perhaps, the feeling of the toothbrush and toothpaste, the aversive feel of water and shampoo being rubbed on one's scalp, the sensation of the sock seam rubbing one's toes, or eating in a noisy or busy environment. When the experiences of daily sensations are uncomfortable or even unbearable, behavior problems may arise in response to what is interpreted as a threat.

Sensory discrimination refers to the ability to derive perceptual meaning from sensory inputs. The understanding of perceptual meaning leads to conceptual understanding of oneself and the environment. To discriminate the qualities of touch and texture allows one to locate the precise place where a mosquito has landed and bit one's skin and recognize whether one's lips have residual food on them. To perceive where one's body ends and the chair begins allows one to recognize where the chair is in relation to oneself in order to sit down. Discrimination of movement fosters an understanding of the internal map of one's body allowing for effective movement through space and occupational performance (e.g., being able to perform the motor actions of brushing teeth on the left and right sides of one's mouth; brushing one's hair, as it is easily seen in the mirror, as well as on the back of one's head). The concepts of front, back, in, out, over, through, and so on, all develop from the capacity to discriminate one's position in space, body position in relation to objects, such as self-care items, furniture, physical spaces, and even other persons. The ability to discriminate the bodies' senses of touch, proprioception and movement through space provides the neural substrate for the development of motor control and engagement with the physical world (Horvat, Croce, & Zagrodnik, 2010). Further, discriminative capacity affords the development of praxis.

Praxis is the three phase capacity to conceptualize, plan, and perform skilled actions to enact task performance. The conceptualization and planning phases require a greater cognitive load, while the action performance phase requires the motoric implementation of the plan. Moreover, all motor incoordination is not due to praxis disorders. The generalized motor incoordination that accompanies intellectual disability may or may not be linked to praxis deficits, although portions of the central nervous system that support such functions may be impaired. The cognitive dimensions of praxis impact the learning and mastery of new and complex tasks, and it is common for individuals to have difficulty learning self-care, vocational, and domestic activities of daily living due to their inability to figure out how to progress through tasks step by step. Implementing task and performance analyses, reinforcing the step-by-step action sequences through forward or backward chaining, and using visual pictorial cues are strategies that often help individuals master the cognitive demands of learning and performing more complex tasks. Therapists should be mindful of the effects of frustration and high cognitive loads on an individual's emotional and behavioral state. When an individual experiences frustration or confusion, SNS and stress responses will impact the individual's learning capabilities, and, in extreme cases, there may be a tendency to react with behavior outbursts or self-injurious behavior (Willner, 2015).

While stressors, including frustration or confusion, are common in daily life, individuals with intellectual disability may experience greater stress than the general population for several reasons: a fragile neurological status; cognitive limitations that impact complex daily life task performance; cognitive and communicative limitations affecting comprehension and social interactions; ineffective

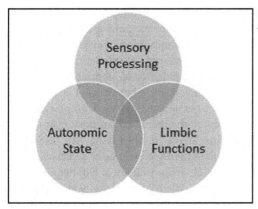

Figure 3-1. Transaction of sensory processing, autonomic, and limbic functions.

sensory processing; the impact of psychiatric conditions and dual diagnoses; a dearth of meaningful occupational engagement; a lack of control over daily routines and occupational choices; and the influence of medications and their side-effects. Moreover, individuals with intellectual disability may have fewer available resources for coping with stress and stressful life events; loss, grief, and pain that cannot be easily communicated (Scott & Havercamp, 2014).

Interplay of Autonomic Systems, Sensory Systems, and Limbic Functions

The three neurobehavioral systems previously discussed are intricately connected through various neurological structures and networks. With its sympathetic and parasympathetic branches, the ANS sets a foundational tone for the rest of the nervous system's functioning, and one's responsiveness to the challenges of daily life situations is dependent on the ANS's state. However, the ANS is directly connected to limbic structures and functions. For example, both the autonomic and limbic systems share responsibility for the regulation of endocrine and hormonal responses to stress through the hypothalamus and the amygdala. An individual who is in an alert, SNS-driven state is likely to experience the emotional responses of anxiety, hypervigilance, irritability, and aggression and may feel the need to escape or withdraw (Willner, 2015). An individual driven by PSNS influences will experience feelings of calmness and contentment (Figure 3-1).

Sensory influences contribute to both the ANS and the limbic functions with resultant reciprocity. Oversensitivity or disordered sensory processing will affect the state or tone of the ANS with concurrent limbic responses of anxiety or irritability. Subsequently, emotional and behavioral outcomes are sequelae to the primal interconnections between sensory, ANS, and limbic functions. In the presence of behavioral challenges, therapists should be thorough in their evaluation of behavioral antecedents and consider potential medical or neurobehavioral causes first and foremost. For example, pain, as a sensory stimulus, will engender SNS activation and increased cortisol production (Willner, 2015). Many individuals with intellectual disability who are unable to convey the presence or impact of their pain using verbal or gestural means may demonstrate increased emotionality, or resort to outbursts, head banging, eye gouging, etc., in an attempt to communicate or manage the pain stimulus, albeit ineffectively (Glaesser & Perkins, 2013; Medeiros, Rojahn, Moore, & van Ingen, 2014; Peebles & Price, 2011). Behavior is observable and often measurable and is always caused by something internal or external. Behavior may be directed toward oneself, as in the case of self-injurious or self-abusive behaviors (e.g., slapping, hitting, biting oneself, poking one's eyes, picking at scabs), directed toward the physical environment through destruction of property, or toward other persons, such as staff (Medeiros et al., 2014).

Consistent with behavioral and psychological theories, behavior problems are often attributed to the individual's motivation to seek attention. However, behavior problems more frequently arise in response to medical needs, psychological distress, and neurosensory considerations. While the detrimental or self-injurious behaviors need to be deterred for the individual's safety, identification of the cause or trigger of the behavior is paramount before interventions are implemented. The simple, linear solution of designing and implementing a behavioral plan of action to manage the behavioral symptoms or sequelae of an underlying problem will not be sufficient, and may be harmful if the cause of the behavior is not determined and responded to appropriately; medical, psychological, or neurosensory concerns may contribute to maladaptive behaviors. For example, behavioral problems may arise in response to one's experience of anxiety and stress in noisy, open spaces when eating lunch. Overresponsivity may be triggered by the increased auditory, visual, and tactile inputs (van den Bosch, Andringa, Baskent, & Vlaskamp, 2016). In this instance, the SNS fight or flight response to entering the busy environment may result in the affective state of panic, fear, and the behavioral response of agitation, resistance or aggression. Often an individual will demonstrate early indicators of stress, such as eye gaze aversion, increased muscle tone or movement, increased respiration, skin color changes, and hand to mouth or face gestures. While these warning signs may be brief and fleeting prior to a behavioral outburst, they signal the beginnings of sensory stress. A therapist who is attuned to the individual with poor sensory processing will ideally attend to these early behavioral indicators and take proactive steps to provide therapeutic or preventative interventions to avert behavior problems and thus protect the individual from emotional distress.

STRENGTHENING PROTECTIVE FACTORS TO INFLUENCE STATE AND EMOTIONAL BEHAVIORAL OUTCOMES

Protective factors refer to those strategies or interventions that reinforce an individual's strengths, prevent weaknesses from impacting one's emotional state, and facilitate effective coping, stress management, and adaptive responses. Protective factors serve to lessen or eliminate perceived risks and enhance the probability of success in the individual's occupational engagement. One of the most salient factors for occupational therapy practitioners is to seek an in-depth understanding of the person with intellectual disability, including his or her responses to environmental and social stressors. Practitioners should consider the many sensory and contextual challenges that trigger anxiety or behavior problems and consider various alternative explanations for poor behavior prior to implementing interventions. Collaboration with the individual and caregivers will foster strong connections and supports for the individual through the development of effective, person-centered strategies designed to build relationships between the parties. The goal is to enhance an individual's emotional and behavioral competence regardless of his or her level of intellectual disability.

Protective factors can also be reinforced using sensory motor techniques to influence an individual's autonomic tone or state. Individuals often utilize their own sensory strategies in response to stress or to provide themselves with comfort or perceptual constancy (Medeiros et al., 2014). Rocking, tapping, chewing, and rubbing are common examples of sometimes stereotypical self-soothing techniques (Joosten & Bundy, 2008). Given this chapter's focus on the ANS and sensory systems, consideration should be given to the provision of meaningful sensory inputs, such as activities that provide proprioceptive, deep touch pressure, and movement inputs to facilitate PSNS activation and promote better emotional stability.

As mentioned earlier in this chapter, the PSNS is responsible for the conservation and restoration of body resources, promoting lowered heart and respiration rates, increased peristaltic activity in the gut, and overall calming of the nervous system. When an individual is influenced by more SNS activity, carefully chosen sensory techniques can be employed to counteract negative effects and influence a PSNS response. The influences of the physical and social environment cannot be overestimated. The type and volume of environmental sounds, caregiver volume of speech and amount of verbal directions, and background sound plays an important role in an individual's ANS state (van den Bosch et al., 2016). Likewise, the amount of visual stimuli, from color, the movement of persons in the room, lighting, and clutter also promote restoration and relaxation or contribute to facilitation and activation of alertness.

Sensory inputs, especially those that involve deep touch pressure and proprioception, are often effective pre-occupation, preparatory strategies to promote PSNS bias. Sitting or lying in a cocoon chair, swing, or wrapping up in a blanket may provide total body pressure, which is relaxing and calming. Wearing snug (not tight) t-shirts or spandex clothing, commonly used in athletic wear, may provide a hug-like sensation, and the deep touch pressure can be calming. Weighted lap pads or blankets can be purchased or fabricated for those individuals for whom deep pressure is calming. Other self-administered tactile inputs for promoting neural cues for calming might include maintained touch to the palms (the namaste or prayer position), maintained touch to the perioral region (trigeminal distribution), and maintained touch to the periumbilical area. Slow linear movement, as when sitting on a glider moving forward and backward, may also be calming and organizing, especially if the movement is slow, rhythmic, and repetitive. These suggestions can ideally be implemented by the individual and, therefore, facilitate efforts toward self-regulation of one's arousal and state. Some individuals find that wearing a weighted shoulder wrap, or a "snake" created from a tube sock filled with uncooked beans or rice, laid upon one's upper trapezius muscles, can be self-administered and promote deep-touch pressure for self-regulation. Care should always be taken with individuals who have neurological, orthopedic, or medical conditions, especially when considering any sensory techniques that involve movement or joint compression.

Techniques involving sensory inputs have not been fully examined with adults with intellectual disability and must never be applied as a "one size fits most" approach (Hoch, Symons, & Sng, 2013). Few studies have specifically examined the relationships of autonomic arousal and self-injury in individuals with intellectual disability. While there may be face validity to therapists' understanding of the relationships between the autonomic, limbic, and sensory systems, one must be cautious in applying such neurobehavioral principles without careful consideration and thoughtful discernment. Moreover, everyone with whom we work has his or her own unique nervous system and life experiences, and their unique needs for care and intervention must be honored.

CONCLUSION

While many of the suggestions in this chapter relate to the consideration of sensory influences for modifying individuals' arousal and emotional states, the intent of this work was to expand therapists' capacity to explore the complexity and interrelatedness of the nervous system functions with a deepened understanding of the individuals we serve. There are excellent resources on sensory-based interventions available that pertain to research on and work with children, but these should be applied carefully to adults with intellectual disability.

With increasing research in the field of intellectual disability from many disciplinary fields, little is known about the work of good occupational therapy with these individuals. Occupational therapy practitioners can bring their professional backgrounds in psychosocial, developmental, neurorehabilitation, and occupation-focused evaluation and intervention to their work with these adults. While more research is certainly needed, the individuals we serve today need each of us to be observant, compassionate, and knowledgeable of their neurobehavior and never assume that their behavior and unique characteristics are related exclusively to their intellectual disability diagnosis. Each person is always more complicated and worthy of in-depth, evidence-informed evaluation processes and interventions.

REFERENCES

Ayres, A. J. (1972). *Sensory integration and learning disorders*. Los Angeles, CA: Western Psychological Services.

Bar-Shalita, T., Granovsky, Y., Parush, S., & Weissman-Fogel, I. (2015). Physiological measures of modulation in individuals with sensory modulation disorder (SMD). *American Journal of Occupational Therapy, 69*(Suppl. 1), 6911505108p1. doi: 0.5014/ajot.2015.69S1-RP202C

Brett-Green, B. A., Miller, L. J., Schoen, S. A., & Nielsen, D. M. (2010). An exploratory event-related potential study of multisensory integration in sensory over-responsive children, *Brain Research, 1321,* 67-77.

Black, P. H. (2002). Stress and the inflammatory response: A review of neurogenic inflammation. *Brain, Behavior, and Immunity, 16,* 622-653.

Bundy, A. C., Lane, S. J., & Murray, E. A. (2001). *Sensory integration: Theory and practice* (2nd ed.). Philadelphia, PA: F. A. Davis.

Cooper, S., McLean, G., Guthrie, B., McConnachie, A., Mercer, S., Sullivan, F., & Morrison, J. (2015). Multiple physical and mental health comorbidity in adults with intellectual disabilities: Population-based cross-sectional analysis. *BMC Family Practice, 16,* 110-121.

Cooper, S., Smiley, E., Morrison, J., Williamson, A., & Allan, L (2007). Mental ill-health in adults with intellectual disabilities: Prevalence and associated factors. *British Journal of Psychiatry, 190,* 27-35.

Csikszentmihályi, M. (1990). *Flow: The psychology of optimal experience.* New York, NY: Harper & Row.

Davidson, R. J. (2003). Affective neuroscience and psychophysiology: Toward a synthesis. *Psychophysiology, 40,* 655-665.

Furniss, F., & Biswas, A. B. (2012). Recent research on aetiology, development and phenomenology of self-injurious behaviour in people with intellectual disabilities: A systematic review and implications for treatment. *Journal of Intellectual Disability Research, 56,* 453-475.

Glaesser, R. S., & Perkins, E. A. (2013). Self-injurious behavior in older adults with intellectual disabilities. *Social Work, 58,* 213-221.

Hoch, J., Symons, F., & Sng, S. (2013). Sequential analysis of autonomic arousal and self-injurious behavior. *American Journal on Intellectual and Developmental Disabilities, 118,* 435-446.

Horvat, M., Croce, R., & Zagrodnik, J. (2010). Utilization of sensory information in intellectual disabilities. *Journal of Developmental and Physical Disabilities, 22,* 463-473.

Janig, W. (2014). Sympathetic nervous system and inflammation: A conceptual view. *Autonomic Neuroscience, 182,* 4-14

Jopp, D. A., & Keys, C. A. (2001). Diagnostic overshadowing reviewed and reconsidered. *American Journal on Mental Retardation, 106,* 416-433

Joosten, A. V., & Bundy, A. C. (2008). The motivation of stereotypic and repetitive behavior: Examination of construct validity of the Motivation Assessment Scale. *Journal of Autism and Developmental Disorders, 38,* 1341-1348.

Kandel, E. R., Schwartz, J. H., Jessell, T. M., Siegelbaum, S. A., & Hudspeth, A. J. (Eds.). (2013). *Principles of neural science.* (5th ed.). New York, NY: McGraw-Hill Companies Inc.

Kinnealey, M., Koenig, K. P., & Smith, S. (2011). Relationships between sensory modulation social supports and health related quality of life. *American Journal of Occupational Therapy, 65*(3), 320-327. doi: 10.5014/ajot.2011.001370

Koopman, F. A., Stoof, S. P., Straub, R. H., van Maanen, M. A., Vervoordeldonk, M. J., & Tak, P. (2011). Restoring the balance of the autonomic nervous system as an innovative approach to the treatment of rheumatoid arthritis. *Molecular Medicine, 17,* 937-948. doi: 10.2119/molmed.2011.00065

Levine, M. (1999). *Developmental variation and learning disorders* (2nd ed.). Cambridge, MA: Educators Publishing Service.

Mahoney, W. J., Roberts, E., Bryze, K., & Parker Kent, J. A. (2016). Occupational engagement and adults with intellectual disabilities. *American Journal of Occupational Therapy, 70,* 7001350030p1-6. doi: 10.5014/ajot.2016.016576

Mason, J., & Scior, K. (2004). "Diagnostic overshadowing" amongst clinicians working with people with intellectual disabilities in the U.K. *Journal of Applied Research in Intellectual Disabilities, 17,* 85-90.

Medeiros, K., Rojahn, J., Moore, L. L., & van Ingen, D. J. (2014). Functional properties of behavior problems depending on level of intellectual disability. *Journal of Intellectual Disability Research, 58,* 151-161.

Moore, K. L., & Persaud, T. V. N. (2015). *The developing human: Clinically oriented embryology* (10th ed.). Philadelphia, PA: Saunders.

Peebles, K. A., & Price, T. J. (2011). Self-injurious behavior in intellectual disability syndromes: Evidence for aberrant pain signaling as a contributing factor. *Journal of Intellectual Disability Research, 56,* 441-452.

Richards, C., Oliver, C., Nelson, L., & Moss, J. (2012). Self-injurious behavior in individuals with autism spectrum disorder and intellectual disability. *Journal of Intellectual Disability Research, 56,* 476-489.

Reiss, S., Levitan, G. W., & Szyszko, J. (1982). Emotional disturbance and mental retardation: Diagnostic overshadowing. *American Journal of Mental Deficiency, 86,* 16-20.

Reynolds, S., Lane, S. J., & Richards, L. (2010). Using animal models of enriched environments to inform research on sensory integration intervention for the rehabilitation of neurodevelopmental disorders. *Journal of Neurodevelopmental Disorders, 2*(3), 120-132.

Roley, S. S., Blanche, E. I., & Schaaf, R. C. (2001). *Understanding the nature of sensory integration with diverse populations.* San Diego, CA: Therapy Skill Builders.

Schaaf, R. C., Benevides, T., Blanche, E. I., Brett-Green, B., Burcke, J. P., Cohn, E. S., … Schoen, S. (2010). Parasympathetic functions in children with sensory processing disorder. *Frontiers in Integrative Neuroscience, 4*, 4.

Schroeder, B. W., & Shinnick-Gallagher, P. (2005). Fear learning induces persistent facilitation of amygdala synaptic transmission. *European Journal of Neuroscience, 22*, 1775-1783. doi: 10.1111/j.1460-9568.2005.04343.x

Scott, H. M., & Havercamp, S. M. (2014). Mental health for people with intellectual disability: The impact of stress and social support. *American Journal on Intellectual and Developmental Disabilities, 119*, 552-564.

Turygin, N., Matson, J. L., & Adams, H. (2014). Prevalence of co-occurring disorders in a sample of adults with mild and moderate intellectual disabilities who reside in a residential treatment setting. *Research in Developmental Disabilities, 35*, 1802-1808.

van den Bosch, K. A., Andringa, T. C., Baskent, D., & Vlaskamp, C. (2016). The role of sound in residential facilities for people with profound intellectual and multiple disabilities. *Journal of Policy and Practice in Intellectual Disabilities, 13*, 61-68.

Willner, P. (2015). The neurobiology of aggression: Implications for the pharmacotherapy of aggressive challenging behaviour by people with intellectual disabilities. *Journal of Intellectual Disability Research, 59*, 82-92.

Zull, J. (2002). *The art of changing the brain: Enriching teaching by exploring the biology of learning.* Sterling, VA: Stylus Publishing.

4

Attitudes and Beliefs That Guide Occupational Therapy Practice for Adults With Intellectual Disability

Kimberly Bryze, PhD, OTR/L

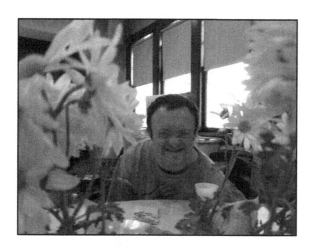

Key Words: attitudes, beliefs, competency, medical model, occupational engagement, occupational therapy, relationship, social model, values

Bryze, K.
Occupational Therapy for Adults With Intellectual Disability (pp. 41-49).
© 2020 Taylor & Francis Group.

The profession of occupational therapy is directed by a philosophic position that outlines the values, beliefs, and attitudes that guide its practices. The American Occupational Therapy Association (AOTA) revises and updates its philosophical position statements on a regular basis, and portions of a current one are offered here:

> Occupations are activities that bring meaning to the daily lives of individuals, families, and communities and enable them to participate in society. All individuals have an innate need and right to engage in meaningful occupations throughout their lives. Participation in these occupations influences their development, health, and well-being across the lifespan. As such, participation in meaningful occupation is a determinant of health. The focus and outcome of occupational therapy are individuals' engagement in meaningful occupations that support their participation in life situations. Occupational therapy practitioners conceptualize occupations as both a means and an end to therapy. That is, there is therapeutic value in occupational engagement as a change agent, and engagement in occupations is also the ultimate goal of therapy. (AOTA, 2011)

Occupational therapy practitioners believe that human beings are occupational in nature, and that they engage in activities that are meaningful and necessary, not only for survival, but for enjoyment, interpersonal communication, productivity, and personal restoration. People are motivated to engage in occupations as they are shaped by personal interests, culture, physical and social contexts, and by opportunities afforded. Moreover, the form and function of occupations change and evolve across ones life span (e.g., playing with clay vs. kneading bread dough), although certain occupations are learned early and refined across time (e.g., using utensils for eating, cutting food to prepare a meal). The occupational therapy practitioner chooses occupations based on the person's interests, abilities, and challenges; the specific task or occupation needed or desired, and the contextual supports or barriers in which the occupational performance takes place.

Specific occupational therapy practices, as they involve evaluation, intervention, and support for adults with intellectual disability, are also shaped by the values and beliefs held by the individual practitioner. Whether tacit or explicit, a practitioner's values direct the choice of questions asked, observations made, theoretical models that guide practice, assessments from which to gather data, etc. The practitioner's values and beliefs are conveyed through these questions, assessments, and interactions to the person served, as well as to other staff or caregivers and, in turn, influence their interactions with and support of the person.

Occupational therapy practice is also guided by conceptual theories and models that facilitate reasoning, decision making, evaluation, and intervention approaches. This chapter will explore essential values and beliefs that have been embraced by occupational therapy, and will emphasize certain tenets that support a competence model, or set of perspectives and beliefs, which can effectively be applied to occupational therapy for adults with intellectual disability. Without sacrificing our technical, scientific, or specialized areas of expertise, this chapter will challenge occupational therapy practitioners to embrace an appreciation for the uniqueness and worth of individuals with intellectual disability and, perhaps, understand them in a different way than the traditional models afford.

VALUES SHAPE OCCUPATIONAL THERAPY'S APPROACH TO PRACTICE

Values are defined as the principles or standards of behavior a person embraces and holds to be right or good. Values underlie the enactment of personal and professional behaviors, philosophies, belief systems, and professional practices, and are strong motivators for decision making and problem solving in everyday life. While they may be implicit and infrequently discussed, a person's values influence one's presence and interactions in the physical and social world.

The value for a person's essential humanity, despite severe and sometimes chronic disease or disability, is central to the practice of occupational therapy. Occupational therapy does not limit its concern only to a person's physical capacity, disease, or conditions, but also to the effects of the environment and goals upon his or her health and well-being. Value for the client or patient, as a collaborative partner, is noted when a practitioner operates from the perspective of what is most important to the person and is used to focus intervention goals and therapeutic efforts. The value for each person's essential humanity is also seen in occupational therapy's efforts in advocacy for disability rights and social justice. Occupational therapy practitioners continue to value the right to the highest quality of life for each person, regardless of the presence of intellectual disability or other disorders. The philosophic and pragmatic approaches of practitioners provide evidence of their concern with health, facilitating, and strengthening the healthy aspects of individuals' lives, and enabling persons to engage in the activities they need and want to pursue.

Occupational therapy emerged from a climate of caring. Its roots were embedded in moral treatment that focused on the ways persons with mental and physical disorders were restored to healthy living. Moral treatment embraced three important facets (1) a firm belief in the dignity of all human beings, despite their immediate condition, (2) a belief that many human problems resulted from a disruption of the habits and routines that structure daily living, and (3) a belief that all human beings, no matter how severely impaired or disorganized, possess some degree of self-control and potential for quality living (Kielhofner & Miyake, 1983). Embracing these facets in occupational therapy for adults with intellectual disability today requires a conceptualization of occupation that is deeper and broader than what is common to practice in many traditional settings.

All persons, regardless of ability, seek to explore and master their world, to perform meaningful activities, and to be in relationships with others. Unfortunately, some people do not actively master, but are mastered by, their world, and are not allowed the opportunity to explore new activities and occupations. Many individuals with intellectual disability are lonely or feel abandoned. Moreover, they feel fear, shame, or anxiety and feel poorly about themselves and others (Vanier, 2010). While skillful practitioners are often needed to solve specific problems of living, it is essential for them to be concerned with the individual as a whole person, and to come alongside and take the persons' experience of his or her world seriously. To serve people holistically, and not just solve problems of behavior, for example, requires a firm commitment to the values and beliefs of occupational therapy at its best. The greatest threat to the worth of occupational therapy today is not lack of technical knowledge, but the loss of an appreciation for the true nature of occupations and the impact of their value and purpose on being human. The foundation of occupational therapy was and should be firmly grounded in a vision of how occupation organizes the human spirit and improves well-being and quality of living. Further, "occupational therapy practitioners must continually redefine and rearticulate the value of a humane practice that transcends scientific validation and bureaucratic understanding" (Peloquin, 1989).

CONSIDERATION OF VARIOUS CONCEPTUAL MODELS

Since the earliest days of occupational therapy, the values and philosophy of the profession have presented themselves through various models where ideas and beliefs are translated into practice. Occupational therapy practice is guided by conceptual theories and models that facilitate reasoning, decision making, evaluation, and intervention approaches.

Historically, practice with adults with intellectual disability was once approached considering the developmental models that were most appropriate for children, who were still in the active process of growth and development, from childhood through adolescence into adulthood. Whether in the psychologist's process of determining the presence of delay or intellectual disability or in occupational therapy's use of various developmental assessments and adaptive behavior measures, the mental or developmental age was often used as a means for interpreting normative testing results. An individual with intellectual disability may have been likened to "having cognitive ability at a 7-year-old level" or "a global mental age of 5 years". While perhaps descriptive, this use of the developmental frame of reference leads to stigmatization, delimits the potential for opportunities, and occupations to be presented to the person, or may provide exposure to occupations that are appropriate for young children rather than for adults. For example, a 7-year-old child may be quite bright, but likely should not independently ride a large metropolitan bus across the city. However, a young adult with intellectual disability can learn to ride the bus to work every day, fostering self-determination, independence, and adult occupational role performance. The practitioner's beliefs or assumptions that the person is like a young child influences and impacts the decisions that are made regarding immediate occupational therapy practice, choice of future occupations, and therapeutic efforts.

Attitudes toward persons with disabilities are historically, culturally, and situationally determined. Just as the developmental model may limit one's professional reasoning, other traditional ways of understanding disability may equally impact a practitioner's decision making. The very definition of intellectual disability in modern times informs people of what is inherently "wrong" with these persons, and the medical and rehabilitation models situate the problem of disability within the person and view their difficulties as the direct and inevitable consequences of impairment. Oliver (1996) described this as personal tragedy theory, in which many professionals and various services are required to enable a person with disabilities to assimilate into non-disabled society, come to terms with their impairments, or to shield/remove them from society if they cannot improve or be "cured" (Oliver, 1996). The medical model inadvertently supports the development of the sick role, where the person with disability places responsibility for decisions onto medical or therapy professionals so they can alleviate their "undesirable" situation (Dewsbury, Clarke, Randall, Rouncefield, & Sommerville, 2004).

Whereas, the sick role is most often a temporary one, the role of one who is impaired or disabled is more permanent and one in which the individual accepts dependency. This medicalized approach is similar to the conceptualization of the rehabilitation role, where the individual must accept their condition, making the most of their efforts and abilities to achieve or regain normality. These medical models of disability have been criticized for the way in which they view persons with disabilities as somehow less than or lacking and unable to assume a full role in society. Medical models also work within the frame of an expert-patient relationship, where the expert seeks to cure, or at least alleviate, the problems or symptoms experienced by the patient's disability.

The medical model perspective supports approaches that reduce the complex problems of those with disabilities to issues of medical prevention, cure, or rehabilitation. The social model, however, is a deliberate attempt to shift the focus away from the functional limitations of individuals with impairments to the problems created or caused by the environmental barriers and cultural practices that "disable" individuals with impairments. Social model thinking is focused on the identification and removal of barriers, independent living, anti-discrimination legislation, and other responses to social oppression. The social model essentially defines disability as oppression and presumes the idea that persons with disabilities are oppressed in particular situations. In its most radical sense, social model advocates may so strongly disavow individual limitations and medical approaches and believe that impairment is not seen as a problem in and of itself. Rather, people are disabled by the actions of society and not by their body's limitations or challenges. Extreme medical interventions to remediate, rehabilitate, or cure impairment are rejected. It holds that the inclusion of all people is vital, yet society, which is constructed by and for non-disabled people, excludes persons with disabilities by its social, attitudinal, and physical barriers. Disability is seen as a constructed concept and, as such, is a responsibility shared by all parties. Further, impairment is distinguished from disability; the former is individual and private, while the latter is structural and public. The real priority of the social model is to accept impairment and to remove disability. However, in practice, public and individual aspects are inextricably linked in the complexity of the lived experience of disability. The reality is that persons with disabilities face both discrimination as well as intrinsic limitations (Shakespeare, 2013).

A thoughtful purview of the social model does not need to deny the importance or value of individually-based medical, rehabilitative, or educational interventions for persons with disability. Occupational therapy's current values are an amalgam of the medical and social models. For example, the values of the medical model include (1) recovery from illness, (2) specialist knowledge and action, and (3) objectivity, analysis, diagnosis, and treatment. The values of the social model include (1) the elimination of disabling environments, barriers, and cultures; (2) acceptance of impairment and removal of disability, which is socially constructed; and (3) inclusion and acceptance of all persons. The relevance of and potential for both models are most evident when considering individuals who experience physical disabilities. However, intellectual disability remains tacitly conceived as a biological deficit or problem of inherent incapacity. A practitioner can adapt environments, construct effective cuing mechanisms for task performance, and advocate for independent living for an adult with intellectual disability, yet, the person's need for social support and physical assistance will remain significant considering the intellectual challenges. More imaginative approaches communicate notions of distributed competence, different abilities and capacities, adaptation, and situational intelligence. While the terms evolve to create varied meanings, the terminologies and labels remain historically, culturally, and situationally determined, with persons with intellectual disability lagging far behind in funding, services, and recognition of individuals' worth and humanity.

Labels are generally imposed rather than chosen by the persons. An example of the challenge to and concern with the use of labels is presented:

> When my daughter was born, we named her Ashlynne. She came early. She was tiny, but she was beautiful, with 10 perfect fingers and 10 perfect toes. She was precious to us. By the end of the first year, she had been given lots of diagnoses: cerebral palsy, spastic quadriplegia, seizure disorder, developmental delay, dysphagia, and even more things people called her. Now Ashlynne is 6 years old. She tools around in a power wheelchair and loves to go fast. She has a great sense of humor. She loves people, is happy almost always, and tries to do almost everything by herself. She is my warrior daughter. She is the joy of my life. (Maya T., personal communication).

As a wise social worker shared with me (the author), "The impact of a parent receiving an official diagnosis for their young child can feel like the end of the world. It is important for us to remind them that the child is still the same child today as he was yesterday. The only thing that changed is that there is now a label, a term. But the same child is here" (T. Copeland, personal communication, 2001).

Competency-Based Model

The foundations for a model based on constructs of competency were originally disseminated in a text that is no longer published (Kielhofner & Miyake, 1983), yet the ideas presented in this original work hold true for occupational therapy practice today. The concept of competency typically signifies a skill set or capacity for some tasks or requirements. Competence focuses on the person-occupation-environment fit, or the interaction between the person and the physical or social environment. It involves occupational performance within the context of one's life and situational perspective. Persons seek to develop competence through making choices, and enacting control over objects and processes that have meaning or purpose for them and that attract interest or serve some personal value. Individuals experience themselves as being competent when they can perform successfully, on their own terms, given situational contexts and life experiences.

Individual competence refers to a person's capacity to adapt to external demands and expectations, as well as to his or her internal world of self or lived experience. The degree to which a person views themselves as being competent is a predicting factor in the actions they will take on in the future. Competent persons believe in their ability to choose and accomplish activities that they can perform effectively. Thus, competence begins with an individual's successful experiences and their personal views on self-efficacy. Individuals who view themselves as competent have access to environments, persons, and materials that allow them to perform well or at least "good enough." Individuals with higher quality of life view themselves in a positive light, as environmental supports afford them various opportunities to perform well. Therefore, having a positive self-assessment, plus adequate social and physical environmental resources, affords the development of competence. Competence and self-determination are related. Competence also recognizes the right of individuals to choose and control their own experiences and areas of performance. Unfortunately, these entitlements are often limited or removed from adults with intellectual disability. While an individual's perception of self is often linked to others' judgments of them, the self-perceptions of individuals with intellectual disability are often largely dependent on others' assessment or perceptions about their performance, capacity, or worth.

Individuals with intellectual disability benefit from the careful and intentional application of a competency-based model. The challenges involved in discovering and nurturing competence in these individuals requires a concentrated effort. The competency model can be used for even the most complicated individuals, as long as the belief in control and meaningful engagement are afforded to the individual.

There are four essential elements of competence:
1. Abilities and limitations of the individual
2. Individual self-assessment
3. Expectations of others for their performance in the situated environment
4. The range of opportunities and resources available to the person within and across environments

Persons with intellectual disability often face an imbalance in these elements, as focus is concentrated on their limitations, while the other elements are not addressed. These four elements should ideally be in balance, and, when ability is limited, the other elements must shift to provide the needed balance. One of the most seriously limiting features of life for a person with intellectual disability is the inability or unwillingness of others to recognize or grant competence to their efforts and performances because they differ from the "normal" or average, and are, therefore, "not good enough." Those who serve persons with intellectual disability must construct a different conceptualization of their competence and afford choices based on belief in their competence as starting points for interventions. For example, maximizing the environment to multiply conditions for control is essential. The opportunity for a person to express choice, even if only to select the texture of clothing they wear, or choose where to sit at the dining table, are simple starting points. There is also competency to be acknowledged in the simplicity of cooperating with dressing procedures or feeding oneself. These types of performances should be elements of recognized competence in individuals with significant intellectual disability. The ability to be competent—and recognized as such—in uncomplicated ways can be personally meaningful to the person.

The mystery of a person's competency in light of significant impairments is described in an early work by Kielhofner (1983), who was studying the daily life adaptation of persons with intellectual disability in the community. He wrote:

> I worked with Paul, a young man with athetoid cerebral palsy, at his group home. I found Paul in the kitchen eating. I sat with him for a while as he ate and said a few things to him from time to time. It is amazing to watch Paul eat. I have the feeling that if I were given his body at this moment, I would be absolutely unable to do anything useful with it. Despite all its writhing and distortions, Paul's body does all the things it has to and the care with which he organizes and executes each movement is striking. Paul is truly a graceful cerebral palsied person. It is near mystery to watch him wind his unruly hands around a cup of tea which is purposefully not too hot so as not to burn him should a sudden involuntary movement dump it into his mouth or over his face. He slowly places one hand toward the cup, nudging it with the other to focus the movement. When his hand is in place, he makes a grasping movement which sends off a whole parade of involuntary contractions throughout his arm. The second hand is still steadying things during all this. Then, the second hand moves just as carefully to embrace the other one. Now, with this two-handed grasp in which his fingers literally encircle and hide the cup, he brings his face and hands to meet halfway and sips the tea with lips and throat that move uncontrollably. The tea spills, he makes

gurgling and loud sipping noises and chokes a bit on the tea. In the midst of all this, Paul remains impeccably calm and dignified. A great spirit of inner calm and strength emanates through a withered, contorted and unruly body. (pp. 83-84)

When given the opportunity and gift of time, individuals with intellectual disability and concurrent motor impairments often acquire the ability to use the "unmanageability" of their bodies to perform tasks that are important to them. This is noted particularly in the purposeful and meaningful occupations enacted in their unique ways within the context of their daily lives. Occupations have an organizational capacity, which exceeds the direct consequences of movements or physical prowess. The purpose of occupations becomes the context for meaning, and meaning is contextually determined by the occupations or actions chosen by the person.

Further, a person's identity, as well as the nature and extent of their participation, is socially-determined. Communicative, cognitive, and behavioral competence should be assessed from the perspective of the person's life situation because recognition and production of competent occupations is often interactional. The competency-based perspective encourages occupational therapy practitioners to ponder, enquire, and discover features of the person's life experiences, capabilities, and circumstances as well as the ways in which the physical and social environments support or constrain participation in occupations. The competency-based perspective requires that practitioners focus on the delicate process of structuring physical and social environments, such that some measure of control may be found, and that provide resources relevant to the perspectives, values, and interests of the person with intellectual disability.

As mentioned earlier in this chapter, the attitudes and values practitioners hold influence practice for adults with intellectual disability. The primary value of the competency-based model includes understanding a person from the emic (insider) perspective. Recognizing that competence is socially determined and constructed allows an appreciation for individual competence that is relative to and understood in terms of the person's ability and limitations. Yet, the constructs of a competency model might not be enough. If the social and interactional context is vital to determining competence, and the physical and social environments are critical for providing support to an individual, the type and extent of supports must be closely examined. The attitudes that inspire the way for essential supports, especially social, to be established must be explored.

Relationship Model: An Example

All humans are relational, social beings. People rely on others for companionship, assistance, direction, and connection, yet, depth of relationship (i.e., friendship) is often challenging to attain. This is a particular concern for persons with intellectual disability who experience relational poverty. Indeed, their identities are constructed from and tethered to others' opinions or perspectives that view them as clients, residents, or consumers but rarely as friends. A relationship model responds to a person's often unspoken, yet purposeful, question, "Will you be my friend?" (Vanier, 2010). Such a model speaks to the need to accept persons as they are, and value their worth and uniqueness with the dignity afforded them in a relational way, as a fellow human being. An example of the relationship model may be clearly seen in the faith-based approach of the L'Arche communities —international, intentional communities of shared living for persons with and without intellectual and developmental disabilities.

A core philosophical belief of L'Arche is the dignity of every person, which demands that those who are marginalized in society, those with intellectual disability, be valued and respected. Core members (those with disabilities) and assistants (those without disabilities) live together in community and find meaning in daily activities, which are often considered to be mundane or ordinary. Each day's importance lies in the presence and interdependence of the members, with less focus given to independent performance. Assistants do not tell core members what to do, nor do they do *to* or *for* core members; there are active attempts to do *with*. Professionals within the community, including occupational therapy practitioners, share their expertise but do not challenge the primary focus of enabling members to live and share their daily lives with others, including doing what one needs and wants to do (occupations). The importance of daily life for the L'Arche members is enriched by this sharing of community—called *sharing life*. Sharing occurs in the preparation and eating of meals together, in chores, in celebrations, and in caring for one another, each member contributing according to their abilities (http://www.larche.org).

In many ways, L'Arche communities represent the world as it could be, as places of diversity, care, and connection. The communities are not utopian, but are authentic home and work settings, with real human beings, all of whom have the challenges that go along with being human. There are members with fears, pain, incapacities, tantrums, irritability, and medical problems. Yet these same members also have acceptance, patience, compassion, generosity, humor, and care to give each other.

An exploration of this type of setting, with its beliefs and attitudes, may be of value to explore for occupational therapy practice. With the focus on doing with, practitioners can come alongside to educate, consult, evaluate, and develop strategies to help core members and assistants do what they want and need to do. The practitioner role becomes one of supporter, collaborator, helper, and friend, rather than instructor, director, doer, or expert. Consistent with the approaches favored in collaboration and coaching models, a practitioner must utilize an authentic approach in evaluation and intervention.

Utilizing this relationship model in occupational therapy practice allows a genuine return to some of the core values and perspectives of early occupational therapy when it was founded on compassion, supports within the environment, and value for the dignity of each person. It can be actualized in approaches where the practitioner comes alongside to listen, help, participate with, and enable individuals. The realization of the relationship model forces a practitioner to slow down, to recognize and appreciate that they are entering the member's cultural space with its temporal, spatial, and interactional uniqueness. The practitioner is not the expert or the supervisor in this context, nor is productivity a primary factor. The pace of shared living is gentler and more natural or authentic than the common medical or residential settings for individuals with intellectual disability.

The relational model, as well as the L'Arche example, embraces the tenets of acceptance of and value for all persons, with or without disabilities. It recognizes the dignity and worth of each person regardless of ability or limitation. The meaningfulness of daily life is seen in the shared daily activities and tasks, no matter how mundane or trivial they may seem. Daily occupations and co-occupations assume a focal position. At face value, co-occupation involves doing with the other person, and the occupations of the other person could not take place without the presence and shared experience of another. Co-occupations involve the shared actions of one person influencing the actions of the other (Pierce, 2003). Further, co-occupations have been explained in terms of two or more persons involved in sharing four elements to varying degrees: shared physicality, emotionality, intentionality, and meaning (Pickens & Pzur-Barnekow, 2009). In a relational context, co-occupation involves doing *with* and alongside the other person, sharing the space, physical actions, and objects. It involves a shared intention that may include the purpose or outcome of a particular task, or may simply be enjoying sharing time together in conversation or leisure pursuits. Emotionality may be seen in shared affect, communication, and social interaction between the two people as they engage and participate in the occupations at hand. The shared meaning of doing occupations *with* another person is part of a bond that forms and strengthens close relationships or friendships. Co-occupation is one way to honor and value the small but important things in daily life and to co-construct meaning.

The search for meaning is a distinct characteristic of being human, including for those with intellectual disability. Each person seeks to make meaning out of their life experiences, values, and the many possibilities embedded in their daily lives. Conversely, meaninglessness is associated with a lack of belief in the value, usefulness, or importance of what one does and, perhaps, who one is. Occupational therapy practitioners focus on the important, yet mostly ordinary activities, of being human within immediate and societal contexts. When those activities or occupations are carried out with mindfulness and care, and in relationship to another valued person, they have an effect far beyond their apparent insignificance. Occupational therapy is concerned with these meaningful and purposeful daily life tasks, as well as the meaning of a disability to the individual, and the meaning of their occupational engagement despite their disability. The types of problems occupational therapy practitioners address transcend weak muscles and clumsy fingers to persons who cannot do what they believe is very important to do for their lives. Rather than seeing impairments or conditions as developmental, neurological, musculoskeletal, or psychiatric disorders, the recommendation is offered here to consider viewing persons' problems in light of occupation and real-life "disorders": caring for one's body, preparing one's lunch, going out for a walk with friend, finishing one's work, etc. This is one reason why occupational therapy is a unique profession. It is what we should do as practitioners, and more importantly, it relates to why we do what we do and with whom.

Occupational therapy practice for adults with intellectual disability would likely be strengthened by centering itself on competency and relation models of care. Our values for practice must build on the technical proficiency of our profession, with care for the persons and the meaning of their occupational engagement. Practitioners must not attempt to "fix" impairments just because they are present, but provide opportunities for occupation, to improve quality of life, and to assist individuals in the dynamic process of living their lives more fully in relation to others. Practitioners provide the art of possibilities for those who are often not seen for the individuals they are, with strengths, interests, compassion, and desires for relationship. It is an incredible role—and even greater responsibility—to work with adults with intellectual disability.

REFERENCES

American Occupational Therapy Association. (2011). The philosophical base of occupational therapy. *American Journal of Occupational Therapy, 65*(Suppl.), S65. doi: 10.5014/ajot.2011.65

Dewsbury, G., Clarke, K., Randall, D., Rouncefield, M., & Sommerville, I. (2004). The anti-social model of disability. *Disability & Society, 19(2)*, 145-158.

Goodley, D. (2001). 'Learning difficulties,' the social model of disability and impairment: Challenging epistemologies. *Disability and Society, 16(2)*, 207-2331.

Kielhofner, G. (1983). A paradigm for practice: The hierarchical organization of occupational therapy knowledge. In G. Kielhofner (Ed.), *Health through occupation: Theory and practice in occupational therapy* (pp. 83-84). Philadelphia, PA: F. A. Davis.

Kielhofner, G., & Miyake, S. (1983). Rose-colored lenses for clinical practice: From a deficit to a competency model in assessment and intervention. In G. Kielhofner (Ed.), *Health through occupation: Theory and practice in occupational therapy* (pp. 257-266). Philadelphia, PA: F. A. Davis.

Oliver, M. (1996). *Understanding disability: From theory to practice.* Basingstoke, United Kingdom: Palgrave.

Peloquin, S. M. (1989), Looking back: Moral treatment. *American Journal of Occupational Therapy, 43*, 534-544.

Pickens, N. D., & Pzur-Barnekow, K. (2009). Co-occupation: Extending the dialogue. *Journal of Occupational Science, 16*, 151-156.

Pierce, D. (2003). *Occupation by design: Building therapeutic power.* Philadelphia, PA: F. A. Davis

Shakespeare, T. (2013). The social model of disability. In L. Davis (Ed.), *The disability studies reader* (pp. 215-227). New York, NY: Routledge.

Vanier, J. (2010). What have people with disabilities taught me? In H. Reinders (Ed.), *The paradox of disability* (pp. 19-24). Grand Rapids, MI: Eerdmans Publishing.

5

Promoting Participation in Context Through Self-Determination

Evan E. Dean, PhD, OTR/L

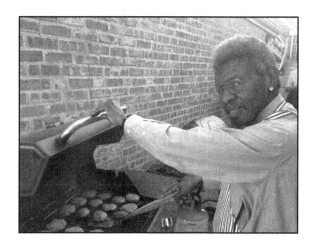

Key Words: adult, context, intellectual disability, participation, self-determination, supports

Bryze, K.
Occupational Therapy for Adults With Intellectual Disability (pp. 51-59).
© 2020 Taylor & Francis Group.

Participation in meaningful, everyday life activities promotes health and well-being (American Occupational Therapy Association [AOTA], 2014). Additionally, engagement in these everyday activities is "a result of choice, motivation, and meaning within a supportive context and environment," (AOTA, 2014).

The first part of this description—that participation in everyday activities are linked to choice, motivation, and meaning—demonstrates a link between participation and self-determination (Dean, Fisher, Shogren, & Wehmeyer, 2016). A self-determined person participates in meaningful, goal-directed, everyday activities that promote health and well-being (Shogren et al., 2015). When we, as occupational therapy practitioners, consider participation in context, in light of self-determination, supporting the people we serve to be self-determined becomes an integral part of the occupational therapy practice. The second piece of the description—that engagement happens in a supportive context and environment—is equally important. While recent models of self-determination acknowledge the role of context, little research has been conducted to demonstrate the role that context can play in supporting self-determination (Shogren, 2013; Shogren et al., 2015).

As discussed in previous chapters, adults with intellectual disability have not consistently been given the opportunity or support to develop skill in self-determination, which has impacted participation. This chapter will describe self-determination as it is conceptualized in the intellectual disability literature and highlight ways that occupational therapists can support self-determination for adults with intellectual disability. This chapter is divided into four sections. The first section will describe self-determination and focus on research highlighting contextual influences on self-determination. Next, self-determination will be linked to occupational therapy practice by defining disability in light of socio-ecological models of disability. The third section will discuss practical ways occupational therapists can promote self-determination in their practice with adults with intellectual disability. Finally, a case example will be provided to highlight promotion of self-determination through occupational therapy intervention.

SELF-DETERMINATION

Self-determination is a personal characteristic possessed by all people that can affect participation in daily life (Wehmeyer, 2005). Self-determined behavior was originally described as being comprised of four characteristics: autonomy, self-regulation, psychological empowerment, and self-realization (Wehmeyer, 1999). A more current definition of self-determined behavior may be offered as "volitional actions that enable one to act as the primary causal agent in one's life and to maintain or improve one's quality of life" (Wehmeyer, 2005). Within this definition, the term *volitional* refers to intentional and conscious choice, and *causal agent* means that a person acts to accomplish a goal or create a change. Put another way, persons are self-determined when they engage in intentional, goal-oriented actions to affect their own quality of life. Self-determination is enhanced when a person uses their strengths and supports to act toward a chosen goal. The environment provides opportunities for self-determined action.

Causal agency theory (Shogren et al., 2015) reconceptualized self-determination to highlight that a self-determined person acts in ways they believe will move them closer to their goals. This theory describes the role context can play in providing opportunities, as well as supports, for self-determined action. Context can also create barriers to participation. In causal agency theory, self-determined action is described as being volitional, agentic, and involving action-control beliefs (Shogren et al., 2015). All of these concepts are related to the four characteristics originally described by Wehmeyer (1999). Volitional action is related to Wehmeyer's (1999) construct of autonomy and is described as intentional and based on a person's preferences. Agentic action is directed by the person in pursuit of a goal (related to self-regulated action in Wehmeyer [1999]). Finally, through action-control beliefs, a person feels the actions they are taking will move them closer to their goal. Action-control

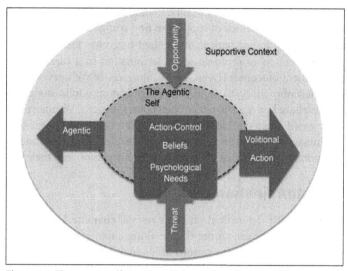

Figure 5-1. The agentic self in context. (Adapted from Shogren, K. A., Wehmeyer, M. L., Palmer, S. B., Forber-Pratt, A., Little, T., & Lopez, S. [2015]. Causal agency theory: Reconceptualizing a functional model of self-determination. *Education and Training in Autism and Developmental Disabilities*, 50, 251-263.)

beliefs are associated with Wehmeyer's (1999) characteristics of psychological empowerment and self-realization.

A separate but related theory about self-determination, self-determination theory (Ryan & Deci, 2000), provides a foundational aspect of causal agency theory, which are psychological needs (Shogren et al., 2015). Self-determination theory describes the role the environment plays in motivation (Ryan & Deci, 2000). This theory describes three psychological needs that are related to motivation: autonomy, competence, and relatedness. These psychological needs can be supported or challenged by contextual factors. As therapists, we are part of the context of the people we serve. We can assist in shaping the environment to meet individuals' psychological needs through intervention in the physical and social environment. For example, we can create opportunities for meaningful activity that increase autonomy and structure those activities to promote competence. These psychological needs are foundational in causal agency theory's conceptualization of the agentic self (Shogren et al., 2015).

Figure 5-1 depicts the dynamics of causal agency theory's self-determined person (called the *agentic-self*) acting in context. A self-determined person has a desire to satisfy psychological and biological needs (autonomy, competence, and relatedness). The environment creates a press (represented by the arrows labeled *opportunity* and *threat*), which is a call to action for the person (acting as an agentic self). The press can either be opportunities or threats to self-determined action. The individual is driven to action if the environmental press matches the person's interests, strengths, and supports. Additionally, the individual believes that action to meet the environmental press will move the person toward his or her freely chosen goals.

As described previously, the context can either be an opportunity for or a threat to action, which could cause the person to act successfully, not act at all, or adjust their plan to meet the demands of the environment. It is important to note that a person can act to meet an environmental demand that will not satisfy his or her psychological needs. This action, while coming from the person, is not coming from the agentic self (i.e., this action may not be in service to a person's freely chosen goals). For example, an adult with intellectual disability who wants to work at a restaurant may be supported by a service agency that only employs individuals in a segregated setting working on an assembly line. The person may work in the sheltered workshop for something to do, but this action may not be agentic if the person desires work in the community. Rather, the action may be motivated by external (environmental) demands, such as a lack of support to find competitive employment.

Self-determination has been linked with many desired outcomes for adults with intellectual disability. For example, intervention to promote self-determination in a career context has also been show to increase employment outcomes (Dean, Burke, Shogren, & Wehmeyer, 2017; Dean, Shogren, Wehmeyer, Almire, & Mellenbruch, 2019). In transition-aged young adults, students with higher levels of self-determination also have better employment outcomes (Shogren, Wehmeyer, Palmer, Rifenbark, & Little, 2013) and increased quality of life (Nota, Ferrari, Soresi, & Wehmeyer, 2007). Given the importance of self-determination, occupational therapy practitioners who serve adults with intellectual disability should incorporate practices that promote self-determination into their work.

What Does Self-Determination Look Like?

As described previously, self-determination is a personal characteristic that is unique for each individual (Wehmeyer, 2005). It means more than making choices, although this is a component. Self-determination will look differently for various individuals, so a unique approach to understanding the individual and their life goals is needed. However, we can know if an adult with intellectual disability is supported in a way that affords them the opportunity to express their self-determination (Agran, Storey, & Krupp, 2010). For example, if a person makes a choice, do we honor that choice? When a person encounters a barrier, do we remove the barrier for him or her, or do we teach the person how to overcome (or go around) the barrier? If a person communicates a choice, but we don't understand his or her communication style, do we teach alternative methods of communication so the person can be understood (Johnson & Bagatell, 2018)?

For people who communicate through action or behavior, understanding a person's interests can be difficult. Do we seek to understand what they are communicating? Do we enter a relationship with the person so that we can fully understand the person's interests based on his or her behavior? Mahoney, Roberts, Bryze, and Parker Kent (2016) describe behaviors that occupational therapists can observe that may indicate interest in activities. By observing individuals with intellectual disability, we can begin to understand a person's interests by noticing what activities the person initiates, the person's affect while engaging, and the person's focused attention on the activity.

Understanding a person's interests is foundational in supporting self-determination and a meaningful life. Professionals can then begin to put in place a system of support to promote engagement in those interests. For example, if an adult who attends a day program seems to be drawn to activities involving water, perhaps he or she would be interested in exploring jobs at a car wash. An occupational therapist can structure car washing to promote learning of the task and begin to assess the person's interest. If an adult is drawn to playing ball games in the day program, maybe he or she can be taught how to play basketball at the community gym. Whether the authentic context is a car wash or community basketball court, prospects for developing friendships and connections based on interest will be enhanced. As the person engages in meaningful activity where other community members also engage in those same activities more opportunities for self-expression and self-determination will ensue.

Finally, it is important to note that self-determination is different from being independent (Wehmeyer, 2005). Self-determination is about making decisions and mobilizing action toward those decisions. A person can be self-determined by directing his or her supports toward their goal. For example, a woman who wants a job but does not know how to read will need help finding available jobs and filling out job applications; however, she can make the decision about whether or not the job is a good fit for her. Conversely, a person can be skilled at many tasks, but if others always prescribe those tasks, the person may not have the opportunity to exercise their self-determination.

Socio-Ecological Models of Participation

Modern conceptualizations of disability describe disability as a mismatch between a person and their environment. One of the first organizations to promote a socio-ecological framework was the World Health Organization (2001) in their *International Classification of Functioning, Disability and Health* (ICF). The ICF highlights the relationship between the environment and person by defining *participation* as a balance between health conditions (e.g., disorders and diseases) and environmental factors. Environmental factors are the physical, social, and attitudinal elements of a person's surroundings, which can either promote or inhibit participation in real-life, social settings. Occupational therapists and other professionals who are concerned with the effects of the person and the environment on participation use similar socio-ecological models to guide their practice (Dunn, Brown, & McGuigan, 1994).

Professionals who support people with intellectual disability developed a model of human functioning that conceptualizes disability in a similar way to the ICF (Schalock et al., 2010). This model, developed by the American Association on Intellectual and Developmental Disabilities (AAIDD), describes disability as a part of the continuum of normal human functioning. Disability is still considered a mismatch between a person's skills, abilities, and the environment; however, the AAIDD model also introduces the concept of supports, which can help bridge the gap between a person and his or her environment.

When participating in a given context, a person requires support when there is a mismatch between the skills, experiences, and interests of the person and the social, physical, and cultural demands of a given context. Support within the physical environment could be adapting the environment, such as the addition of a tool to complete a task, or the removal of an obstacle to allow a person to move from one place to another. Additionally, a training program could alter the social environment of a person with intellectual disability for caregivers designed to place more importance on the interests and goals of the person with intellectual disability.

AAIDD has conceptualized the term *supports* to mean "resources and strategies used to promote the development, education, interests and well-being of a person and to enhance individual functioning," (Luckasson et al., 2002). Supports are used to lessen the gap between a person and his or her environment so that he or she can participate more fully (Thompson et al., 2009). While supports can be used to build capacity within an individual, such as providing education, they are generally thought of as environmental modifications designed to align the demands of the environment with a person's strengths. Using this definition, professionals who want to support a person, to minimize the effect of a condition or impairment, can support the person by building capacity in either the person or the environment. Many times, it is in the person's best interest for professionals to focus their interventions on the environment rather than the person (Dunn et al., 1994). For example, a person who exhibits behavioral issues in a segregated setting can be supported to work in a different environment without first needing to change his or her behavior in the segregated environment.

Related to self-determination, context and supports can promote or inhibit self-determined action (Shogren, 2013). One way the context can support self-determination is through providing an opportunity to express self-determination. Adults with developmental disabilities who transitioned from a more to less restrictive environment (e.g., moving from a group home where staff is always present and the person has several roommates to his or her own home) became more self-determined (Wehmeyer & Bolding, 2001). Similarly, people with developmental disabilities who lived in less restrictive housing arrangements had more personal control than people who lived in more restrictive housing (Stancliffe, Abery, & Smith, 2000) and more opportunities to make choices (Neely-Barnes, Marcenko, & Weber, 2008).

Promoting Self-Determination

Occupational therapists can promote self-determination by building component skills of self-determination, such as goal setting, choice making, and problem solving (Wehmeyer & Shogren, 2016). Opportunities to build these skills are inherent in authentic participation contexts. This section will define each of these component skills and discuss how occupational therapy intervention can promote development of these skills.

Goal setting is a critical component of self-determination. Setting a goal requires a person to know what they want to do and understand the barriers they may face. Experience participating in the activities for which an individual is setting a goal is key to this process. For example, a person who wants a job in a restaurant has many options. They may want to cook or work more closely with customers. Both of these positions require a different set of skills and present different barriers. Gaining experience performing different duties related to different positions in a restaurant will help the person narrow their focus on setting goals to obtain a restaurant job.

Adults with intellectual disability had historically little opportunity to set goals for themselves, therefore, affording the person the opportunity to set goals becomes an important step in the therapeutic process. Occupational therapists can create environments where adults are supported in setting goals and working to achieve those goals (Krammer, Roemer, Liljenquist, Shin, & Hart, 2014).

Providing more opportunity for self-direction can increase a person's self-determination. Heller, Miller, and Factor (1998) and Heller, Miller, and Hsieh (2002) studied the impact of support systems on the participation of adults with intellectual disability. They found that people who lived in smaller settings, as well as settings where residents could make decisions about the arrangement and decoration of living spaces and activity planning, had a higher level of community integration. These findings are consistent with the self-determination literature. Researchers have demonstrated that by only changing a person's living or working environment, a person can become more self-determined (Stancliffe et al., 2000; Wehmeyer & Bolding, 2001). Participants in these studies had the opportunity to make decisions for themselves and they responded by making those decisions.

Problem solving involves working through barriers to achieve a desired outcome. To solve a problem, a person must understand the problem, develop possible solutions, decide on a course of action, and evaluate the outcome of their action related to the problem (Wehmeyer & Shogren, 2016). When learning how to problem solve, it is important to remember that unsuccessful attempts to solve a problem can be just as beneficial as successful attempts. An important component of occupational therapy, for adults with intellectual disability, is to let the person decide which action to take to solve the problem. If they are unsuccessful, this is a time to process the experience with the person and support them to set a new course of action.

Occupational therapists need to enhance goal-setting and problem solving with their clients. The Cognitive Orientation to daily Occupational Performance (CO-OP; Polatajko & Mandich, 2004) is a client-centered, performance-based approach developed in Canada, supported by evidence, and applied worldwide with children and adults who experience problems with daily activities. In this model, a client sets a goal and then learns a problem-solving routine designed to promote self-regulated performance (Missiua, Mandich, Polatajko, & Malloy-Miller, 2001). This intervention has typically been used in children to address difficulties in motor-learning; however, the elements of client-directed goal setting and self-regulated problem solving make CO-OP a promising intervention to promote aspects of self-determination in adults with intellectual disability as well.

For adults with intellectual disability, occupational therapists have collaborated with special educators to implement the Self-Determined Career Development Model (SDCDM). The SDCDM promotes goal setting and problem solving related to employment. During the intervention, a facilitator supports a job seeker through three problem-based phases to address barriers to employment (Wehmeyer & Palmer, 2003). In the first phase, the job seeker is supported to set an employment-related goal. In phase two, the job seeker develops and implements a plan designed to meet the goal identified in phase one. Finally, in phase three, the job seeker reflects on his or her progress toward the goal, which could result in modifying the goal or developing a new goal. The SDCDM has been successful in supporting career development and self-determination for individuals with disability (Dean et al., 2017; Dean et al., 2019).

Occupational therapists can act as facilitators during the process or can support the process by creating opportunities for the job seeker to gain the needed experience to navigate the problem-solving phases. For example, if a person is setting a goal related to obtaining employment but has little experience with employment, the occupational therapist may set up shadowing experiences in different job sectors so the person can understand what is required of them in specific jobs. The following case example will demonstrate how an occupational therapist can support self-determination related to employment.

CASE EXAMPLE

Caroline is a 30-year-old woman who sought support from an occupational therapist at her community support agency (CSA) for adults with intellectual disability. The occupational therapist leads the employment program at the CSA and Caroline wanted a job. Caroline's support team was concerned about her looking for employment because she came into the CSA with poor personal hygiene and dirty clothes. The therapist agreed to assess Caroline's morning routine while he helped her look for a job.

Discovering Interests/Making Choices

During the home visits with Caroline, the occupational therapist noticed that Caroline loved to talk about her clothes and got satisfaction from arranging them in her closet. This observation was in contrast to her daily appearance. Caroline frequently wore the same clothes for multiple days and did not bathe regularly. When asked why she didn't wear her nice clothes every day, she shrugged and said, "I don't see anyone during the day." Based on Caroline's interest in clothes, the occupational therapist began talking with Caroline about a job with clothing retailers.

Setting a Goal

Caroline said she would be interested in a job in a clothing store. The occupational therapist supported Caroline to set goals related to her employment interests. Caroline set goals related to developing interview skills and learning what the potential job demands would be. She also indicated that she would need support to find and apply for jobs because she did not have access to a computer or reliable transportation.

Putting a Plan in Motion

The occupational therapist contacted a clothing retail store near the CSA where Caroline spent her day. The store had an opening and was interested in interviewing Caroline. Meanwhile, Caroline began practicing her interview skills. Caroline developed a series of questions that she thought the employer would ask during an interview. She then began practicing responses to those questions. The occupational therapist conducted mock interviews to give Caroline a chance to practice being asked questions. At the same time, the occupational therapist tried various behavioral and environmental interventions to address Caroline's hygiene and dressing routines. The therapist learned that Caroline understood the routines she needed to complete but did not complete them. No change in these routines occurred until Caroline learned that she was going to visit the store and they were hiring. The following day, Caroline came into the CSA bathed and dressed in clean clothes. She was smiling and telling everyone she had an interview. When Caroline visited the store, she shadowed employees to learn more about their jobs. The occupational therapist debriefed Caroline after these visits to help her analyze her strengths related to the jobs and also her support needs. Caroline got the job after her successful interview.

Role of Context With Daily Routine

The day after Caroline found out she had an interview, she came into the program with her teeth brushed, hair washed, and dressed professionally. The therapist complemented Caroline on her appearance and asked what caused the change. Caroline replied, "I have an interview." Caroline continued with her hygiene and dressing routine and eventually found out she got the job at the clothing retailer. She has continued washing and dressing nicely. In the end, Caroline's context needed to be altered for her to complete the hygiene routine. That is, the expectations of appropriate dress in the workplace prompted Caroline to change her hygiene and dressing routines. When she got the interview, she was no longer a day program member but a job seeker. She understood the expectations of being a job seeker and began meeting those expectations.

CONCLUSION

This chapter has described self-determination for adults with intellectual disability and described ways that occupational therapists can support self-determination in practice. Through supporting self-determination, we are also supporting participation in self-chosen, meaningful activities that are central to the health and well-being of all people. As this chapter points out, context can play a large role in supporting self-determination, especially through providing opportunities to make choices, problem solve, and attain goals.

REFERENCES

American Occupational Therapy Association. (2014). Occupational therapy practice framework: Domain and process, 3rd edition. *American Journal of Occupational Therapy, 68*(Suppl. 1), S1-S48.

Agran, M., Storey, K., & Krupp, M. (2010). Choosing and choice making are not the same: Asking "what do you want for lunch?" is not self-determination. *Journal of Vocational Rehabilitation, 33*, 77-88.

Benitez, D. T., Lattimore, J., & Wehmeyer, M. L. (2005). Promoting the involvement of students with emotional and behavioral disorders in career and vocational planning and decision-making: The self-determined career development model. *Behavioral Disorders*, 431-447.

Dean, E. E., Burke, K. M., Shogren, K. A., & Wehmeyer, M. L. (2017). Promoting self-determination and integrated employment through the Self-Determined Career Center Development model. *Advances in Neurodevelopment and Disorders, 1*(2), 55-62. doi: 10.1007/s41252-017-0011-y

Dean, E. E., Fisher, K. W., Shogren, K. A., & Wehmeyer, M. L. (2016). Participation and intellectual disability: A review of the literature. *Intellectual and Developmental Disabilities, 54*(6), 427-439.

Dean, E. E., Shogren, K. A., Wehmeyer, M. L., Almire, B., & Mellenbruch, R. (2019). Career design and development for adults with intellectual disability: A program evaluation. *Advances in Neurodevelopment and Disorders, 3*(2), 111-118.

Devlin, P. (2008). Enhancing the job performance of employees with disabilities using the self-determined career development model. *Education and Training in Developmental Disabilities*, 502-513.

Dunn, W., Brown, C., & McGuigan, A. (1994). The ecology of human performance: A framework for considering the effect of context. *American Journal of Occupational Therapy, 48*, 595-607.

Heller, T., Miller, A. B., & Factor, A. (1998). Environmental characteristics of nursing homes and community-based settings, and the well-being of adults with intellectual disability. *Journal of Intellectual Disability Research, 42*, 418-428.

Heller, T., Miller, A. B., & Hsieh, K. (2002). Eight-year follow-up of the impact of environmental characteristics on well-being of adults with developmental disabilities. *Mental Retardation, 40*, 366-378.

Johnson, K. R., & Bagatell, N. (2018). "No! You can't have it": Problematizing choice in institutionalized adults with intellectual disabilities. *Journal of Intellectual Disabilities*, 1-16.

Kramer, J. M., Roemer, K., Liljenquist, K., Shin, J., & Hart, S. (2014). Formative evaluation of Project TEAM (Teens Making Environment and Activity Modifications). *Intellectual and Developmental Disabilities, 52*, 258-272.

Luckasson, R., Borthwick-Duffy, S., Buntinx, W. H. E., Coulter, D. L., Craig, E. M., Reeve, A., ... Tasse, M. J. (2002). *Mental retardation: Definition, classification, and systems of supports* (10th ed.). Washington, D.C.: American Association on Mental Retardation.

Mahoney, W. J., Roberts, E., Bryze, K., & Parker Kent, J. A. (2016). Occupational engagement and adults with intellectual disabilities. *American Journal of Occupational Therapy, 70*, 7001350030.

Missiuna, C., Mandich, A. D., Polatajko, H. J., & Malloy-Miller, T. (2001). Cognitive Orientation to daily Occupational Performance (CO-OP) part I—Theoretical foundations. *Physical & Occupational Therapy in Pediatrics, 20*, 69-81.

Neely-Barnes, S., Marcenko, M., & Weber, L. (2008). Does choice influence quality of life for people with mild intellectual disabilities? *Intellectual and Developmental Disabilities, 46*, 12-26.

Nota, L., Ferrari, L., Soresi, S., & Wehmeyer, M. (2007). Self-determination, social abilities and the quality of life of people with intellectual disability. *Journal of Intellectual Disability Research, 51*, 850-865.

Polatajko, H., & Mandich, A. (2004). *Enabling occupation in children: The Cognitive Orientation to daily Occupational Performance (CO-OP) approach*. Ottawa, ON, Canada: CAOT Publications.

Ryan, R. M., & Deci, E. L. (2000). Self-determination theory and the facilitation of intrinsic motivation, social development, and well-being. *American Psychologist, 55*, 68-78.

Schalock, R. L., Borthwick-Duffy, S. A., Bradley, V. J., Buntinx, W. H., Coulter, D. L., Craig, E. M., ... Reeve, A. (2010). *Intellectual disability: Definition, classification, and systems of supports* (Vol. 26). Washington, D.C.: American Association on Intellectual and Developmental Disabilities.

Shogren, K. A. (2013). A social-ecological analysis of the self-determination literature. *Intellectual and Developmental Disabilities, 51*, 496-511.

Shogren, K. A., Wehmeyer, M. L., Palmer, S. B., Forber-Pratt, A., Little, T., & Lopez, S. (2015). Causal agency theory: Reconceptualizing a functional model of self-determination. *Education and Training in Autism and Developmental Disabilities, 50*, 251-263.

Shogren, K. A., Wehmeyer, M. L., Palmer, S. B., Rifenbark, G., & Little, T. (2013). Relationships between self-determination and postschool outcomes for youth with disabilities. *Journal of Special Education, 48*(4), 256-267.

Stancliffe, R. J., Abery, B. H., & Smith, J. (2000). Personal control and the ecology of community living settings: Beyond living-unit size and type. *American Journal on Mental Retardation, 105*, 431-454.

Thompson, J. R., Bradley, V. J., Buntinx, W. H. E., Schalock, R. L., Shogren, K. A., Snell, M. E., ... Yeager, M. H. (2009). Conceptualizing supports and the support needs of people with intellectual disability. *Intellectual and Developmental Disabilities, 47*, 135-146.

Wehmeyer, M. L. (1999). A functional model of self-determination describing development and implementing instruction. *Focus on Autism and Other Developmental Disabilities, 14*, 53-61.

Wehmeyer, M. L. (2005). Self-determination and individuals with severe disabilities: Re-examining meanings and misinterpretations. *Research and Practice for Persons with Severe Disabilities, 30*, 113-120.

Wehmeyer, M. L., & Bolding, N. (2001). Enhanced self-determination of adults with intellectual disability as an outcome of moving to community-based work or living environments. *Journal of Intellectual Disability Research, 45*(5), 371-383.

Wehmeyer, M. L., & Palmer, S. B. (2003). Adult outcomes for students with cognitive disabilities three-years after high school: The impact of self-determination. *Education and Training in Developmental Disabilities, 38*, 131-144.

Wehmeyer, M. L., & Shogren, K. A. (2016). Self-determination and learners with autism spectrum disorders. In R. Simpson & B. S. Myles (Eds.), *Educating children and youth with autism: Strategies for effective practice* (3rd ed.). Austin, TX: ProEd.

World Health Organization. (2001). *International classification of functioning, disability and health* (ICF). Geneva, Switzerland: Author.

6

The Human-Ness of Relationships

Mariana D'Amico, EdD, OTR/L, FAOTA

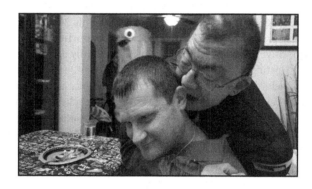

Key Words: childbearing, child raising, friendships, identity, marriage, roles, sexuality, social skills

Bryze, K.
Occupational Therapy for Adults With Intellectual Disability (pp. 61-72).
© 2020 Taylor & Francis Group.

Human beings are inherently relational, beginning before birth and predisposed toward seeking connection and interaction with others. Even in the face of significant communication, sensory, and cognitive impairments, human beings are social, seeking relationships with others. Literature supports the importance of early relationships as foundational for health, well-being, and a long life (Anderson & Anderson, 2003; Friedman & Martin, 2011; Gladwell, 2000). Therefore, it is important that these first relational foundations are healthy and positive. Occupational therapy practitioners should consider and address the importance of social relationships and interactions in their work with persons with intellectual disability across their life span. This chapter will address issues related to relationships within family contexts, between teacher and student, friendships, romantic relationships, and the social skills that support social interactions, which build and support relationships.

FAMILY AS PRIMARY CAREGIVER AND RELATIONSHIP

Family may include one or two parents, siblings, extended family members, such as grandparents, aunts, uncles, and cousins, and friends chosen as family members. These primary family relationships are important in setting the foundation for other future relationships beyond childhood, such as friendship, romantic love, marriage, family, and community participation. Parents of children with intellectual disability experience both sadness and joy with their children, with most parents reporting positive emotions that balance negative experiences (Bostrom, Broberg, & Hwang, 2010; Giallo & Gavidia-Payne, 2006; Hastings, Allen, McDermott, & Still, 2002). Many parents of children with intellectual disability provide love and understanding, opportunities for personal and family growth, generation of positive attitudes, and engagement of family and friends as supports (Giallo & Gavidia-Payne, 2006; Hastings et al., 2002). Such healthy, positive parental relationships are important for all children, including those with intellectual disability, as this first relationship sets up the foundation for future relationships with siblings, friends, teachers, community members, and significant others. Children develop self-esteem and emotional health through this first relationship (Roberts & Bengtson, 1993). Therefore, it is extremely important to provide support or identify resources in the community and family for parents of children with and without disabilities.

Families with strong, positive marital relationships and parent-child relationships demonstrate less conflict and dysfunction between family members and siblings (Schuntermann, 2007). Thus, they provide a more nurturing and loving experience for their child with intellectual disability as well as their other children. They identify their children as a source of joy, spiritual growth, and family unity, and this carries over to the siblings of the child with intellectual disability as they also learn those skills and develop similar relationships with their sibling and their parents (Choi, 2013; Floyd, Purcell, Richardson, & Kupersmidt, 2009; Giallo & Gavidia-Payne, 2006; Schuntermann, 2007). The child with intellectual disability also learns what comprises a loving, nurturing relationship. While having a child with intellectual disability may be a source of stress for the family, many things can ameliorate that stress, such as loving relationships and supports. External supports of grandparents, friends, and other relatives may provide buffers to unhealthy family dynamics and stressors, and promote prosocial behaviors and wellness of the family and the child with special needs. Loving relationships provide the secure attachment needed for safely engaging in the world. Regardless of the severity of the intellectual impairment, a human being recognizes and responds to loving and caring.

Family routines provide another mechanism for providing a stable, secure experience for children, especially for the child with intellectual disability. As family behaviors and interactions are consistent within the child's world, learning can take place. Consistent family routines also help siblings adjust to life challenges around a sibling with intellectual disability (Giallo & Gavidia-Payne, 2006). Clear behavioral expectations of family interactions, modeled well by parents as role models, assist with role and skill development within the family unit and set a foundation for future relationships. Something as simple as expectations for completing chores or home maintenance, such as picking up toys, eating together, and playing together, help establish routines and patterns of behavior. Finding ways to engage the child with intellectual disability in the family routines, regardless of their level of performance, is important for all members of the family and provides lessons in perseverance, coping, gentleness, understanding, and love. Confident parenting, paired with appropriately high expectations, results in responsiveness from all children, especially when expectations are clear and explicit (Platt, Roper, Mandleco, & Freeborn, 2014). Parents who promote positive sibling relationships and include the typical sibling in sharing the care for their child with intellectual disability provide opportunity for the development of empathy and overall positive family dynamics. Life rituals, whether familial, spiritual, religious, or community-based, provide opportunity for identity, growth, and belonging for all family members, including the child with intellectual disability. Life celebrations and transitions are part of family routines and engender expected patterns of behavior (Platt et al., 2014).

Children with intellectual disability raised in neglectful or abusive homes, or who have severe sensory deficits, may manifest significantly impaired behavior and ineffective relationships with others or themselves. These behavioral challenges may range from odd and illogical to harmful or detrimental to self and others, such as self-injurious or aggressive behaviors (McEwen, 2003). Often children from neglectful or abusive homes manifest emotional and physical scars, may be malnourished, diagnosed with failure to thrive, or depression, or present with aggression and hostility (McEwen, 2003). These unsuccessful initial family relationships result in poor attachment and trust, fear, and anger. Skills learned are often inappropriate but develop as attempts toward survival. Socially inappropriate behaviors may emerge that provide some solace or protection in a chaotic or unsafe home environment, such as rocking or other stereotypies, but will be unacceptable elsewhere. Negative life experiences change the biochemistry of the mind and body (McEwen, 2003); emotional and physical dysregulation will impair the child's ability to relate to others and find comfort in their presence. Greater understanding and concerted efforts to work together, as part of health care/educational teams, may be required for acquiring the skills to assist such fragile children successfully. Sensory-based interventions may assist those individuals with intellectual disability who have sensory sensitivity or sensory-seeking behaviors. Sensory-based interventions may deter the individual engaging in self-stimulatory or harmful behaviors. Those who are hypersensitive may need some gentle, incremental exposure to sensory experiences. Guided learning and/or behavior modification programs may assist some individuals in developing basic skills. Creating a safe, consistent, trustworthy environment will be vital for learning essential skills for relationship building with an individual who has severe behaviors and sensitivities.

SIBLINGS

Sibling relationships are the second most significant family relationship for children with intellectual disability. Positive sibling relationships are important for both the siblings with and without intellectual disability. Siblings provide a significant foundation for learning how to relate to others in a prosocial manner, perceive negative interactions, and negotiate play skills for peer engagement (Floyd et al., 2009). Sibling relationships may be positive or negative and provide opportunities for growth and development, as well as learning to love and care for others, develop a sense of purpose, responsibility, and maturity. Non-disabled siblings experience challenges with their siblings who learn slower, have difficulty learning and adhering to social rules and behavior, and who demonstrate disruptive behaviors (Graff et al., 2012). The siblings may develop a closeness with their brother or sister with intellectual disability, which may result in becoming the caregiver and protector in later life. However, during adolescence, some siblings may find the sibling with disabilities more challenging to care for and have peer relationships with (Graff et al., 2012). Healthy parental relationship and interactions, as well as external supports, may mediate sibling conflicts and distress (Choi, 2013).

Sibling gender may influence the relationship as well, as girls and boys relate differently to their sibling with intellectual disability. Boys tend to see their disabled sibling as a playmate and may challenge them to develop play skills and teach them how to play. Girls, on the other hand, often emulate the mother in the caregiving role and provide direction and instruction on behavioral expectations (Floyd et al., 2009). Both boys and girls view their sibling with intellectual disability as a friend and see themselves as future care providers (Graff et al., 2012). Siblings with and without disabilities benefit from positive, warm, affectionate sibling relationships with better mental health and emotional states (Gass, Jenkins, & Dunn, 2007). Their relationships influence their ability to mediate stress, have friendships, and relationships with others through their shared co-occupations of play, family activity, and community engagement.

TEACHER-STUDENT RELATIONSHIP

Teacher student relationships are important, as are those of family and friends, especially during the developmental years. Similar to the relationships between parent and child, the relationship between teacher and student influences self-esteem and agency and is also important for developing the skills of social communication and working with others. Influences that affect adjustment to school and non-school environments include poor behavioral control, social disengagement, and low academic success, which influences their relationships with teachers (Eisenhower, Baker, & Blacher, 2007). While students with intellectual disability require more assistance for adjustment and success in school, a good relationship with the teacher can mediate and improve the outcomes for these students (Eisenhower et al., 2007). Teacher-student relationships may be challenged when a student's needs are high or the student has significant behavioral challenges (McGrath & Van Bergen, 2015; Nurmi, 2012; Pianta, Hamre, & Allen, 2012). Thus, it becomes important to equip teachers with the skills and supports to create a warm, flexible environment for students with intellectual disability. The teacher who can help the child self-regulate and adapt to the school environment can also help their peers engage with the student with intellectual disability successfully and mitigate conflicts and disruptions. Children spend a quarter of their waking hours in school and positive teacher-student relationships and personal interactions improve agency and peer relationships for all children. Again, engagement, whether through technology assistance, bodily means, peer assistance, or adaptive assistance, in mutually enjoyable activities with others, promotes healthy behavior, mood, sociability, and student learning outcomes (McGrath & Van Bergen, 2015; Nurmi, 2012; Pianta et al., 2012). Given the proper environment and warm teacher-student interactions, all students can learn and flourish.

FRIENDSHIP

Friendship is where one learns what it is to be in trusting relationships outside the family, and how these first relationships develop (Duguay, 2011). Friendship is the foundation of most relationships—sibling, peer, and romantic. Friendships form through repeated mutual engagement in co-occupations. Within the context of occupations, warmth, affection, and trust develop between those engaged in the occupational processes. A friend is a person with whom one has a bond of mutual affection and respect. Friendship can range in degrees of intensity, from acquaintances to best friends, and with whom one shares secrets, hopes, dreams, and life experiences. Acquaintances can become friends by frequently meeting at the same place at the same time, such as bus friends, lunch friends, or library friends. These relationships may begin tentatively, and then deepen as the frequency and sharing becomes more automatic and comfortable. It is important to teach individuals with intellectual disability about the different levels of friendship with something like a circle of people or friends diagram. Those who are closest are friends, while those who are furthest away may be acquaintances or strangers.

Friendships and interconnections form the basis for community, and communities built on healthy relationships have sustained their livelihood, growing and prospering together by hunting, gathering food, farming together, working out differences, and valuing each other's contributions (Pontzer, 2017). Social networks are life sustaining and provide emotional and physical supports; persons who are socially supported and connected with others will live longer, healthier lives despite an existing disability or poor health conditions (Anderson & Anderson, 2003; Gladwell, 2000). This human connectedness is what sustains people through childhood, adolescence, adulthood, and later adulthood.

Parents want their children to have friends and engage socially, regardless of disability, condition, or health challenges (Cohn, Miller, & Tickle-Degnan, 2000; Mactavish & Schleien, 2004: Parkinson, Rice, & Young, 2011). Loneliness is often a precursor to depression and feeling disenfranchised by society, such as having classmates that are friendly but not really friends (Duguay, 2011). Having a social network of friends is perceived to be a sign of health and happiness for both children and adults (Anderson & Anderson, 2003). Sharing experiences, thoughts, and activities is part of relationship and friendship. One such effort of building intensive relationships and friendships is encompassed by the Circle of Friends Program (http://www.circleoffriends.org). In the program, which begins for young children in school and continues through graduation from high school, students with and without disability eat lunch and spend time together, conversing and playing games, creating circles of friends.

A parallel in adulthood is the Best Buddies Program (www.bestbuddies.org). This program's main purpose is to allow volunteers to be paired with a buddy with intellectual disability and provide them with a friend. Best Buddies is dedicated to ending the social, physical, and economic isolation of people with intellectual disability.

Having friends and participating in activities with peers favor the development of dating, romantic relationships, and sexual activity (Wiegerink et al., 2010). Having friends feeds the soul and the heart, no matter what life brings or the challenges people face. Friends bring joy, share sadness, provide support, encouragement, and guidance. Friends provide people with a sense of value and belonging. Friends are people with whom one can be free in the fullness of one's personhood. From friendship, love and romantic relationships develop.

All people have a desire for intimate relationships. Individuals with intellectual disability have the same human desires and drives for love as everyone else. Fulfilling love relationships include friendships, passion, playfulness, support, and compatibility of values, finances, raising family, and interaction with others. Many individuals hope to marry someone who is not only their life partner, spouse, and lover, but also best friend. Higgins (2010) states that relationships and social networks are intricately linked to sexual well-being and human rights. People are born with the innate drive for connection with others and this is no different for people with intellectual disability. They also desire friendship, relationship, romantic love, to marry, and have families. While parents, teachers, and society may view this population differently, needing protection, as asexual, or limited in capability (Higgins, 2010; Howard-Barr, Rienzo, Pigg, & James, 2005; Swango-Wilson, 2010, 2011; Wilkenfeld & Ballan, 2011), this is a misperception that is being challenged.

SOCIAL SKILLS AND BOUNDARIES

Adults with intellectual disability experience all life's emotions but may not always have the words to communicate their feelings in socially acceptable ways. This is an area where much training is required for some individuals so they can understand themselves and others (Noonan & Taylor Gomez, 2011). Social skills are the framework in which friendships and other relationships exist, whether work, community, family, parenting, or romantic relationships. Social skills training must often be explicit; some skills may be learned implicitly but most will need to be learned explicitly with pictures, words, and experiences. Self-protection and personal advocacy should be part of this training. Learning which actions of others are safe and which are dangerous and what boundaries exist within relationships to maintain safety and dignity are important for children and adults with or without disabilities. Children and adults with intellectual disability are often susceptible to sexual and physical abuse by others, including caregivers (Higgins, 2010; McCarthy 2014).

ROLES AND IDENTITY

Individuals with and without disabilities develop roles that shape identity throughout their life span. Beginning in childhood, a person identifies as male or female regardless of birth gender, and as a family member, takes on roles taught or expected within the family context. Individuals' roles include child, parent, worker, friend, lover, and caretaker and the roles will change over time as the environmental press influences the physical, technological, and social dimensions of one's life. Role expectations within family relationships are important for the person with intellectual disability. The individual then understands to whom they belong, develops identity as a human being of value, and develops skills that support their role expectations. Gaining responsibility and mastering behavioral expectations help the person evolve into more advanced roles as they grow into adolescence and adulthood. Gender roles are classic identifiers based on culture, societal expectations, and family biases. Other life roles evolve from relationships and opportunities, such as daughter, son, student, worker, friend, adult, wife, husband, spouse, significant other, volunteer, Girl or Boy Scout, and team member.

Providing opportunities for role development and exploration is essential for all persons. Persons with intellectual disability may need extra training or supports to develop skills associated with roles or to identify roles they want to pursue. Opportunities should be afforded early in life within the family, with responsibilities for chores and inclusion in family activities. Parents often need to seek out or create opportunities in their communities where their family member with disabilities can participate, especially in activities where persons without disabilities are involved. Occupational therapists can create programs, such as dance, sports, social events, and volunteer activities within the community. For example, including a student with intellectual disability as a member of a team or club and providing the instruction they need to participate, or educating other team members how to provide direction and be inclusive can be a role an occupational therapy practitioner can assume. Consider other opportunities, such as learning to shop with family and friends, participating in social outings with peers from school, church, or the neighborhood, will further contribute to a person's role development. Persons with intellectual disability will need to learn to self-advocate within schools, communities, and industries for opportunities to engage and be included. Learning how to communicate assertively and be able to discern which people or experiences are hurtful or dangerous need to be part of social skills development for these individuals (Dukes & McGuire, 2009; McCarthy, 2014).

The development of social and parenting roles for individuals with intellectual disability require support from service providers and community agencies (www.thearc.org). Fostering self-efficacy with emerging role development is important for these individuals, as they are frequently mistreated by systems, including learning to be dependent on others, fearing authority figures, limited training in self-sufficiency, maltreatment by caregivers or service providers, stigmatization, and overwhelming life circumstances (Green & Cruz, 2000). Supports should include "resources and strategies that promote the development, education, interests, and personal well-being of a person and enhance individual functioning" (Lightfoot & LaLiberte, 2011). Role development and identity are essential for anyone growing from adolescence to adulthood and roles assumed and desired by individuals with intellectual disability are the same as those without disabilities.

SEXUALITY AND MARRIAGE

Identity as a sexual being is a natural part of one's identity and having intimate relationships is a basic human drive. Affection that begins in friendship may develop into a loving relationship and manifest in the desire to be physically close to someone, hold them, hug them, touch them, or kiss them. Touch is the first major sensory system by which we meet the world in utero and immediately after birth. As a person grows, learning to touch and be touched in a positive, healthy way develops from that first parent-child, safe and loving touch into other relationships.

"Sexuality is an integral part of the personality of everyone: man, woman and child. It is a basic need and an aspect of being human that cannot be separated from other aspects of human life," (Langfelt & Porter, cited in Richards, Miodrag, & Watson, 2006). Sexuality is part of personal identity and includes sexual orientation and preferences. Sexual exploration is part of normal development. Sexual engagement connects the pleasure centers of the mind and body, and is often part of a loving relationship (Richards et al., 2006). However, sexuality is still a taboo subject for many teachers, caregivers, parents, and even occupational therapy practitioners (Duguay, 2011).

Society has only recently begun to recognize that people with intellectual disability are sexual beings who have the same needs for affection, intimacy, and sexual relationship as those without disabilities (Richards et al., 2006; Shakespeare, 2000). Studies support that individuals with developmental disabilities are not seen as sexual beings by their teachers and parents (Higgins, 2010; Swango-Wilson, 2008, 2010, 2011) until inappropriate behaviors manifest in the home, classroom, or community. Isler, Beytut, Tas, and Conk (2009) emphasized it is crucial that parents who have a child, adolescent, or adult with special needs be informed and educated by health care professionals about sexual development. As intellectual and developmental disabilities exist in a wide range of functions and challenges, different individuals will require different interventions. However, those individuals with intellectual disability and inability to read social cues have the most difficult time addressing sexually related behaviors (McGuire & Bayley, 2011). Valencia and Cromer (2000) identified that teenagers with disabilities engage in sexual activity early due to the perception that sex is a normalizing teenage behavior and activity. Shandra and Chowdhury (2012) found that girls with challenging conditions or disabilities are more likely to want a pregnancy at the first sexual intercourse because of their desire for love and bonding with someone who cares for them. Having friends and participating in activities with typical peers favors development of dating, romantic relationships, and sexual activity (Wiegerink, et al., 2010).

The percentages of preference for sexual orientation is the same for people with and without intellectual disability (Bedard, Zhang, & Zucker, 2010). Thus, it is important to provide support and education about same sex attraction and relationships, including sexual health needs (Higgins, 2010; Noonan & Gomez, 2010). People with intellectual disability identify as heterosexual and as LGBTQ (lesbian, gay, bisexual, trans, and queer) and thus, require support and information about healthy ways to express their sexuality, regardless of relationship.

Unfortunately, people with disability are a vulnerable population when considering gender-based discrimination and sexually-based victimization (Duguay, 2010; Higgins, 2010; McGuire & Bayley, 2011). Both adults and children with intellectual disability are at greater risk for sexual assault, violence, and exploitation than people without disability (Sullivan & Knutson, 2000). Caregivers, familiar individuals, co-residents, family members, and facility staff are included in the potential perpetrators of such incidences (Bowman, Scotti, & Morris, 2010; Higgins, 2010; McCarthy, 2014). Individuals with intellectual disability may require more explicit education for protection and require greater vigilance on the part of parents, teachers, caregivers, and care providers. It is extremely important to educate providers, parents, teachers, and caregivers about sexual abuse awareness and prevention (Bowman et al., 2010; Isler et al., 2009; Higgins, 2010, McCarthy, 2014).

Self-pleasuring, through masturbation, is an activity that may begin in childhood as part of typical developmental exploration. Parents need to address this as they see fit, in accordance with their values. The challenge comes when children continue to engage in self-gratification at unacceptable locations and times, such as in the classroom during the school day. The response to such challenges should involve school personnel and family to create a plan for learning and behavior management. Additionally, the student may need direction on how to manage their pleasure and the pleasure of their chosen sexual partners and relationships (Beber & Biswis, 2009; Hellemans, Roeyers, Leplae, Dewaele, & Deboutte, 2010). Individuals with intellectual disability, especially women, will need to become knowledgeable and empowered in their ability to choose to engage sexually or not. Sexual education requires simple language, pictures, time, modeling of behaviors, social skills training, and supportive environments (McCarthy, 2014; Schaafsma, Kok, Stoffelen, & Curfs, 2014). One resource exists in the Florida Department for Developmental Disabilities (www.fddc.org) with its workbook for parents and teachers to address sexuality across the life span; other states may have similar resources located in their Departments of Disabilities or Education. Every parent and health care provider should avail themselves of resources about sexuality and all its expressions, as teaching our adolescents and adults with intellectual disability to engage in safe sexual behaviors is vital for their health and well-being. Such education also provides the opportunity for addressing life stages related to marriage and family development.

Some health care providers and parents have opted to have their daughters with intellectual disability sterilized or utilize various forms of birth control (McCarthy, 2011; Stefansdottir & Hreinsdottir, 2013). In its more severe ideology, the documented history of intellectual disability includes the atrocities of the eugenics movement of the early 20th century in the United States. Legislators, medical professionals, and even social reformers developed and enacted sterilization laws, which were motivated by the theory that certain undesirable genetic traits were the underlying causes of such social deficiencies as "feeblemindedness," "mental disturbance," "sexual deviance," and "criminology." Advocates of forced sterilization were persuasive and promoted reproductive surgery as a public health service to ensure that society would then be free from the genetic possibility of generating children who also had mental illness, mental deficiency, or other undesirable genetic characteristics (Stern, 2015). While many parents may still choose to have their young, adult daughters with intellectual disability use birth control devices or medication to avoid unwanted pregnancies (Grover, 2011), women with intellectual disability are physically capable of childbearing and may desire to have their own children. Men and women with disabilities have the same desires for family and loving relationships.

Many, if not most, children, regardless of disability, dream about and desire marriage and to live with their significant other. As individuals live within family, church, and community contexts, life rituals, such as marriage, are experienced. Strong personal identity and supportive family can encourage and assist in the process of planning a wedding and entering married life. Marriage for individuals with intellectual disability was once a greater concern but is now becoming a more acceptable and common reality, as these individuals are being viewed as having the same needs for friendship, love, and marriage. Recent publications and media presentations have conveyed portrayals of persons with Down syndrome or autism. In the United States and the United Kingdom, persons with mild intellectual disability tend to marry, some cultures expect marriage regardless of disability status, and other cultures even believe that marriage is a cure for the disability. Individuals with intellectual disability may often marry another person with disabilities (Beber & Biswis, 2009).

Marriage is an important and complex relationship that exceeds the sexual expectation to include love, caring, and gentleness (Dukes & McGuire, 2009; McCarthy, 2014; Schaafsma et al., 2014). Learning to cook, prepare meals together, maintain a home, clean, shop, and manage money are all skills needed to live in society and as a married couple. Sharing responsibilities with each other is important and may require training and education about the structuring of time and tasks. Some of these skills are learned in the home, school, or through community activities and opportunity. Some couples may need external support and guidance from community agencies and families to complete these tasks successfully.

PARENTING

Parents with intellectual disability can be successful raising their own children (The Arc, 2008; Beber & Biswas, 2009; Lightfoot & LaLiberte, 2011), although they may require significant supports in raising their child, such as education related to child care (e.g., feeding, clothing, health monitoring, safety). Occupational therapy practitioners could take the lead to provide supports to parents with intellectual disability for this educational and skill training. Through the Looking Glass is a nonprofit organization in Berkeley, California that is renowned for advocating and supporting parents with a variety of disabilities, providing advocacy, support, education, research, and services to families, professionals, and other organizations (http://lookingglass.org). In the United States, it is still common for children of parents with intellectual disability to be removed from the home and placed in other living situations (The Arc, 2008). The socioeconomic status and parenting capacity are both areas of concern. The United Nations Convention on the Rights of Persons with Disabilities supports keeping families intact by ensuring that a child not be separated from their parents based on disability. Helping parents access public benefits effectively, such as early intervention, nutritional resources, and crisis intervention services, are some ways community agencies can provide support. The American Association on Intellectual and Developmental Disability has advocated for providing parental supports for parents with intellectual disability to raise their own children, resulting in some states requiring child welfare agencies and the court system to consider the provision of parental supports; unfortunately funding for such programming remains limited (Lightfoot & LaLiberte, 2011).

Literature regarding the outcomes for children raised by parents with intellectual disability remains mixed. Some studies identify children as doing as well as others in development and success in school and as adults, while others identify children not being successful, requiring intervention (Collings & Llewellyn, 2012; Llewellyn, McConnell, Honey, Mayes, & Russo, 2003; McGaw, Ball, & Clark, 2002). Support groups for parents with intellectual disability promote the parents' well-being (McGaw et al., 2002). Providing home-based intervention may be beneficial and create better outcomes for the parents and their children (Llewellyn et al., 2003). Lastly, the importance of attachment and loving relationship bodes well for all children, despite having a parent with intellectual disability (Collings & Llewellyn, 2012; McGaw et al., 2002).

SPIRITUALITY

Individuals with intellectual disability have spiritual relationships within the faith traditions of one's family. These relationships within the faith community may become sources of support, a means of making friends, and a way to engage in the mission of the community. Spiritual communities become an outlet for social engagement, learning, kindness, and provide opportunity for individuals to live their faith practices. Faith traditions provide structure and routine and thus become nurturing in their own way. Such opportunities offer the development of social skills, work skills, volunteer activities, caretaking, and community integration, while feeding the soul, heart, and mind. Individuals belong, become, and do within the community through all life stages.

CONCLUSION

Relationships are essential for health and well-being. Positive, loving relationships promote a sense of being, belonging, and engagement in family, school, and the community for individuals with intellectual disability. Individuals desire engagement in loving relationships with a significant other. They can have healthy, intimate relationships and raise healthy children. Supports may be necessary to assist individuals with disability to live successful, loving lives and have enriched relationships and friendships.

REFERENCES

Anderson, N. B., & Anderson, P. E. (2003). *Emotional longevity: What really determines how long you live*. New York, NY: Penguin Books.

The Arc. (2008). Position statement: Parents with intellectual and/or developmental disabilities. Retrieved from www.thearc.org/who-we-are/position-statements/life-in-the-community/parents-with-idd

Beber, E., & Biswas, A. (2009). Marriage and family life in people with developmental disability. *International Journal of Culture and Mental Health, 2*(2), 102-108. doi: 10.1080/17447140903205317

Bedard, C., Zhang, H., & Zucker, K. (2010). Gender identity and sexual orientation in people with developmental disabilities. *Sexuality and Disability, 28*, 165-175.

Bostrom, P. K., Broberg, M., & Hwang, P. (2010). Parents' descriptions and experiences of young children recently diagnosed with intellectual disability. *Child: Care, Health, and Development, 36*, 93-100. doi: 10:10.1111/j.1365-2214.2009.01036.x

Bowman, R., Scotti, J., & Morris, T. (2010). Sexual abuse prevention: A training program for developmental disabilities service providers. *Journal of Child Sexual Abuse, 19*, 119-127.

Choi, H. (2013). Siblings of children with Down syndrome: An integrative review. *American Journal of Maternal Child Nursing, 38*(2), 72-78.

Cohn, E., Miller, L. J., & Tickle-Degnan, L. (2000). Parental hopes for therapy outcomes: Children with sensory modulation disorders. *American Journal of Occupational Therapy, 54*, 36-43.

Collings, S., & Llewellyn, G. (2012). Children of parents with intellectual disability: Facing poor outcomes or faring okay? *Journal of Intellectual & Developmental Disability, 37*(1), 65-82. doi: 10.3109/13668250.2011.648610

Duguay, L. (2011). Sexuality: Still a taboo subject? *Exceptional Parent Magazine*, 16-17.

Dukes, E., & McGuire, B. (2009). Enhancing capacity to make sexuality-related decisions in people with an intellectual disability. *Journal of Intellectual Disability Research, 53*(8), 727-734. doi: 10.1111/j.1365-2788.2009.01186.x

Eisenhower, A. S., Baker, B. L., & Blacher, J. (2007). Early student teacher relationships of children with and without intellectual disability: Contributions of behavioral, social, and self-regulatory competence. *Journal of School Psychology, 45*, 363-383. doi: 10.1016/j.jsp.2006.10.002

Floyd, F., Purcell, S. Richardson, S., & Kupersmidt, J. (2009). Sibling relationship quality and social functioning of children and adolescents with intellectual disability. *American Journal of Intellectual and Developmental Disability, 114*(2), 110-127.

Friedman, H. S., & Martin, L. R. (2011). *The longevity project*. New York, NY: Penguin Books.

Gass, K., Jenkins, J., & Dunn, J. (2007). Are sibling relationships protective? A longitudinal study. *Journal of Child Psychology and Psychiatry, 48*(2), 167-175.

Gladwell, M. (2000). *The tipping point*. Boston, MA: Little, Brown & Company.

Giallo, R., & Gavidia-Payne, S. (2006). Child, parent, and family factors as predictors of adjustment for siblings of children with disability. *Journal of Intellectual Disability Research, 50*(12), 937-948.

Graff, C., Mandleco, B., Dyches, T., Coverston, C., Roper, S., & Freeborn, D. (2012). Perspectives of adolescent siblings of children with Down syndrome who have multiple health problems. *Journal of Family Nursing, 18*(2), 175-199.

Green, N., & Cruz, V. (2000). *Working with families with children/parents with developmental disabilities*. Denver, CO: The Social Work Program, Metropolitan State College of Denver.

Grover, S. (2011). Gynaecological issues in adolescents with disability. *Journal of Paediatrics and Child Health, 47*, 610-613.

Hastings, R., Allen, R., McDermott, K., & Still, D. (2002). Factors related to positive perceptions in mothers of children with intellectual disabilities. *Journal of Applied Research in Intellectual Disabilities, 15*, 269-275.

Hellemans, H., Roeyers, H., Leplae, W., Dewale, T., & Deboutte, D. (2010) Sexual behavior in male adolescents and young adults with autism spectrum disorder and borderline/mild mental retardation. *Sexuality and Disability, 28*, 93-104.

Higgins, D. (2010). Sexuality, human rights and safety for people with disabilities: The challenge of intersecting identities. *Sexual and Relationship Therapy, 25*(3), 245-257. doi: 10.1080/14681994.2010.489545

Howard-Barr, E., Rienzo, B., Pigg, M., & James, D. (2005). Teacher beliefs, professional preparation and practices regarding exceptional students and sexuality education. *Journal of School Health, 75*(3), 99-104.

Isler, A., Beytut, D., Tas, F., & Conk, Z. (2009). A study on sexuality with the parents of adolescents with intellectual disability. *Sexuality and Disability, 29*, 229-237.

Lightfoot, E., & LaLiberte, T. (2011). Parental supports for parents with intellectual and developmental disabilities. *Intellectual and Developmental Disabilities, 49*(5), 1-7.

Llewellyn, G., McConnell, D., Honey, A., Mayes, R., & Russo, D. (2003). Promoting health and home safety for children of parents with intellectual disability: A randomized controlled trial. *Research in Developmental Disabilities, 24*, 405-431. doi: 10.1016/j.ridd.2003.06.001

Mactavish, J. B., & Schleien, S. J. (2004). Re-injecting spontaneity and balance family life: Parents' perspectives on recreation families that include children with developmental disability. *Journal of Intellectual Disability Research, 48*, 123-141.

McCarthy, M. (2011). Prescribing contraception to women with intellectual disabilities: General practitioners' attitudes and practices. *Sexuality and Disability, 29*, 339-349.

McCarthy, M. (2014). Women with intellectual disability: Their sexual lives in the 21st century. *Journal of Intellectual and Developmental Disability, 39*(2), 124-131. doi: 10.3109/13669250.2014.894963

McEwen, B. S. (2003). Early life influences on life-long patterns of behavior and health. *Mental Retardation and Developmental Disabilities Research Reviews, 9*, 149-154. doi: 10.1002/mrdd.10074

McGaw, S., Ball, K., & Clark, A. (2002). The effects of group intervention on the relationships of parents with intellectual disabilities. *Journal of Applied Research in Intellectual Disabilities, 15*, 354-366.

McGrath, K. F., & Van Bergen, P. (2015). Who, when, why and to what end? Students at risk of negative student-teacher relationships and their outcomes. *Educational Research Review, 14*, 1-17. doi: 10.1016/j.edurwev.2014.12.001

McGuire, B. E., & Bayley, A. A. (2011). Relationships, sexuality and decision-making capacity in people with an intellectual disability. *Current Opinion in Psychiatry, 24*, 398-402. doi: 10.1097/YCO.0b013e328349bbcb

Noonan, A., & Taylor Gomez, M. (2011). Who's missing? Awareness of lesbian, gay, bisexual and transgender people with intellectual disability. *Sexuality and Disability, 29*, 175-180.

Nurmi, J. (2012). Students' characteristics and teacher—child relationships in instruction: A meta-analysis. *Educational Research Review, 7*, 177-197. doi: 10.1016/j.edurev.2012.03.001

Parkinson, K., Rice, H., & Young, B. (2011). Incorporating children's and their parents' perspectives into condition specific quality of life instruments for children with cerebral palsy: A qualitative study. *Values in Health, 14*, 705-711. doi: 10.1016/j.jval.2010.12.003

Pianta, R. C., Hamre, B. K., & Allen, J. P. (2012). Teacher-student relationships and engagement: Conceptualizing measuring, and improving the capacity of classroom interactions. *Handbook of Research on Student Engagement*, 365-386. doi: 10.1007/978-1-4614-2018-7_17

Platt, C., Roper, S. Mandleco, B., & Freeborn, D. (2014). Sibling cooperative and externalizing behaviors in families raising children with disabilities. *Nursing Research, 63*(4), 235-242.

Pontzer, H. (2017). The exercise paradox. *Scientific American, 316*(2), 26-31.

Richards, D., Miodrag, N., & Watson, S. (2006) Sexuality and developmental disability: Obstacles to healthy sexuality throughout the lifespan. *Developmental Disabilities Bulletin, 34*(1 & 2), 137-155.

Roberts, R. E. L., & Bengtson, V. L. (1993). Relationships with parents, self-esteem, and psychological well-being in young adulthood. *Social Psychology Quarterly, 56*(4), 263-277.

Schaafsma, D., Kok, G., Stoffelen, J., & Curfs, L. (2014). Identifying effective methods for teaching sex education to individuals with intellectual disabilities: A systematic review. *Journal of Sex Research, 52*(4), 412-432. doi: 10.1080/00224499.2014.919373

Schuntermann, P. (2007). The sibling experience: Growing up with a child who has pervasive developmental disorder or mental retardation. *Harvard Review of Psychiatry, 17*(5), 297-314. doi: 10.1080/10673220701432188

Shakespeare, T. (2000). Disabled sexuality: Towards rights and recognition. *Sexuality and Disability, 19*, 263-282.

Shandra, C., & Chowdhury, A. (2012). The first sexual experience among adolescent girls with and without disabilities. *Journal of Youth and Adolescence, 41*, 515-532.

Stefansdottier, G., & Hreinsdottier, E. (2013). Sterilization, intellectual disability and some ethical and methodological challenges: It shouldn't be a secret. *Ethics and Social Welfare, 7*(3), 302-308. doi: 10.1080/17496535.2013.815792

Stern, A. M. (2015) *Eugenic nation: Faults and frontiers of better breeding in modern America*. Oakland, CA: University of California Press.

Sullivvan, P. M., & Knutson, J. F. (2000). Maltreatment and disabilities: A population based epidemiological study. *Child Abuse and Neglect, 24*(10), 1257-1273.

Swango-Wilson, A. (2008). Caregiver perceptions and implications for sex education for individuals with intellectual and developmental disabilities. *Sexuality and Disability, 26*, 167-174. doi: 10:1007/s11195-008-9081-0

Swango-Wilson, A. (2010). Systems theory and development of sexual identity for individuals with intellectual/developmental disability. *Sexuality and Disability, 28*, 157-164.

Swango-Wilson, A. (2011). Meaningful sex education programs for individuals with intellectual/developmental disabilities. *Sexuality and Disability, 29*, 113-118.

Valencia, L., & Cromer, B. (2000) Sexual activity and other high risk behaviors in adolescents with chronic illness: A review. *Journal of Pediatric and Adolescent Gynecology, 13*, 53-64.

Wiegerink, D., Roebroeck, M., Van Der Slot, W., Stam, H., Cohen-Kettenis, P., & the Southwest Netherlands Transition Research Group (2010). Importance of peers and dating in the development of romantic relationships and sexual activity of young adults with cerebral palsy. *Developmental Medicine & Child Neurology, 52*, 576-582.

Wilkenfeld, B. F. & Ballan, M. S. (2011). Educators' attitudes and beliefs towards the sexuality of individuals with developmental disabilities. *Sexual Disability, 29*, 351-361. doi: 10.1007/s11195-011-9211-y

ADDITIONAL RESOURCES

Florida Developmental Disabilities Council | www.fddc.org

Florida Developmental Disabilities Council has workbooks for parents to assist them in developing skills and thinking about how to teach their children with developmental disabilities about puberty and sexuality. These workbooks are in Spanish also. Workbook titles include *Sexuality Education for Children and Adolescents with Developmental Disabilities* and *Sexuality Across the Lifespan.*

The Arc | www.thearc.org

The Arc began as a group of parents of children with intellectual and developmental disabilities to a national organization with statewide chapters. They provide advocacy, resources, and efforts toward state and national legislation on behalf of people with disabilities.

Through the Looking Glass | http://lookingglass.org

Through the Looking Glass is a nationally recognized center that has pioneered research, training, and services for families in which a child, parent, or grandparent has a disability or medical issue. They offer several resources related to parenting with intellectual and other disabilities.

Oak Hill | www.oakhillcrse.org

The Center for Relationship & Sexuality Education at Oak Hill empowers people with developmental disabilities through programs about relationship and sexuality.

7

Evaluation of Occupational Performance and Engagement

Kimberly Bryze, PhD, OTR/L

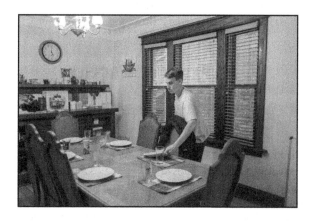

Key Words: adaptive behavior, Assessment of Motor and Process Skills (AMPS), dynamic assessment, Evaluation of Social Interaction (ESI), occupational profile, performance assessment

Bryze, K.
Occupational Therapy for Adults With Intellectual Disability (pp. 73-86).
© 2020 Taylor & Francis Group.

Evaluation is a dynamic process by which an occupational therapy practitioner utilizes critical and ethical reasoning, based on current best evidence, to gather specific and needed information about an individual. Evaluation may be used to identify a person's strengths and needs, determine eligibility for occupational therapy services, or, specifically, to design and initiate interventions to improve occupational performance, occupational engagement, and facilitate participation in everyday living (Kramer & Hinojosa, 2009). The occupational therapy practitioner gathers relevant information about an individual's interest in and performance of occupations—the ordinary and familiar things that people need, want, and have to do to take care of themselves, the home environment, and to interact with others. The evaluative process may include the administration of specific assessments, targeted interviews, and formal observations to gather systematic or objective data. Evaluations should also include informal observations and interactions in various circumstances to gather qualitative, contextual information about the individual. The practitioner must be vigilant to employ skill when administering specific assessments and must use care to avoid reliance only on one's previous experiences and opinions. Further, both objective and informal means of information gathering must be balanced against evidence-based decision making.

This chapter will provide the practitioner with occupation-focused approaches for collecting essential information about individuals' performance across contexts and in interaction with others. Formal and informal methods of evaluation will be presented and additional resources will be offered. Given the complexity of gathering accurate information from and about individuals with differing abilities, who may not be able to communicate or perform in expected or standardized ways, ideas related to dynamic assessment will be woven throughout the chapter.

OCCUPATIONAL PROFILE

The initial step in an evaluation process is to begin constructing the person's occupational profile through person-centered narratives of their occupational history, experiences, and routines. An individual's interests, daily activities, and habits are essential to gather from the individual and significant others. In the course of interviewing and listening to the individual and caregivers, the practitioner collects information about the individual's strengths and concerns related to performing various occupations. Identifying existing supports and barriers for the individual is also part of the occupational profile process. With the increased focus placed on productivity and time constraints in traditional occupational therapy practices, practitioners may be tempted to assume a problem solving, linear means of gathering "just enough" information about a person referred for evaluation. However, by restricting one's focus on the problem-based referral and gathering only the immediate information to solve specific concerns it may ultimately impact the variety and benefits of interventions afforded to that individual. The best occupational therapy assumes a holistic, thorough understanding of an individual's occupational life.

Adults with intellectual disability may not be able to communicate or demonstrate clearly to the practitioner the facets of their occupational lives. Whether due to challenges with communication, opportunities afforded to them, or others' assumptions about their potential, an occupational therapy practitioner should invest the time needed to observe, learn, listen, and reflect on the individual's occupational life trajectory. While the information may not be easily obtained, a thorough occupational profile will offer the greatest assistance when designing strategies to an individual referred for evaluation. The construction of the occupational profile is an ongoing process and proceeds into and through the next step of the evaluation process; the analysis of the individual's occupational performance.

Occupational Performance

In most direct terms, occupational therapy practitioners help individuals engage in the tasks they want, need, and have to do in their daily lives (occupations) and which facilitate participation in everyday living (Fisher, 1998; Wilcock & Hocking, 2015). Therefore, one of the most important evaluative tasks a practitioner can perform is assessment of an individual's occupational performance. While it is true that other professionals are concerned with and address the ability to do tasks or activities, the occupational therapy practitioner should ideally enact a performance analysis, rather than relying on another service provider's interpretation of their task performance. The occupational therapy practitioner incorporates foundational and related knowledge and skills in activity analysis, performance analysis, fluency with specific assessments, and clinical reasoning for data interpretation and construction of appropriate occupation-based interventions.

The evaluation of occupational performance requires performance assessment and analysis (Fisher, 2009). Performance assessment requires the actual observation of an individual performing a task in its natural context. It requires the practitioner to observe and take notes on the person doing the task, then identify the strengths and areas of concern related to his or her performance. The practitioner must also take into account the contextual physical and social supports and barriers to the person's performance. Performance assessment occurs within the natural context for the task performance (e.g., brushing one's teeth in the washroom where they typically brush their teeth, making a sandwich in the kitchen where food preparation typically takes place).

There are few gold standard assessments of occupational performance (Gillen, 2013), especially those well-suited to adults with intellectual disability. Gold standard assessments should be occupation focused and should utilize observation as the method of assessment. The practitioner observes the person performing the occupations and is focused on the occupation and the person's performance. However, some of the commonly used performance assessments attempt to measure the perceived impact of the person's cognitive or perceptual skills on their performance; while observation of occupational performance is the method for assessment, the practitioner's focus is on the underlying cognitive-perceptual capabilities, at the level of person factors and body function (Fisher, 2013). For example, the Árnadóttir OT-ADL Neurobehavioural Evaluation (A-ONE; Árnadóttir, 1990), was designed to evaluate the impact of neurobehavioral impairments on the functional performance of activities of daily living (ADLs) in persons with cognitive-perceptual dysfunction. The A-ONE is well-developed, valid (Gardarsdóttir & Kaplan, 2002), and occupation-based, but its focus is on identifying the underlying cognitive-perceptual impairments that are assumed to influence ADL performance. Likewise, the Executive Function Performance Test (EFPT; Baum, Morrison, Hahn, & Edwards, 2003) was designed to evaluate cognitive abilities through an occupation-based assessment process. The EFPT requires individuals to complete specific ADLs, such as hand washing, preparing oatmeal, telephone skills, taking medication, and paying bills. The practitioner's focus is directed toward determining the amount of assistance an individual requires for completing tasks and identifying which executive functions influence the ADL performances. From the data gathered, the practitioner then judges the individual's capacity for independent functioning. The assessment is reliable (Baum et al., 2008) and occupation based (i.e., the individual is observed actually performing certain ADL tasks), but is focused on determining which executive functions interfere with ADL performance. Both the A-ONE and the EFPT focus on body functions or client factors, such as the cognitive, sensory, neuromuscular, attentional, and movement-related functions—capacities that reside within the person and that converge to enable the development of performance skills (Fisher & Jones, 2014).

Performance skills, however, are universal, observable skills that are key components of enacting successful occupations, such as ADL/instrumental activity of daily living (IADL) tasks and social interactions. Performance skills are learned and goal-directed. There are two occupation-based and occupation-focused performance assessments that are highly relevant for persons with intellectual disability: the Assessment of Motor and Process Skills (AMPS; Fisher & Jones, 2014), and the

Evaluation of Social Interaction (ESI; Fisher & Griswold, 2015). Both assessments are valid and reliable and are sensitive to measuring change in performance over time. Each assessment is constructed upon the principal occupation performance skills articulated in the current version of the American Occupational Therapy Association (AOTA) *Occupational Therapy Practice Framework: Domain and Process, Third Edition* (AOTA, 2014). The motor and process performance skills are the essential components of the AMPS, and the social interaction skills are the essential components of the ESI.

The AMPS allows an occupational therapy practitioner to evaluate a person's quality of performance of personal or complex/IADLs. The AMPS is comprised of 16 motor and 20 process performance skills that are observable, goal-directed actions enacted by a person doing a task in the context of an appropriate environment for that task. The practitioner observes the person performing tasks that are relevant to, chosen by, and familiar to the individual being assessed. The practitioner observes and takes notes of the person's performance and actions in time, and then uses the observational notes to rate each of the 36 motor and process skills consistent with the AMPS manual specifications for quality of performance (i.e., competent, questionable, ineffective, severely limited). The ordinal scores for each skill are then entered into the Occupational Therapy Assessment Package (OTAP) software from which criterion ability measures of motor and process ADLs can be derived. As precise calculations of ADL performance ability, the criterion ability measures can be used to ascertain the need for supervision and indicate the individual's level of independence and safety in occupational performance. An example of using the AMPS as a sensitive, standardized measure is presented at the end of this chapter in the section entitled, "Do Interventions Based on Adaptive Occupations Improve Occupational Performance?"

Likewise, the ESI (Fisher & Griswold, 2015) is designed to evaluate a person's quality of social interaction during natural social exchanges with social partners. The ESI is an observational assessment in which the practitioner observes the person interacting with another person and, as with the AMPS, observes and takes notes of the social interaction. The practitioner then uses the observational notes to rate each of the 27 social interaction skills consistent with the ESI manual specifications for quality of social interaction (i.e., competent, questionable, ineffective, severely limited). The ordinal scores for each skill are then entered into the Occupational Therapy Assessment Package software from which criterion ability measures of social interaction can be derived. Similarly, the ability measures may be used for outcomes measurement and the identification of the need for additional services or supervision.

The AMPS and ESI are both utilized in the practitioner's implementation of a true performance analysis of a person's task performances. The practitioner will identify and describe the actions the person does and does not perform effectively, and consider the interactions of the various skills on each other as they influence task performance. Moreover, the practitioner can examine the performance skills that cluster together to develop goals and plan intervention for the person.

The validity and reliability of the AMPS with individuals with intellectual disability has been studied (Bryze, 1991; Kottorp, Bernspang, & Fisher, 2003; Kottorp, 2008), and it has been shown to be an excellent assessment for measuring ADL and IADL occupational performance. However, persons with significant cognitive or language impairments may have difficulty or may not be able to engage in the interview and task contract phases of administering a standardized AMPS process. The practitioner should collaborate with a staff or family member who knows the person well to identify potential tasks that are relevant and meaningful for the individual to perform for the assessment process. Further, many persons with intellectual disability have not had the opportunity to learn or practice certain occupations, such as food preparation or housekeeping tasks, given their residential or living situations. With the more than 100 ADL/IADL potential tasks used with the AMPS, which range in difficulty from very easy to much harder than average, the practitioner can use many tasks of appropriate challenge and relevance to administer this performance assessment to individuals with intellectual disability. While some modifications may need to be made to administer the AMPS to persons with intellectual disability, the practitioner can still assess the client by allowing them to first perform the tasks that will be observed to provide the opportunity to learn and practice the tasks.

It should be noted, however, that modifying the AMPS process significantly may create a less-than-standardized situation, and legitimate ability measures may not be able to be derived. However, the motor and process skills are universal and observable in any occupational performance. Observing the person's performance with the performance skills in mind will afford the practitioner invaluable, qualitative information about his or her performance capabilities in natural contexts, as they enact relevant and meaningful ADLs.

Sometimes conversing with a person with intellectual disability is not possible because of speech-language difficulties, even though the person is social and interested in interacting with his or her social partners where he or she lives and works. In such a case, the practitioner may choose to interview the person's caregiver to initially learn about his or her strengths and challenges with social interaction and identify the natural settings for the person where social interactions can be observed for the assessment. Even when difficulties with expressive, verbal language are present, a practitioner can utilize the ESI as an assessment of social interaction, provided the person attempts to communicate and expresses spoken or signed words in social interactions. The ESI is a sensitive tool to enable practitioners to plan effective interventions that will support the person's social interactions. The social interaction performance skills can also be used in observational performance assessment in unstandardized contexts. Again, the practitioner will not be able to derive ability measures, but may gain qualitative insight into the person's relative strengths and areas of weakness in social interaction.

While the AMPS and ESI were designed to assess a person's occupational performance in a standardized manner, the motor, process, and social interaction performance skills are also universally employed as the person performs a wide variety of tasks, including vocational or work and leisure pursuits (AOTA, 2014). Practitioners can develop proficiency in observing the performance skills across different areas of occupation and contexts. Learning to see these universal skills in action, and to remain focused on occupation, helps the practitioner appreciate the performance skills' contributions to a person's occupational performance in daily life. Rather than relying on assumptions and interpretations of underlying impairments and body functions, the use of the performance skills to identify a person's strengths and areas of need further support a dynamic, occupation-focused assessment process.

Dynamic Assessment

Dynamic assessment focuses on the transaction between assessment and intervention within relevant contexts. Dynamic assessment processes seek to measure to what extent a person can perform the skills and behaviors integral to functional tasks given authentic environmental modifications. One of the most unique characteristics of dynamic assessment is the inclusion of intervention as an integral aspect of the assessment process. Dynamic assessment relies less on standardized assessment procedures and directs more focus on changes in the person's performance of tasks given environmental or social supports (Lidz, 1996). It allows the practitioner to identify which skills a person is capable of learning or improving, which intervention strategies are most effective, and which types of intervention will be most likely to transfer or generalize to everyday situations (Kolakowsky, 1998).

Dynamic assessment approaches emphasize the importance of the direct, observational assessment of actual competencies to identify a person's potential for change. Dynamic assessment supplements traditional outcome-oriented methods. Outcome-oriented approaches measure whether the person can or cannot perform particular skills or behaviors and are often used in occupational therapy to evaluate more global constructs, such as developmental skills or adaptive behavior. Such traditional assessment of persons with intellectual disability has been based on the assumption that measures of existing aptitudes and traits can predict future behavior, subsequent learning, performance, and adjustment. The results of such assessment practices often underestimate a person's potential. However, the integration of dynamic assessment can afford the practitioner a process-oriented approach to understanding a person's strengths and limitations in the context of authentic performances.

One approach to dynamic assessment involves modifying the test administration procedures or the task materials to measure the person's performance under optimal learning conditions. This approach seeks to identify what physical or human resources (e.g., supervision, reinforcement, adaptive materials, environmental adaptation) are required for the person to attain a certain level of performance. For example, consider assessing a person's performance of eating soup with a soup spoon. Given the person's arthritis, the practitioner observes their performance with the traditional spoon but then provides a spoon with a built-up handle and observes whether their performance improves using the adapted utensil. Another example might be the use of visual cues/schedules, as used by various professionals and caregivers for individuals with autism spectrum disorders, perhaps more often than for adults with intellectual disability. The benefits of using visual cues should be considered for inclusion as a dynamic method for the assessment processes. An individual's deficits in receptive language or attention may hinder his or her understanding and appropriate response to directions or other verbal cues, and the provision of visual cues or photos may appropriately prompt the person to the next step or task to be performed. Some individuals with intellectual disability may perceive actual photographs better than line drawings or symbols, such as those used in Boardmaker software (Tobii Dynavox LLC). Further, arranging the visual cues in a vertical, top-to-bottom arrangement may also be more effective than a left-to-right arrangement for some persons with intellectual disability who may have visual field impairments or other visual perceptual deficits.

Another approach to dynamic assessment involves the use of task analysis for the functional analysis of behavior under natural life situations (i.e., less than optimal learning conditions). Most tasks are comprised of consecutive steps, or sets of specific behaviors. For example, a task analysis for preparing a peanut butter and jelly sandwich would include such steps as (1) obtaining the necessary supplies (i.e., bread, peanut butter, jelly, knife, spoon, and plate), (2) removing two slices of bread from the package, (3) opening the peanut butter and jelly jars, and (4) spreading peanut butter on one slice of bread, etc. Analysis of this task would require identification of which steps the person had difficulty performing or was unable to complete, and requires the practitioner to consider possible reasons why the person did not effectively complete the particular steps. Ideally, the practitioner observes the task performance and thinks in terms of the performance skills, then considers the impact of the ineffective steps on the total task. Task analysis may be used within an informal or ongoing assessment process, and may also be used in intervention for the training of specific functional tasks.

Dynamic assessment can be a powerful adjunct to an occupation-based, performance assessment of person-centered, relevant tasks within appropriate contexts. Dynamic assessment can assist with identifying a person's strengths and challenges, and gaining an in-depth understanding of what contextual supports are needed to enhance overall occupational performance.

Assessment of Adaptive Behavior

As noted in Chapter 1, the diagnosis of an intellectual disability is determined by the combination of intelligence tests and measures of adaptive behavior. When a person's intelligence (i.e., intelligence quotient [IQ]) falls significantly below the average range and parallel concurrent limitations in adaptive behavior are identified, a diagnosis of intellectual disability can be determined (American Psychiatric Association, 2013; Schalock et al., 2015). Adaptive behavior has been defined as "the collection of conceptual, social, and practical skills that have been learned and are performed by people in their everyday lives" (Tasse et al., 2012, p. 659). Adaptive behaviors change and develop as the person transitions through childhood and adolescence into adulthood, evolves in response to life settings and social constructs, and is modified based on both personal values and the expectations of other important people. Adaptive behavior is assessed to determine how well a person is able to function in the areas of personal, social, community, educational, or vocational daily life.

Adaptive behavior measures are used for diagnostic purposes, primarily by psychologists. Occupational therapy practitioners may also utilize adaptive behavior scales to provide specific data relevant for services eligibility and to estimate successful adjustment to the residential living setting. Adaptive behavior is contextual and many adults with intellectual disability are challenged to generalize skills and behaviors across contexts. However, adaptive behavior scales are not designed to predict success or failure in alternative placements or settings. Some of the most common adaptive behavior scales for use with adults with intellectual disability include Vineland Adaptive Behavior Scales (Sparrow, Cicchetti, & Balla, 2005), the Adaptive Behavior Assessment System (Harrison & Oakland, 2003), and the Scales of Independent Behavior–Revised (Bruininks, Woodcock, Weatherman, & Hill, 1996). The reliability and validity of these tools have been determined to be strong, and while they are most commonly used for diagnosing and identifying children's and adolescents' needs for intervention services, they have included in their normative sample persons up to 80 years of age. Most adaptive behavior scales compare the person's abilities to those of similar age and tend to be designed as outcome assessments, seeking to identify if a person can perform a particular task. The Scales of Independent Behavior–Revised is an exception because it seeks to determine not only whether the person can or cannot perform a particular task, but also the frequency by which tasks are performed to determine the person's capability and also willingness to participate in life skill task performance.

The Inventory for Client and Agency Planning (ICAP; Bruininks, Hill, Weatherman, & Woodcock, 1986) is another assessment designed to measure adaptive and maladaptive behavior. In many states, it is widely used in adult service agencies to determine a person's eligibility for services, identify potential areas for goal development, and individual service planning and reporting. The ICAP's greatest use for occupational therapy practitioners is its compatibility with the Checklist of Adaptive Living Skills (CALS; Morreau & Bruininks, 1991), a criterion-referenced measure of almost 800 specific adaptive living skills across four domains of adaptive behavior and the supplemental curriculum, the Adaptive Living Skills Curriculum (ALSC; Bruininks, Morreau, Gilman, & Anderson, 1991). The categories identified in the CALS and the ALSC include areas within personal living skills (e.g., eating, grooming, toileting, dressing, health care, sexuality, socialization), home living skills (e.g., clothing care, meal planning and preparation, home cleaning, home maintenance, home safety), community living skills (e.g., mobility and travel, time management, money management, shopping, community safety, community leisure, community participation, social interaction), and employment skills (e.g., job search, job performance and attitude, employee relations, job safety).

The items that comprise the CALS have been rigorously studied on persons with and without disabilities, and have been analyzed using Rasch measurement to ensure that the skills progress in difficulty (Morreau & Bruininks, 1991). For example, of the 51 items subsumed under the category of dressing, the level of item difficulty ranges from "relaxes or extends arms and legs while being helped to dress and undress" (Item 1.5.1.) to "buttons or snaps a shirt, blouse, or coat" (Item 1.5.24.) to "ties a necktie" (Item 1.5.51.). For each category, the items range from easy and appropriate for young children or persons with significant intellectual disability, to more difficult and appropriate for adults without disabilities. Moreover, each skill in the CALS is cross-referenced with that particular skill in the ALSC, to afford a practitioner specific strategies to teach that skill during intervention or to provide habilitation staff, as they work with the person. A range of creative methods and activities are provided for each item within the ALSC for developing the particular performance, as well as appropriate goals and precise training objectives. While there are more than 800 items represented in the CALS and ALSC, the practitioner need only convert a person's ICAP scores into the CALS to determine a functional range, or working level, of skills for that person. Skills that fall below the working level are likely already mastered and are too easy for the person, while skills that fall above the working level are likely not yet mastered and may provide the next "just right challenge" for targeted intervention. The ICAP, CALS, and ALSC can be obtained from the Houghton Mifflin Publishing Company (www.hmhco.com).

Sensory Contributions to Performance and Behavior

Sensory contributions to one's quality of living and engagement in daily life can be significant, whether visual or auditory impairments, paresthesia secondary to neurological conditions, or dysfunction of sensory processing. Sensory abilities should be considered in assessment processes and efforts should be taken to interpret results in light of extant sensory disorders. Individuals with intellectual disability frequently present with visual impairments (Warburg, 2001), including nearsightedness, strabismus, cataracts, keratoconus, glaucoma, and other ophthalmological disorders that may impact the ease with which they negotiate their environment and enact occupational performance. The process of examining the extent of visual impairment is complicated by the presence of intellectual disability, and many persons are underserved in this area of health care. Certain behaviors or symptoms may indicate the presence of low vision to caregivers and practitioners, including but not limited to squinting, eye redness or irritation, hesitancy to step from one surface to another (e.g., from carpeting to tiled flooring), holding objects close to one's face to view, glancing at objects from the side rather than directly, and over- or under-reaching for objects. With increasing visual impairment, an individual may appear to be disinterested or unmotivated to participate in activities. While withdrawal from engagement may suggest other behavioral concerns, the person's vision may be a cause of disinterest and change in participation.

One's ability to accurately perceive environmental and social contexts is highly dependent on accurate sensory inputs. When deficits or dysfunction are present, a person may experience functional limitations in performing ADLs and may well experience diminished emotional safety and security across various contexts and in social situations. Such sensory-perceptual deficits may confound assessment efforts and impact the results of the assessment process. Communication with a person who has visual impairments may be more difficult, especially in face-to-face encounters. Human beings rely on nonverbal dimensions of communication more so than verbal communication alone. For example, one's facial expression, body language, use of gestures, and nonverbal communication of varying intensity and meaning can account for the majority of our communication and interaction, especially with individuals whose receptive and expressive language skills are impaired (Bialistock, 2005).

Sensory processing and its effect on daily life task performance was presented earlier in this textbook. As noted, dysfunction in processing sensory information can influence a person's comfort with and ability to manage daily tasks, including social interaction. The presence and resultant impact of sensory processing dysfunction in adults with intellectual disability is dependent largely on the practitioner's knowledge and thorough understanding of this construct, and involves careful observation across contexts. Formal assessments for identifying sensory processing disorder in adults with intellectual disability are few; most tools are designed for use with children. Two assessments designed for use with adults rely on self-reporting during a semi-structured interview, which becomes complicated in the presence of communication skill deficits. The Sensory Integration Inventory–Revised (Reisman & Hanschu, 1992) is a tool that can help structure a practitioner's observations, provide areas for inquiry when interviewing caregivers, and highlight potential influences of sensory processing dysfunction in adults with intellectual disability. The Adolescent/Adult Sensory Profile (Brown & Dunn, 2002) is another assessment designed for use with adults. However, reliability is strengthened when used with individuals who can effectively self-report. Evaluation of sensory processing, therefore, requires a skillful and observant practitioner who understands the neurobehavioral foundations and the theory of sensory integration on human occupation and can carefully apply these principles to persons with intellectual disability.

Sensory processing disorders that present as sensory modulation dysfunction, especially sensory overresponsivity, are likely to have a great impact on daily life performance in persons with intellectual disability. While not all behavior or occupational performance difficulties can or should be attributed to sensory processing dysfunction, a skillful practitioner should carefully identify the sensory contributions to a person's difficulty with task performance. For example, as most of our personal self-care tasks involve considerable tactile input (e.g., showering, toileting, washing hair, brushing teeth, dressing), dysfunction in processing tactile inputs will likely be noticeable as avoidance or behavioral problems in the context of performing core ADL tasks. With tactile hypersensitivity, a person may avoid touching or holding certain objects due to its tactile characteristics. An individual may become increasingly agitated or irritated as the task continues and the tactile inputs seemingly accumulate. Further, a skilled practitioner may observe a person's insistence on the presence of certain sensory comfort items (e.g., a stuffed animal, a weighted blanket) and increasing agitation if those items are put aside in order to participate in other activities. Considering this behavior in light of sensory needs, rather than just labeling it a misbehavior, is possible when one uses knowledge of neurosensory processing in the critical reasoning process. The presence of picky eating or avoidance of certain textures of foods may also indicate sensory hypersensitivity, or the more serious difficulties with chewing, managing food within the mouth, or deficits in swallowing, which would then require further evaluation in conjunction with other professionals.

Additional Approaches to Assessment

The Volitional Questionnaire (VQ) is a standardized, observational tool designed to rate 14 behavioral indicators of volition and motivation (de las Heras, Geist, Kielhofner, & Li, 2007). The VQ allows an occupational therapy practitioner a method to systematically gather information about the ways a person reacts to and acts within his or her environment. From the observations and ratings, the practitioner gains insight into a person's inner motives, and identifies ways the environment enhances or diminishes volition. de las Heras was especially interested in individuals with severe intellectual disability who resided in large care facilities as many were nonverbal and unable to report their interests and choice of activities. Through observation of an individual's participation and engagement in various daily activities, the practitioner rates each item on the VQ according to an ordinal rating scale: No Opportunity to Observe; Passive; Hesitant; Involved; and Spontaneous. From these results the practitioner infers the volitional contributions to occupational engagement in relevant daily life or leisure tasks.

The Activity Card Sort (ACS), Second Edition (Baum & Edwards, 2008) is an occupation-focused assessment in which a practitioner can gather a person's occupational history and interests, and identify possibilities for enhanced occupational engagement. The ACS consists of 89 photographs of adults performing IADL, leisure, and social activities and, in conversation with the person who chooses specific activities, the practitioner can calculate the percentage of activity an individual performs and retains across time. While the ACS is not typically utilized for adults with intellectual disability, it could be an effective resource for gathering the history and interests of an individual who may have difficulty conversing fully in a narrative conversation or interview. The motoric requirements are minimal and involve pointing to or placing each card on the table. The photographs can be presented as limited choices (e.g., only the low-demand physical leisure activities) for individuals with need for fewer choices to be presented.

FINAL CONSIDERATIONS

It is important to re-emphasize that the evaluation process is a vital facet of occupational therapy practice. When evaluating adults with intellectual disability, the practitioner needs to be responsive and observant, attend to small increments of improvement, and celebrate successes regularly. Individuals with intellectual disability are often challenging to assess in traditional and standardized ways, and practitioners are required to be creative, thoughtful, and patient as the traditional methods for assessment may not provide them with accurate results. A practitioner will need to interview caregivers (e.g., staff, family members) and closely listen to the examples or stories provided as explanations. These narratives often offer important information for evaluation data.

Practitioners need to evaluate adults with intellectual disability thoroughly. The practitioner should observe, interview, and listen carefully and use one's therapeutic, affective skills thoughtfully. While these are the knowledge and skills sets of occupational therapy practice, practitioners need to embrace an attitude of not automatically choosing the most obvious solutions or interpretations for individuals with intellectual disability. The adults served by occupational therapy practitioners may not be able to communicate easily or effectively and may not be able to show us directly the ways we can come alongside to support, enhance, and assess their occupational capabilities.

An example, from the author's consultation practice, is provided as the case of Andy. While an unusual case, it may offer some insight into listening for and observing what is perhaps most important:

> Andy was a 61-year-old man diagnosed with Down syndrome. He lived in a large intermediate care facility. The case manager (qualified intellectual disability professional), remarked off-handedly that staff members had complained about Andy "not wanting to feed himself lately." While the meals often included many of his favorite foods, Andy was not eating very much. I inquired further and learned that the past 2 weeks had been increasingly more challenging, and plans were made to contact the behavior therapist to help the staff address Andy's "stubbornness" regarding mealtimes.
>
> I observed the dinner hour when the individuals from the unit sat in their self-chosen seats at various round tables. Staff members helped them serve themselves from family-style bowls of food and offered assistance to those who required physical help to eat their meals. Andy's plate was placed in front of him, and he sat at the table with his forearms on the table and his spoon in his right hand. Andy looked at the food on his plate, and mumbled something to a nearby staff member who encouraged him to eat his food. As I watched his movements, I noted that he hunched his shoulder up and forward when attempting to lift the spoon to the plate to scoop his food, then thrust his neck forward to meet the spoon as he brought it to his mouth. After a couple of bites of food, Andy paused to rest, seemingly tired from these exaggerated movements. After several more attempts, a staff member helped Andy by feeding him several bites of food while informing him that he certainly should do this himself, that he can do this, etc. I continued to watch the progression of the meal, with Andy attempting to feed himself but using obvious and exaggerated compensatory movements to do so.
>
> I asked the staff member if Andy was experiencing difficulty with other activities, such as putting on his shirt or washing his face. The staff member replied, "Now that you mention it, he does seem to need more help lately. We think he is being lazy or stubborn. You know they can get that way."
>
> I noted that Andy demonstrated ineffective performance of several motor skills, such as reaches, lifts, grips, manipulates, calibrates, flows, endures, and paces. While many process skills were also deficient (i.e., continues, terminates, heeds, accommodates, benefits), the obvious performance difficulties lay with motor ability. I spent time with Andy to gather additional data and contributing factors related to body functions and performed informal assessments of functional strength and sensation. I learned that he was quite weak in both arms and did not feel me pinch his ventral and dorsal upper arms when he did not see me pinching him. I explained my findings to the qualified intellectual disability professional, relating that this certainly was not a "behavior" or laziness concern, and that he needed to be examined by a physician very soon.
>
> As information unfolded within the next couple of days, it was learned that Andy had a tumorous growth at the C6–C7 level that impacted both sensory and motor functions. He was referred to a neurologist who then began the process of arranging for surgery and subsequent rehabilitation. Following rehabilitation, Andy was able to resume his level of ADL performance (i.e., feed and dress himself), although with somewhat lessened strength, upon his return to his unit in the care facility. If I had not explored thoroughly and settled

TABLE 7-1. TOOLS AND STRATEGIES FOR ADAPTIVE OCCUPATION	
OCCUPATION	ADAPTIVE TOOLS INTRODUCED
Bathing	Grab bars, tub transfer bench, non-skid mats
Eating	Large-handled utensils, plate guard
Meal preparation	Rocker knives, food processor
Mobility	Ramps for door thresholds, high-visibility stair tapes
Home care	Long-handled broom/dust pan, bed rails
Dressing	Elastic shoelaces, storage containers

for the simple explanation that Andy's problem was "just behavior," the true problem might not have been discovered and Andy might not have had such a successful outcome.

CASE EXAMPLE

This study examined the impact of occupational therapy intervention methods, focused on adaptive occupation, and education/teaching on the daily life task performance of adults with intellectual disability. Do interventions based on adaptive occupations improve occupational performance? Participants included 9 adults with intellectual disability (ages 26 to 73) who lived in community with 10 live-in assistants. Individual interviews were conducted with each of the participants to obtain their perspectives of those ADL/IADL tasks the participants with intellectual disability were and were not able to perform well in their daily lives. Special focus was placed on inquiring about tasks the individuals wanted to perform more independently or safely. The AMPS was administered to evaluate occupational performance. Qualitative data included field observations, interviews, and conversations with participants during intervention sessions. Conversations with participants and results of the AMPS guided the specific interventions for the core members. Individualized interventions were developed based on each core member's specific strengths and needs and were implemented across 6 months' time. Consultation and recommendations were provided to assistants for carry-over of interventions for the participants with intellectual disability and use of adaptive equipment and strategies.

The AMPS was administered during the first and last weeks of interventions and used as a pre- and post-test measure. ADL motor and process ability are reported in logits and represent the overall measure of a person's ADL task performance. Changes in pre- to post-test scores of greater than 0.5 logits for motor skills and 0.4 logits for process skills represent a statistically significant improvement (Fisher & Jones, 2014). Data analysis included qualitative descriptive analysis of notes and observations, which were triangulated with the gain scores derived from pre- and post-test AMPS data.

Data analysis revealed improvements in participants' performance of daily life tasks. ADLs were targeted for intervention and included tasks addressing food and meal preparation, house cleaning, and caring for pets. Table 7-1 illustrates some of the adaptations and adaptive equipment utilized during this study. Participants reported some of the most significant gains were made in their confidence, engagement, and generalization of their newfound competence in tasks across other aspects of their daily lives.

Table 7-2 illustrates the participants' motor and process ability measure, reported as logits, obtained during the pre- and post-test evaluation sessions. Collectively there was not a significant change in motor skills from pre-test (M = 1.13, SD = 0.50) to post-test (M = 1.26, SD = 0.54);

TABLE 7-2. PARTICIPANTS' PRE- AND POST-TEST MOTOR AND PROCESS SKILL ABILITY MEASURES

MOTOR SKILLS

Participant	Gender	Age	Pre-Test	Post-Test	Gain Score
A	F	26	1.5	1.5	0.0
B	M	44	1.7	1.7	0.0
C	M	39	1.5	1.7	0.2
D	M	37	1.1	1.3	0.2
E	M	45	0.1	0.0	-0.1
F	M	38	0.9	0.9	0.0
G	F	48	0.7	1.2	0.5**
H	M	26	1.2	1.3	0.1
I	M	73	1.5	1.7	0.2

PROCESS SKILLS

Participant	Gender	Age	Pre-Test	Post-Test	Gain Score
A	F	26	-0.3	0.1	0.4*
B	M	44	0.6	1.0	0.4*
C	M	39	0.1	0.8	-0.2
D	M	37	0.8	1.1	0.3
E	M	45	0.1	0.3	0.2
F	M	38	-0.4	0.3	0.7**
G	F	48	0.6	0.8	0.2
H	M	26	1.0	1.2	0.2
I	M	73	0.8	1.5	0.7**

*Indicates clinical significance/observable difference
**Indicates statistical significance

$t(8) = 2.052$, $P = 0.074$. There was, however, a significant change in core members' process skills from pre-test ($M = 0.37$, $SD = 0.51$) to post-test ($M = 0.77$, $SD = 0.47$); $t(8) = 5.696$, $P = 0.000$.

While some direct interventions were implemented for participants to acquire specific skills or techniques, adaptive methods enabled the participants to perform tasks more effectively and generalize performance to other environments and activities. While measurable improvements were made in the participants' ability to perform personal and complex ADLs that were important and meaningful to them, most participants continued to rely on supports provided by the assistants, such as verbal cues and help with initial set-up of materials. All participants demonstrated greater initiation of tasks, improved quality of task performance, increased safety, and greater independence.

This study supports the use of adaptive occupation as an effective method for supporting performance of adults with intellectual disability. The study also supports previous research that implicates the AMPS, and especially the process skills ability scale, as a sensitive measure of change in a person's ADL performance (Fisher & Jones, 2014). Further, the use of the AMPS is an effective and authentic assessment for adults with intellectual disability, and a sensitive outcome measure, especially when used in the context of adaptive occupation strategies for intervention. It is important to link the results of assessment directly to intervention for this population. Therefore, this study contributes to the small body of literature supporting occupational therapy with adults with intellectual disability (Bryze & Kiraly-Alvarez, 2018).

REFERENCES

American Occupational Therapy Association. (2014). Occupational therapy practice framework: Domain and process, 3rd edition. *American Journal of Occupational Therapy, 68*(Suppl. 1), S1-S48.

American Occupational Therapy Association. (2017). Vision 2025. *American Journal of Occupational Therapy, 71,* 7103420010p1.

American Psychiatric Association (2013). *Diagnostic and statistical manual* (5th ed.). Washington, D.C.: Author.

Árnadóttir, G. (1990). *Brain and behavior: Assessing cortical dysfunction through activities of daily living (ADL).* St. Louis, MO: Mosby.

Baum, C. M., Connor, L. T., Morrison, T., Hahn, M., Dromerick, A. W., & Edwards, D. F. (2008). Reliability, validity, and clinical utility of the Executive Function Performance Test: A measure of executive function in a sample of people with stroke. *American Journal of Occupational Therapy, 62,* 446-455.

Baum, C., & Edwards, D. (2008). *Activity Card Sort.* Bethesda, MD: American Occupational Therapy Association.

Baum, C. M., Morrison, T., Hahn, M., & Edwards, D. F. (2003). *Test manual: Executive Function Performance Test.* St. Louis, MO: Washington University.

Bialistock, R. (2005). Towards better communication for the blind and visually impaired. *International Congress Series, 1282,* 793-795.

Bryze, K., & Kiraly-Alvarez, A. (2018). *The impact of occupational therapy intervention on the performance of daily life tasks of adults with intellectual disability.* Poster presentation, Midwestern University Suarez Research Day. Downers Grove, IL: Midwestern University.

Bryze, K. A. (1991). *Functional assessment of adults with developmental disabilities.* Unpublished master's thesis, University of Illinois at Chicago, Chicago, IL.

Brown, C. E., & Dunn, W. (2002). *Adolescent/Adult Sensory Profile.* San Antonio, TX: Pearson Education Inc.

Bruininks, R. H., Hill, B. K., Weatherman, R. F., & Woodcock, R. W. (1986). *Inventory for Client and Agency Planning.* Chicago, IL: Riverside.

Bruininks, R. H., Morreau, L. E., Gilman, C. J., & Anderson, J. L. (1991). *Adaptive Living Skills Curriculum.* Chicago, IL: Riverside Publishing.

Bruininks, R. H., Woodcock, R., Weatherman, R., & Hill, B. (1996). *Scales of Independent Behavior—Revised.* Chicago, IL: Riverside Publishing.

de las Heras, C. G., Geist, R., Kielhofner, G., & Li, Y. (2007). *A user's guide to the Volitional Questionnaire* (V. 4.1). Chicago, IL: University of Illinois at Chicago.

Fisher, A. G. (1998). Uniting practice and theory in an occupational framework. *American Journal of Occupational Therapy, 52,* 509-521.

Fisher, A. G. (2009). *The Occupational Therapy Intervention Process Model: A model for planning and implementing top-down, client-centered, and occupation-based interventions.* Fort Collins, CO: Three Star Press.

Fisher, A. G. (2013). Occupation-centered, occupation-based, occupation-focused: Same, same or different? *Scandinavian Journal of Occupational Therapy, 20,* 162-173.

Fisher, A. G., & Griswold, L. A. (2015). *Evaluation of Social Interaction* (3rd ed.). Fort Collins, CO: Three Star Press.

Fisher, A. G., & Jones, K. B. (2014). *Assessment of Motor and Process Skills* (8th ed.). Fort Collins, CO: Three Star Press.

Gardarsdótir, S., & Kaplan, S. (2002). Validity of the Árnadóttir OT-ADL Neurobehavior Evaluation (A-ONE): Performance in activities of daily living and neurobehavioral impairments of persons with left and right hemisphere damage. *American Journal of Occupational Therapy, 56,* 499-508.

Gillen, G. (2013). A fork in the road: An occupational hazard? (Eleanor Clarke Slagle Lecture). *American Journal of Occupational Therapy, 67,* 641-652.

Harrison, P. L., & Oakland, T. (2003). *Adaptive Behavior Assessment System* (2nd ed.). San Antonio, TX: Harcourt Assessment.

Kolakowsky, S. A. (1998). Assessing learning potential in patients with brain injury: Dynamic assessment. *NeuroRehabilitation, 11,* 227-238.

Kottorp, A. (2008). The use of the Assessment of Motor and Process Skills (AMPS) in predicting need of assistance for adults with mental retardation. *Occupational Therapy Journal of Research, 28,* 72-80.

Kottorp, A., Bernspang, B., & Fisher, A. G. (2003). Validity of a performance assessment of activities of daily living (ADL) for persons with developmental disabilities. *Journal of Intellectual Disability Research, 47,* 567-605.

Kramer, P., & Hinojosa, J. (2009). *Frames of reference for pediatric occupational therapy* (3rd ed.). Philadelphia, PA: Lippincott Williams & Wilkins.

Lidz, C. S. (1996). Dynamic assessment approaches. In D. P. Flanagan, J. L. Genshaft, & P. L. Harrison, *Contemporary intellectual assessment: Theories, tests and issues.* New York, NY: Guilford Press.

Morreau, L. E., & Bruininks, R. H. (1991). *Checklist of Adaptive Living Skills.* Chicago, IL: Riverside

Reisman, J. E., & Hanschu, B. (1992). *Sensory Integration Inventory—Revised: For individuals with developmental disabilities*. Stillwater, MN: PDP Products

Schalock, R. L., Borthwick-Duffy, S. A., Bradley, V. J., Buntinx, W. H. E., Coulter, D. L., Craig, E. M., ... Yeager, M. H. (2010). *Intellectual disability: Diagnosis, classification, and systems of supports* (11th ed.). Washington, D.C.: American Association on Intellectual and Developmental Disabilities.

Sparrow, S. S., Cicchetti, D. V., & Balla, D. A. (2005). *Vineland II: Vineland Adaptive Behavior Scales* (2nd ed.). Minneapolis, MN: Pearson Assessments.

Tasse, M. J., Schalock, R. L., Balboni, G., Bersani, H., Borthwick-Duffy, S. A., Spreat, S., ... Zhang, D. (2012). The construct of adaptive behavior: Its conceptualization, measurement, and use in the field of intellectual disability. *American Journal on Intellectual and Developmental Disabilities, 117*, 291-303.

Warburg, M. (2001). Visual impairment in adult people with intellectual disability: Literature review. *Journal of Intellectual Disability Research, 45*, 424-438.

Wilcock, A. A., & Hocking, C. (2015). *An occupational perspective of health* (3rd ed.). Thorofare, NJ: SLACK Incorporated.

8

Promoting Participation and Occupational Engagement

Wanda J. Mahoney, PhD, OTR/L

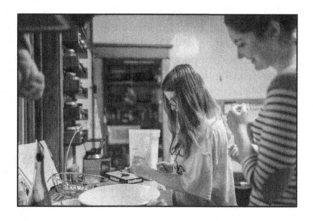

Key Words: active support, adapted occupation, intensive interaction, learned helplessness, occupational engagement, occupational participation, participation, promoting routines, quality of life, self-determination, well-being

Bryze, K.
Occupational Therapy for Adults With Intellectual Disability (pp. 87-98).
© 2020 Taylor & Francis Group.

This chapter is organized into three major sections:

1. Ways to describe the occupational lives of adults with intellectual disability and the link to occupational therapy evaluation and outcomes
2. Major factors that affect the occupational lives of adults with intellectual disability and the implications for occupational therapy evaluation and intervention
3. Information about interventions occupational therapy practitioners can implement to promote participation, occupational performance, and occupational engagement among adults with intellectual disability

OCCUPATIONAL LIVES OF ADULTS WITH INTELLECTUAL DISABILITY

Adults with intellectual disability, regardless of the severity level of their disability, can be active and involved members of society through community and home participation, and occupational engagement. Participation is linked with higher quality of life and sense of well-being (Bigby, Knox, Beadle-Brown, & Bould, 2014; Gjermestad, Luteberget, Midjo, & Witsø, 2017; Talman, Wilder, Stier, & Gustafsson, 2019). Quality of life and well-being are important outcomes for occupational therapists, direct service providers, families, and the adults with intellectual disability. For adults with intellectual disability to participate (i.e., to be involved in life situations in home and community environments; World Health Organization [WHO], 2001), they need appropriate supports that meet their needs. Because of this need for support, which can be extensive at times, it can be helpful to consider different ways to describe the occupational lives of adults with intellectual disability. This may be important from a practical standpoint when determining assessments and outcome measures and also from a broader concern of how to respect adults with intellectual disability, especially those with more severe disabilities, as occupational beings and capture their occupational lives. Three related concepts are helpful to distinguish when describing the occupational lives of adults with intellectual disability: participation, occupational performance, and occupational engagement. Although these terms are sometimes used interchangeably in occupational therapy and infrequently explicitly defined, distinguishing between them can be useful when considering which different aspects of the clients' occupational lives to address.

Participation

Participation is a broad occupational construct with many definitions. Occupational therapists most often use the *International Classification of Functioning, Disability and Health* definition of participation as "involvement in a life situation" (WHO, 2001, p. 10). Although widely used, this broad concept can be difficult to measure, and it is helpful to consider practical aspects of what participation consists of. There is not a comprehensive participation assessment for adults with intellectual disability, and many of the participation assessments for adults with other disabilities may be difficult to administer to this population, or may be more relevant for individuals with recently acquired disabilities (Resnik & Plow, 2009). Assessing participation with adults with intellectual disability may include some or all of the following aspects, informed by research with this population and participation assessments for children with disabilities (Arvidsson, Granlund, Thyberg, & Thyberg, 2014; Crowe, Salazar Sedillo, Kertcher, & LaSalle, 2015; King et al., 2004):

- Variety of activities one participates in (i.e., intensity of participation)
- Frequency of activity participation
- Duration of activity participation
- Satisfaction with activity participation

- Variety of locations where participation occurs (i.e., community inclusion)
- With whom participation occurs (i.e., social inclusion)

Routines are how individuals organize their occupations and link them together in structured ways; so, it may be helpful to consider routines as one way that participation is organized. Routines can be promoting or damaging for one's health, and occupational therapy can foster promoting routines (American Occupational Therapy Association [AOTA], 2014). The routines of adults with intellectual disability may support diverse, intense participation in a variety of environments or enable flexibility to create this. In contrast, routines for some adults with intellectual disability may be so restrictive and structured that change is difficult and requires analysis of person and environmental factors affecting the issue to determine the best way to create incremental change. When the adult's desire for consistency and predictability is the cause of the restrictive routines, helping caregivers to implement picture or written schedules with opportunities for changes may be one way to address this. If caregivers or service agency policies are the source of the restrictive routine, additional analysis into those causes are necessary to determine an appropriate action (Johnson & Bagatell, 2017). The occupational therapy practitioner's strategies need to be different based on the situation. Such situations may involve caregivers not having the knowledge and skills to provide flexible routines, caregivers believing that they need to control every aspect of the environment, or caregivers having an overly structured routine to decrease job stress.

Adults with intellectual disability are at risk of participation restrictions and may spend a large amount of time "doing nothing" (Arvidsson et al., 2014; Crowe et al., 2015; Iacono, Bould, Beadle-Brown, & Bigby, 2019; Mansell & Beadle-Brown, 2012). Therefore, it is appropriate for occupational therapy to focus on participation during evaluation and intervention and as an outcome with adults with intellectual disability.

Occupational Performance

Occupational performance entails doing and accomplishing occupations, and is often discussed in terms of the transaction of the person, environment, and occupation (AOTA, 2014; Law et al., 1996). An essential feature of occupational performance is the quality of performance. Whether that quality is measured objectively or subjectively, occupational performance includes how well the person carries out the occupation. Occupational performance is the construct that is most useful when discussing how much assistance an adult with intellectual disability requires in order to complete necessary occupations. It is the most appropriate outcome to consider when addressing skill development for adults with intellectual disability.

Routines are also related to occupational performance. Many adults with mild intellectual disability have routines for their daily activities that support their independent, occupational performance that have been developed with support during adolescence and early adulthood. Similar to other populations, they may only require occupational therapy services if there is a major life disruption.

Individuals with moderate to severe/profound disabilities often require another person to assist them to perform many occupations, so their routines involve multiple people. In group homes or other settings with groups of adults with intellectual disability, routines allow staff members to coordinate the assistance they offer and ensure that necessary occupations are completed. Staff members may feel overwhelmed by this responsibility and focus on trying to get everything done during their shift. In addition, they may not have sufficient skills to grade assistance or enable adults with intellectual disability to perform occupations, and may not view the adults as capable. Staff members may feel that it is their responsibility to ensure that necessary occupations are completed, so they do the occupations *for* the adults with intellectual disability instead of helping do the occupation *with* them. Occupational therapy practitioners need to consider these complex factors with routines and ensure they have evaluated the situation and its underlying causes before providing recommendations, which may be perceived as another source of caregiver stress.

Occupational Engagement

Occupational engagement is one of the most common terms in occupational therapy, and although it is rarely explicitly defined, it is usually used in a broad sense to refer to doing occupations (Mahoney & Austin, 2014). However, building on the work of occupational therapists and occupational scientists, and attempting to better describe the occupational lives of individuals with severe cognitive disabilities, Mahoney and Austin (2014) proposed a definition of occupational engagement as, "a range of subjective states of being involved or engrossed in meaningful, everyday activity." The following information draws from that presentation. A key question that an occupational therapy practitioner targeting occupational engagement in this way would consider is "How engrossed is the client in this occupation?" When working with adults with intellectual disability, the occupational therapy practitioner may be watching for indicators that the person is getting into the activity (similar to how Csikszentmihályi [1998] describes flow), if they are only half-heartedly involved in the activity or actively avoiding the activity. When conceptualized in this way, occupational engagement is a moment-to-moment phenomenon, and the subjective nature means that the individual experiencing the occupation defines the engagement. It is possible to observe adults with intellectual disability and make inferences about their subjective occupational engagement. One research article describes behaviors associated with high occupational engagement in day program activities (Mahoney, Roberts, Bryze, & Parker Kent, 2016). Occupational therapy practitioners can work to increase the individual's level of engagement in an occupation, as well as increase the amount of engagement or opportunities for occupational engagement the person has. Addressing occupational engagement in this way with adults with intellectual disability, especially those with the most severe disabilities, respects them as occupational beings, captures their passions in their occupational lives, and builds on their strengths. Fostering increased occupational engagement can be a useful way to help caregivers consider how they offer assistance and set up activities differently so they help adults with intellectual disability get into activities.

Occupational Life Summary

When working with adults with intellectual disability with significant occupational challenges independent occupational performance is rarely the targeted occupational therapy outcome. Therefore, although it is unusual to differentiate participation, occupational performance, and occupational engagement to the degree discussed in this chapter, it is useful with this population. Occupational therapy practitioners can consider what factor of the occupational life of the adult with intellectual disability to focus evaluation and intervention on and what to target as an appropriate occupational outcome of intervention.

PERSON-ENVIRONMENT TRANSACTIONS AFFECTING OCCUPATIONAL LIFE

Occupational therapy practitioners recognize that all components of one's occupational life are affected by characteristics of the person, the environment, and the occupation (AOTA, 2014; Law et al., 1996). These factors transact in such a way that while it is possible to assess or discuss aspects of a person's skills or the environment in isolation, both influence each other and occupational performance, engagement, or participation to such a degree that they can never be completely separated. The following sections will discuss major person-environment influences on the occupational lives of adults with intellectual disability, which occupational therapy practitioners should consider. These major factors include the occupational skills of the adult with intellectual disability, volition, self-determination, and social environment. General suggestions for factors affecting occupational life are offered for assessment of adults with intellectual disability, although actual determinations about what the occupational therapy practitioner will assess should be determined based on specific client needs.

Occupational Skills

Occupational skills, also called *performance skills*, are observable, goal-directed actions that occur during occupational performance, and, by definition, include aspects of the person interacting with the environment to do an occupation (AOTA, 2014). The major categories include motor, process, and social interaction skills (AOTA, 2014).

Adults with intellectual disability may exhibit barriers with motor and process skills affecting their occupational performance (Fisher, Griswold, Munkholm, & Kottorp, 2017; Kottorp, Bernspång, & Fisher, 2003). Research indicates that process skills may predict the amount of assistance adults with mild to moderate intellectual disability require for community living (Kottorp, 2008). This may be an important area for occupational therapy to target for assessment and potential intervention.

Adults with intellectual disability may also exhibit barriers with social interaction skills affecting their occupational performance (Fisher et al., 2017). The quality of social interaction skills depends on both the adult with intellectual disability and the social partners. Interacting with peers, staff members, individuals in the community, or family members require different social interaction skills depending on the amount of support the social partner offers (Nijs & Maes, 2014). Caregivers and adults with intellectual disability having fun with each other is an important aspect of social interaction (Johnson, Douglas, Bigby, & Iacono, 2012; Mahoney et al., 2016). The quality and type of social interactions and social interaction skills between adults with intellectual disability and caregivers may be a major factor affecting occupational life.

Volition

Volition is how a person feels about, thinks about, and decides on one's activities and is one's motivation for engaging in occupation (de las Heras, Geist, Kielhofner, & Li, 2007; Lee & Kielhofner, 2017). Volition relates to how a person chooses occupations and ascribes meaning to those occupations. Volition is a personal characteristic, but recognizing the person-environment transaction, volition is also strongly influenced by and cannot be completely separated from aspects of the environment and occupation (de las Heras et al., 2007; Lee & Kielhofner, 2017).

Occupational therapy practitioners recognize the influence of personal meaning, sense of self-efficacy, and interests on occupational experiences. Assessing volition with adults with intellectual disability can provide useful information about their occupational engagement (Mahoney et al., 2016). Further, adults with intellectual disability may have occupational histories that have led to volitional barriers. For example, adults with intellectual disability may have limited occupational experiences that led to a decreased understanding of current activities from which to choose. They may have a history of limited occupational success that has led to decreased volition and a sense of learned helplessness, and providing a choice of an activity may not be sufficient to enable their occupational engagement. It may be necessary to assess the occupational opportunities an adult with intellectual disability has had in the past, to the extent possible, in addition to current occupational experiences, to understand how volition impacts the individual's occupational life.

Self-Determination

Self-determination is a complex construct that involves a person making choices, causing things to happen in one's life, and having some control in aspects that are personally important (Abery & Stancliffe, 2003; Vicente, Guillén, Gómez, Ibáñez, & Sánchez, 2019). It is easy to misinterpret and discount the importance of self-determination for individuals with more severe disabilities, but self-determination is relevant for all individuals and exists on a continuum (Abery & Stancliffe, 2003;

Wehmeyer, 2005). Self-determination involves a combination of personal skills, attitudes, knowledge, and environmental opportunities and support (Abery & Stancliffe, 2003).

Self-determination is an important aspect of occupational therapy, in general, and particularly in the lives of adults with intellectual disability (Angell et al., 2019; AOTA, 2014; Dean, Dunn, & Tomchek, 2015). Self-determination most directly relates to an individual's participation because it broadly relates to a person's life; however, self-determination can also influence a person's occupational performance and occupational engagement.

Self-determination is a developmental phenomenon that builds with experiences to exert choice and control in one's life on small and large scales (Abery & Stancliffe, 2003). Adults with intellectual disability with higher level skills to make choices, solve problems, and advocate for themselves may have significant environmental barriers in terms of opportunities to assert self-determination. Individuals with limited opportunities to express self-determination may develop a sense of learned helplessness. One's attitudes, including self-worth and volition, also influence self-determination. An adult with intellectual disability may have the capability and opportunity to make choices and influence their occupational life, but other attitudinal aspects of self-determination may be a barrier to participation. In one study, many individuals with intellectual disability age 40 and older felt they did not have control over their lives, caused by a variety of self-determination factors (Strnadová & Evans, 2012).

Social Environmental Support

A supportive social environment that meets the needs of adults with intellectual disability is one of the most important factors to ensure optimal occupational performance, occupational engagement, and participation. Caregivers who provide assistance and set up activities for adults with intellectual disability are important factors affecting occupational experiences. Environmental factors significantly impact the opportunities adults with intellectual disability have to access different occupations and affects their quality of life (Beadle-Brown et al., 2015; Belva & Matson, 2013; Gjermestad et al., 2017). For example, a research study demonstrated that adults with profound intellectual disability, living in a large developmental center (i.e., institutional setting), had significantly low performance with instrumental activities of daily living, influenced by the nature of opportunities in the institutional environment as much as the individual's actual skills (Belva & Matson, 2013). Staff members' attitudes toward the adults with intellectual disability and how they interact and provide support can act as a facilitator or a barrier to participation, occupational performance, and occupational engagement (Gjermestad et al., 2017; Johnson et al., 2012; Mahoney & Roberts, 2009; Talman et al., 2019). When staff members have fun with adults with intellectual disability, recognize their individuality, and interact with them respectfully, it supports the occupational experience for the adult with intellectual disability and can result in more work satisfaction for the staff member (Johnson et al., 2012a; Mahoney & Roberts, 2009). The staff members' knowledge, skills, attitudes, and relationships with adults with intellectual disability influence the effectiveness of the support they provide.

Factors Affecting Occupational Life Summary

After prioritizing occupational performance, participation, and/or occupational engagement issues, occupational therapy practitioners consider facilitators and barriers affecting occupational life. For adults with intellectual disability, common barriers include occupational skills, volition, self-determination, and social environment. Each of these issues involves person-environment transactions that can affect occupational therapy intervention.

OCCUPATIONAL THERAPY INTERVENTION

The main role of occupational therapy for adults with intellectual disability is to address occupational outcomes, which may include participation, occupational performance, and/or occupational engagement. To do this, occupational therapy practitioners may address the skills of the adults with intellectual disability directly; however, it is more common that they collaborate with individuals providing support to ensure there is an effective, supportive environment to enable maximal participation and occupational engagement. This may involve a combination of intervention strategies including caregiver training, environmental modification, adapting occupations, and addressing skill development, whether targeting the skills of the adult with intellectual disability or his or her caregiver.

It is more common for occupational therapy practitioners to work with paid staff members who are caregivers for adults with intellectual disability in residential or day centers, although most adults with intellectual disability live with family caregivers (Braddock et al., 2015). Most of the existing intervention research evidence involves work with staff members; therefore, that is the focus of the information in this chapter. However, the information may also be relevant when working with family caregivers. If working with family members, occupational therapy practitioners have to consider potentially long-standing family role dynamics. Whether working with family or staff members, occupational therapy practitioners need to address caregivers' willingness to change. An important way to get caregiver buy-in is to address issues that are important to the caregiver. If the adult with intellectual disability exhibits challenging behavior, an often concerning matter for caregivers, it can be helpful to explain how to provide support for engagement and participation in occupations to decrease challenging behavior.

Habilitation Approach

Occupational therapy practitioners may use a habilitation approach when working with adults with intellectual disability, especially when the targeted outcome is improved occupational performance. There is research-based evidence that occupational therapy intervention can improve activities of daily living performance and process skills in individuals with mild and moderate intellectual disability (Bathje, Lannoye, Mercier, & Panter, 2018; Hallgren & Kottorp, 2005; Waldman-Levi, Golisz, Swierat, & Toglia, 2019). If addressing skill development, occupational therapy practitioners may find it helpful to review performance skill level hierarchies (Kottorp, et al., 2003). Although Kottorp et al. (2003) is an older research article, it includes practical information about how to use a performance skill hierarchy when prioritizing which skills to focus on during occupational therapy intervention with adults with intellectual disability.

Habilitation may also be an appropriate approach to foster occupational engagement when volition is an underlying barrier, although it will likely involve environmental strategies as well. The Remotivation Process offers theoretical and practical intervention guidelines for improving volition (de las Heras, Llerena, & Kielhofner, 2003). This may be a useful intervention resource when working with adults with intellectual disability with limited occupational experiences.

Addressing issues with self-determination affecting occupational life often requires a combination of habilitation and environmental approaches. Occupational therapy practitioners may work with adults with intellectual disability on decision making, emotional self-regulation, problem solving, and self-advocacy in the context of occupational concerns. Because self-determination exists on a continuum and is a developmental process, occupational therapy practitioners may find it helpful to adapt resources designed for children and adolescents, especially when working with older adults with intellectual disability, who may have limited experiences expressing self-determination. In addition, it is necessary to ensure that the individuals regularly offering social support to the adults with intellectual disability do so in a way that fosters self-determination and maximizes occupational experiences. Although occupational therapy practitioners foster and enable activity choices among adults with intellectual disability, there are times when it is appropriate and desirable to coax people to engage in activities they may not actively choose. This is an important skill and distinction to discuss with caregivers (Mansell & Beadle-Brown, 2012). This does not only apply to necessary self-care occupations, where caregivers often understand the need to coax participation. However, when adults have limited occupational experiences and low self-determination, they may need additional support to make choices and encouragement to support participation. In addition, adults with intellectual disability may have limited communication skills that do not allow them to give nuanced answers, such as "not right now" or "after I finish this." It is important to help staff members understand that even if an adult with intellectual disability indicates that they do not want to do an activity, it does not mean they should never be offered the activity again. There is a risk that staff members can interpret "no" responses too definitively, and this can be a delicate balance when working to foster respectful relationships.

Environmental Support

Staff members need to provide adults with intellectual disability opportunities for choices and sufficient support for engagement and participation, and they need knowledge, respectful attitudes, and confidence to do this effectively (Flynn et al., 2018; Talman et al., 2019; Zakrajsek, Hammel, & Scazzero, 2014). Occupational therapy practitioners often address staff members' skills and knowledge, and it is also important to attend to the psychosocial aspects of the relationship to support the occupational lives of adults with intellectual disability. Staff members may be most comfortable when the adult with intellectual disability can perform the activity independently or with set up or when the staff member provides full assistance for the activity (Mahoney & Roberts, 2009; Mansell & Beadle-Brown, 2012). As adults with intellectual disability often have a limited repertoire of activities that they can perform independently, staff members need a variety of strategies for providing support. Staff members may require explicit instruction about ways to grade activities and the support they offer. When determining how to provide this type of intervention, meta-analysis research evidence supports "the combination of in-service with coaching-on-the-job [as] the most powerful format," (van Oorsouw, Embregts, Bosman, & Jahoda, 2009, p. 503).

Occupational therapy practitioners can use evidence from other professions to guide their intervention with adults with intellectual disability. One evidence-based program that is consistent with occupational therapy and focuses on ensuring that adults with intellectual disability have sufficient environmental support is active support. Active support is a program designed for individuals with severe to profound intellectual disability (Mansell & Beadle-Brown, 2012), although it may also be appropriate for individuals with moderate disabilities. There are many research articles about active support (Beadle-Brown et al., 2015; Beadle-Brown, Hutchinson, & Whelton, 2012; Flynn et al., 2018; Iacono et al., 2019). Occupational therapy practitioners who want to implement this program would benefit from consulting the book *Active Support: Enabling and Empowering People with Intellectual Disabilities* (Mansell & Beadle-Brown, 2012), which provides practical information.

There are benefits of active support for both adults with intellectual disability and their caregivers. Outcomes of the program for adults with intellectual disability include increased participation, more time spent doing purposeful activities, more opportunities for decision making, and decreased challenging behavior (Beadle-Brown et al., 2012; Flynn et al., 2018; Mansell & Beadle-Brown, 2012). Staff members report increased job satisfaction, which is an important outcome because staff turnover can be high (Beadle-Brown et al., 2012; Mansell & Beadle-Brown, 2012). To work most effectively, the program requires system changes and organizational support (Mansell & Beadle-Brown, 2012), but it is possible to start implementation on a small scale.

The primary mechanism for change with the active support program is fostering positive relationships with caregivers and facilitating caregivers' skills to provide appropriate levels of assistance to enable participation (Mansell & Beadle-Brown, 2012). This change involves the caregivers' attitudes about individuals with intellectual disability, as well as skills. There are four essential principles of active support that consider areas that must be addressed when implementing the program:

1. Recognizing that every moment has the potential for engagement and participation.
2. Providing short experiences and frequent opportunities, especially for new experiences; what the program calls "little and often" (Mansell & Beadle-Brown, 2012, p. 59).
3. Developing skills to provide a range of assistance with errorless learning.
4. Ensuring that adults with intellectual disability assert choice and control in their lives; enabling caregivers to be a supportive social environment for self-determination.

Depending on the needs of the adults with intellectual disability and the caregivers, different areas may require more emphasis. Because the focus is on supporting more frequent and consistent participation, program implementers need to understand the amount of assistance that staff members offer may increase, especially during initial implementation. Increased frequency of support would be a positive consequence of this program if it led to increased participation; so, it is important to choose outcome measures with this in mind. One professional may be able to start implementing small changes in a single home, program, or even with a small group of staff members. In order to fully implement the program, organizational support is necessary for leadership modeling and follow through, and system changes may be required.

Occupational therapy practitioners may use relationship-based interventions to enable social support for participation and occupational engagement for adults with intellectual disability. Recent research provides support for educational interventions to promote positive relationships between adults with intellectual disability and staff members (Johnson et al., 2017). Intensive interaction is a strategy for practitioners and caregivers to work with those with significant communication impairments and involves matching body language and emotional tones for communication (Caldwell, 2013). Based on parent-infant interactions and used primarily with individuals with autism who may have a co-existing intellectual disability intensive interaction may be a useful strategy for fostering positive relationships between adults with intellectual disability and caregivers (Hutchinson & Bodicoat, 2015). Caldwell (2013) offers case examples and information about training videos for additional information regarding this strategy. Occupational therapy practitioners may use the techniques to build rapport with adults with intellectual disability and severe communication impairments, and they can model how to respectfully and reciprocally communicate, while offering support for occupational experiences.

Occupational therapy practitioners may implement other types of staff training or environmental strategies based on the needs of the adults with intellectual disability and their caregivers. This may include helping the caregivers to structure a routine that maximizes participation for the adult with intellectual disability, while still providing flexibility. When providing suggestions or teaching skills to caregivers, occupational therapy practitioners need to monitor for understanding, buy-in, and follow-through. Regardless of the environmental changes targeted, it is important to monitor outcomes to ensure that suggestions and modifications have an impact on the occupational lives of the adults with intellectual disability.

CONCLUSION

Occupational therapy intervention with adults with intellectual disability should result in improved participation, occupational performance, and/or occupational engagement, which can lead to enhanced quality of life and well-being. Whether occupational therapy practitioners target increased involvement in occupational life, improved quality of performance, or more opportunities for engagement in activities that have a depth of personal meaning, passion, or excitement, it is essential to focus on enhancing the occupational lives of adults with intellectual disability. Occupational therapy practitioners consider the person-environment transactions impacting the occupational lives of adults with intellectual disability and determine whether a habilitation, environmental, or combination approach would better meet their clients' needs. Whether the focus of intervention is on improving the skills of the adult with intellectual disability or the skills of the caregivers providing support, the occupational therapy practitioner needs to implement teaching strategies to foster skill development and monitor their effectiveness.

REFERENCES

Abery, B. H., & Stancliffe, R. J. (2003). A tripartite ecological theory of self-determination. In M. L. Wehmeyer, B. H. Abery, D. E. Mithaug, & R. J. Stancliffe (Eds.), *Theory in self-determination: Foundations for educational practice* (pp. 43-78). Springfield, IL: Charles C. Thomas Publisher, Ltd.

American Occupational Therapy Association. (2014). Occupational therapy practice framework: Domain and process, 3rd edition. *American Journal of Occupational Therapy, 68*(Suppl. 1), S1-S48.

Angell, A. M., Carroll, T. C., Bagatell, N., Chen, C., Kramer, J. M., Schwartz, A., ... Hammel, J. (2019). Understanding self-determination as a crucial component in promoting the distinct value of occupational therapy in post-secondary transition planning. *Journal of Occupational Therapy, Schools, and Early Intervention, 12*(1), 129-143. doi: 10.1080/19411243.2018.1496870

Arvidsson, P., Granlund, M., Thyberg, I., & Thyberg, M. (2014). Important aspects of participation and participation restrictions in people with a mild intellectual disability. *Disability and Rehabilitation, 36*(15), 1264-1272. doi: 10.3109/09638288.2013.845252

Bathje, M., Lannoye, M., Mercier, A., & Panter, K. (2018). A review of occupation-based life skills interventions for adults with neurodevelopmental disorders. *Occupational Therapy in Mental Health, 34*(2), 165-180. doi: 10.1080/0164212X.2017.1360168

Beadle-Brown, J., Hutchinson, A., & Whelton, B. (2012). Person-centred active support—Increasing choice, promoting independence and reducing challenging behaviour. *Journal of Applied Research in Intellectual Disabilities, 25*(4), 291-307. doi: 10.1111/j.1468-3148.2011.00666.x

Beadle-Brown, J., Leigh, J., Whelton, B., Richardson, L., Beecham, J., Baumker, T., & Bradshaw, J. (2015). Quality of life and quality of support for people with severe intellectual disability and complex needs. *Journal of Applied Research in Intellectual Disabilites, 29*(5), 409-421. doi: 10.1111/jar.12200

Belva, B. C., & Matson, J. L. (2013). An examination of specific daily living skills deficits in adults with profound intellectual disabilities. *Research in Developmental Disabilities, 34*(1), 596-604. doi: 10.1016/j.ridd.2012.09.021

Bigby, C., Knox, M., Beadle-Brown, J., & Bould, E. (2014). Identifying good group homes: Qualitative indicators using a quality of life framework. *Intellectual and Developmental Disabilities, 52*(5), 348-366. doi: 10.1352/1934-9556-52.5.348

Braddock, D., Hemp, R., Rizzolo, M. C., Tanis, E. S., Haffer, L., & Wu, J. (2015). *The state of the States in intellectual and developmental disabilities* (10th ed.). Washington, D.C.: American Association on Intellectual and Developmental Disabilities.

Caldwell, P. (2013). Intensive interaction: Using body language to communicate. *Journal on Developmental Disabilities, 19*(1), 33-39.

Crowe, T. K., Salazar Sedillo, J., Kertcher, E. F., & LaSalle, J. H. (2015). Time and space use of adults with intellectual disabilities. *The Open Journal of Occupational Therapy, 3*(2), 2. doi: 10.15453/2168-6408.1124

Csikszentmihályi, M. (1998). *Finding flow: The psychology of engagement with everyday life.* New York, NY: Basic Books.

de las Heras, C. G., Geist, R., Kielhofner, G., & Li, Y. (2007). *A user's guide to the Volitional Questionnaire* (V. 4.). Chicago, IL: MOHO Clearinghouse.

de las Heras, C. G., Llerena, V., & Kielhofner, G. (2003). *A user's manual for remotivation process: Progressive intervention for individuals with severe volitional challenges.* Chicago, IL: MOHO Clearinghouse.

Dean, E. E., Dunn, W., & Tomchek, S. (2015). Role of occupational therapy in promoting self-determination through consumer-directed supports. *Occupational Therapy in Health Care, 29*(1), 86-95. doi: 10.310907380577.2014.958887

Fisher, A. G., Griswold, L. A., Munkholm, M., & Kottorp, A. (2017). Evaluating domains of everyday functioning in people with developmental disabilities. *Scandinavian Journal of Occupational Therapy, 24*(1), 1-9. doi: 10.3109/11038128.2016.1160147

Flynn, S., Totsika, V., Hastings, R. P., Hood, K., Toogood, S., & Felce, D. (2018). Effectiveness of active support for adults with intellectual disability in residential settings: Systematic review and meta-analysis. *Journal of Applied Research in Intellectual Disabilities, 31*(6), 983-998. doi: 10.1111/jar.12491

Gjermestad, A., Luteberget, L., Midjo, T., & Witsø, A. E. (2017). Everyday life of persons with intellectual disability living in residential settings: A systematic review of qualitative studies. *Disability and Society, 32*(2), 213-232. doi: 10.1080/09687599.2017.1284649

Hallgren, M., & Kottorp, A. (2005). Effects of occupational therapy intervention on activities of daily living and awareness of disability in persons with intellectual disabilities. *Australian Occupational Therapy Journal, 52,* 350-359. doi: 10.1111/j.1440-1630.2005.00523.x

Hutchinson, N., & Bodicoat, A. (2015). The effectiveness of intensive interaction, A systematic literature review. *Journal of Applied Research in Intellectual Disabilities, 28*(6), 437-454. doi: 10.1111/jar.12138

Iacono, T., Bould, E., Beadle-Brown, J., & Bigby, C. (2019). An exploration of communication within active support for adults with high and low support needs. *Journal of Applied Research in Intellectual Disabilities, 32*(1), 61-70. doi: 10.1111/jar.12502

Johnson, H., Bigby, C., Iacono, T., Douglas, J., Katthagen, S., & Bould, E. (2017). Increasing day service staff capacity to facilitate positive relationships with people with severe intellectual disability: Evaluation of a new intervention using multiple baseline design. *Journal of Intellectual and Developmental Disability, 42*(4), 391-402. doi: 10.3109/13668250.2016.1246656

Johnson, H., Douglas, J., Bigby, C., & Iacono, T. (2012). A model of processes that underpin positive relationships for adults with severe intellectual disability. *Journal of Intellectual & Developmental Disability, 37*(4), 324-336. doi: 10.3109/13668250.2012.732221

Johnson, K. R., & Bagatell, N. (2017). Beyond custodial care: Mediating choice and participation for adults with intellectual disabilities. *Journal of Occupational Science, 24*(4), 546-560. doi: 10.1080/14427591.2017.1363078

King, G., Law, M., King, S., Hurley, P., Rosenbaum, P., Hanna, S., ... Young, N. (2004). *Children's Assessment of Participation and Enjoyment.* San Antonio, TX: Harcourt Assessment, Inc.

Kottorp, A. (2008). The use of the Assessment of Motor and Process Skills (AMPS) in predicting need of assistance for adults with mental retardation. *Occupational Therapy Journal of Research, 28*(2), 72-80.

Kottorp, A., Bernspång, B., & Fisher, A. G. (2003). Activities of daily living in persons with intellectual disability: Strengths and limitations in specific motor and process skills. *Australian Occupational Therapy Journal, 50,* 195-204.

Law, M., Cooper, B., Strong, S., Stewart, D., Rigby, P., & Letts, L. (1996). The person-environment-occupation model: A transactive approach to occupational performance. *Canadian Journal of Occupational Therapy, 63,* 9-23. doi: 10.1177/000841749606300103

Lee, S. W., & Kielhofner, G. (2017). Volition. In R. R. Taylor (Ed.), *Kielhofner's Model of Human Occupation: Theory and application* (5th ed., pp. 38-56). Philadelphia, PA: Wolters Kluwer.

Mahoney, W. J., & Austin, S. (2014). Theoretical perspective of occupational engagement. In *Conference Proceedings: Society for the Study of Occupation 13th Annual Research Conference* (pp. 74-75). Minneapolis, MN: SSO:USA.

Mahoney, W. J., & Roberts, E. (2009). Co-occupation in a day program for adults with developmental disabilities. *Journal of Occupational Science, 16*(3), 170-179. doi: 10.1080/14427591.2009.9686659

Mahoney, W. J., Roberts, E., Bryze, K., & Parker Kent, J. A. (2016). Occupational engagement and adults with intellectual disabilities. *American Journal of Occupational Therapy, 70,* 7001350030p1-6. doi: 10.5014/ajot.2016.016576

Mansell, J., & Beadle-Brown, J. (2012). *Active support: Enabling and empowering people with intellectual disabilities.* London, United Kingdom: Jessica Kingsley Publishers.

Nijs, S., & Maes, B. (2014). Social peer interactions in persons with profound intellectual and multiple disabilities: A literature review. *Education and Training in Autism and Developmental Disabilities, 49*(1), 153-165.

Resnik, L., & Plow, M. A. (2009). Measuring participation as defined by the *International Classification of Functioning, Disability and Health*: An evaluation of existing measures. *Archives of Physical Medicine and Rehabilitation, 90*(5), 856-866. doi: 10.1016/j.apmr.2008.11.010

Strnadová, I., & Evans, D. (2012). Subjective quality of life of women with intellectual disabilities: The role of perceived control over their own life in self-determined behaviour. *Journal of Applied Research in Intellectual Disabilities, 25*(1), 71-79. doi: 10.1111/j.1468-3148.2011.00646.x

Talman, L., Wilder, J., Stier, J., & Gustafsson, C. (2019). Staff members and managers' views of the conditions for the participation of adults with profound intellectual and multiple disabilities. *Journal of Applied Research in Intellectual Disabilities, 32*(1), 143-151. doi: 10.1111/jar.12516

van Oorsouw, W. M. W. J., Embregts, P. J. C. M., Bosman, A. M. T., & Jahoda, A. (2009). Training staff serving clients with intellectual disabilities: A meta-analysis of aspects determining effectiveness. *Research in Developmental Disabilities, 30*(3), 503-511. doi: 10.1016/j.ridd.2008.07.011

Vicente, E., Guillén, V. M., Gómez, L. E., Ibáñez, A., & Sánchez, S. (2019). What do stakeholders understand by self-determination? Consensus for its evaluation. *Journal of Applied Research in Intellectual Disabilities, 32*(1), 206-218. doi: 10.1111/jar.12523

Waldman-Levi, A., Golisz, K., Swierat, R. P., & Toglia, J. (2019). Scoping review: Interventions that promote functional performance for adolescents and adults with intellectual and developmental disabilities. *Australian Occupational Therapy Journal, 66*, 458-468. doi: 10.1111/1440-1630.1257

Wehmeyer, M. L. (2005). Self-determination and individuals with significant disabilities: Examining meanings and misinterpretations. *Research and Practice for Persons with Severe Disabilities, 30*(3), 113-120. doi: 10.2511/rpsd.30.3.113

World Health Organization. (2001). *International classification of functioning, disability and health (ICF)*. Geneva, Switzerland: Author.

Zakrajsek, A. G., Hammel, J., & Scazzero, J. A. (2014). Supporting people with intellectual and developmental disabilities to participate in their communities through support staff pilot intervention. *Journal of Applied Research in Intellectual Disabilities, 27*(2), 154-162. doi: 10.1111/jar.12060

9

Home Life

Kimberly Bryze, PhD, OTR/L

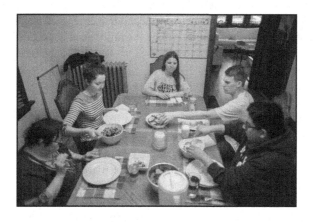

Key Words: active support, co-occupation, group homes, home, intermediate care facility, quality of life

Bryze, K.
Occupational Therapy for Adults With Intellectual Disability (pp. 99-108).
© 2020 Taylor & Francis Group.

Providing care and professional services to adults with intellectual disability is a responsibility shared by all health care professionals; however, the occupational therapy scope of practice offers unique contributions to this population. Our profession is instrumental in serving these individuals from a person-centered approach to occupational performance, participation, and quality of life, through efforts directed toward education, advocacy, and therapeutic alliances with family, direct care staff, and other professionals. Occupational therapy is uniquely suited to serve this population in many settings, including in the clinic, at work, in the community, and, more importantly, in their homes.

The use of the word *home* suggests meanings that are deeper and more complex than the commonplace use of the term, whether as a noun, verb, or adjective. Home may represent the residence or house where one lives, whether a physical or institutional residence. Home may also embody the presence of and interrelationship with others, carrying emotions, memories, and contextual significance. Home may elicit impressions or memories of being cared for, supported, and emotional safe, yet, home may also elicit feelings of dread, fear, or memories of pain, confusion, or a desire to avoid "that place." While for some home may represent a place of comfort or safety and may include other persons, family members, or even pets, for other individuals with intellectual disability, home may only represent where one spends time and sleeps, with different caregivers coming and going. Home is a complex topic to cover, and as occupational therapy practitioners, we value the importance of these physical, emotional, and relational places.

This chapter will address several important areas of practical and critical considerations of home life for individuals with intellectual disability, salient occupations, and their contributions to meaningful participation and quality of life. Issues of independence/dependence and relationships with others will be highlighted. A common thread will be the multifaceted issue of living with supports.

THE FIRST OR PRIMARY HOME

Family is a fundamental unit of society, comprised of individuals who are related by birth, marriage, formalized relationship, and may include nuclear and extended family members. Family may also be comprised of individuals who care for and are committed and dedicated to each other without specific familial or blood ties. Within a family, children are cared for and live with their parents or family members until, and often into, young adulthood. Oftentimes, adults with intellectual disability remain with their parents or family members far into adulthood. Family is the primary context where children learn the personal, social, and complex life skills that allow them to function within the community and society. Further, each family has its own culture, routines, and traditions. Children learn the values, rules, and behaviors for living in society from their family's ways of living.

Each member of a family has certain roles and responsibilities, and family life is enacted through habits and traditions. Demonstrations of care for each other, expressions of their values, and indications of respect are emphasized in a variety of ways. Whether celebrating family members' birthdays, attending religious services or celebrations, or a family's monthly breakfast food for dinner nights, each member of the family becomes part of the rhythm and flow of family routines and traditions. Specifically, celebrations provide a way to honor and enjoy each family member, which may involve preparing and eating a special treat, giving and receiving presents, or preparing for a seasonal tradition. Through special occasions, as well as routine and contextualized ways of living, families co-construct meaningful events where each family member has a place or role. Each member of the family may assume responsibility for certain tasks that support the whole family. For instance, the head of the family may work to provide the source of financial income. Another member of the family may be primarily responsible for the acquisition and preparation of food, and most, if not all, family members contribute to the upkeep of the home. All family members, including children, may assume tasks or chores that support the daily life and family routines, such as feeding the family dog, picking up toys, or taking out the garbage. However, for those with intellectual disability, expectations for contributing to the family through task performance may be neglected or minimized.

As a person with intellectual disability learns to perform a task, they need a parent or caregiver to come alongside and provide support, or to perform the task with another as a co-occupational experience. In family life, especially with younger children and those with intellectual disability, *doing with* the other person is an effective way of ensuring task completion, while supporting the person's performance as needed. For example, caregivers frequently allow a person to begin the task of brushing his or her own teeth but will then make sure all the teeth are cleaned well. In another example, the individual with intellectual disability will help by pouring in pre-measured ingredients or will help mix the dough. The caregiver will perform steps of the task that are more challenging, such as placing the cookie sheet into the hot oven to bake or measuring a teaspoon of vanilla. Such co-occupation is an inherent facet of everyday life, and touches on the interdependence of all family members within the home. These contextualized situations of sharing time and activities with others provide depth of meaning to the construct of home for everyone.

While some individuals with intellectual disability live in their family home into adulthood and then transition to supported community living, a proportion of individuals reside in institutional living environments for most of their adult lives. Children in the 19th and 20th centuries were often placed in institutional care early in life, where they lived with few resources and opportunities. Deinstitutionalization efforts in the mid-1900s prompted the social and ethical responsibilities of supporting individuals with intellectual disability to engage in more active roles within society. Issues related to housing, habilitation, and individualized supports became areas of focus, as alternative placements were found, or homes were created for individuals leaving larger institutions. Nearly 30,000 individuals with intellectual disability continue to live in state-operated institutions. Although the Olmstead Decision required states to eliminate segregated housing for individuals with intellectual disability, 37 states continue to maintain state-operated institutions (Braddock, et al., 2015). While some institutions exist today, they are less in number and house fewer individuals overall than those in the early 20th century.

There currently exist several different settings for individuals who transition from their family home to more independent living. Of the 5.1 million persons with intellectual disability in the United States accounted for in 2015 (Braddock et al., 2015), the majority (71% or 3.6 million) lived with family caregivers while 13% (680,851) lived in supervised residential settings, and 16% (794,164) lived alone or with a roommate. Of those living with family caregivers, 41% (1.5 million) were aged less than 41 years, whereas 35% (1.3 million) were age 41 to 50 years, and 24% (872,042) were 60 or more years of age. Facilities for housing seven or more individuals with intellectual disability exist as nursing facilities, state institutions, private or public intermediate care facilities (ICF/IDs), or other residential arrangements. Smaller, less than six person arrangements, include supported or supervised residential settings (e.g., public or private ICF/ID homes), or settings in which individuals live independently or with a roommate (Braddock, et al., 2015). ICF/IDs intend to provide quality personal care and services for diagnosing, treating, and rehabilitating individuals with intellectual disability in order to enhance their functional capabilities. These services may include, but are not limited to, ongoing psychological and psychiatric care, nursing, occupational therapy, physical therapy, speech and language services, and vocational training (Johnson & Bagatell, 2017).

Placements outside of the family home are often prompted by caregivers' declining health, increasing behavioral challenges of the person with intellectual disability, and with the medical challenges or increased needs of those with disabilities as they age (McConkey, Kelly, Mannan, & Craig, 2011; Woodman, Mailick, Anderson, & Esbensen, 2014). As understood from child development experts and psychologists, family relationships have an important influence on the initial social, psychological, and emotional well-being of a child, and this holds true for individuals with intellectual disability. Adaptive behavior, physical and mental health, and social interaction have been identified as factors that are highly influenced by early familial relationships (Hamilton, Sutherland, & Isacono, 2005; Wehmeyer & Bolding, 2001). Further, as individuals' transition to community living outside the home, family involvement continues to be an important factor to ease the persons transition to more independent living (Heller, Miller, & Hsieh, 2002).

Occupations Are Learned and Performed Within the Home

Occupational therapy practitioners are often called upon to evaluate and design interventions to facilitate skill mastery in areas of daily living, which typically take place within the home. Regardless of where one lives or from whom one learns to perform life skills tasks, which are necessary and relevant, such tasks are an important part of daily life for adults with or without intellectual disability. Certain tasks, such as personal self-care, eating, dressing, and home upkeep, need to be done, either by oneself or by another person. From an early age, children learn from their family members how to care for themselves, their material belongings and living spaces, and how to care for others in their family. The family is responsible to care for and teach children with or without disabilities those life skills, which eventually lead to independence and self-determined living.

The presence of intellectual disability, however, influences the ease and methods by which the child will learn these essential daily living skills. Children without disabilities tend to learn daily living tasks effortlessly and within age-appropriate timelines, while children with disabilities may require more practice, different approaches to performing tasks, and additional supports to learn and accomplish necessary tasks. Family members may also struggle with the additional time and responsibility required for training their children with disabilities, and may resort to doing for the child rather than allowing and supporting the child to, for example, dress themselves before school, as it often takes less time to just "get them dressed." Time and effort are not the only factors involved, and parental disappointment or grief may also interfere. Moses (1987) called this *loss of a dream*, which refers to the grieving process a parent experiences when their initial dreams of a healthy, "normal" child are not realized. Such grief may present itself as depression, anger, and other symptoms of this emotional undercurrent, and each parent and family may react differently. The child with intellectual disability may be treated differently than other children in the family, and overcompensation or over-protection of the child may be the behavioral outcome. Over-protectiveness may result in doing for the individual with intellectual disability and prevent the child or adolescent from learning those personal, social, and complex activities of daily living (ADLs). School personnel will often build these life skills into the student's individualized education plan. Transition plans that are developed for adolescents with intellectual disability often include life skill goals and interventions.

Active Supports and Co-Occupation

Adults with intellectual disability can and should be responsible for their personal self-care, as well as those instrumental activities of daily living (IADLs) that support self-maintenance, care of one's home and immediate environment, and interaction with others in their home. Living life fully in one's home environment implies a certain amount of responsibility for engaging in tasks that need to be accomplished during a given time span. While generalization of task performance across settings is often a challenge for persons with intellectual disability, they will require additional assistance or active supports to perform their personal self-care, home management, and other IADLs. For adults without disabilities, typical daily and weekly life is filled with home tasks to accomplish (e.g., preparing meals, cleaning the kitchen, laundering clothing and household towels and bedding, straightening rooms, dusting and vacuuming, caring for the pet). For individuals with intellectual disability, however, these home care tasks are often relegated to "the staff," with minimal assistance from those persons who reside in the home. Lessened expectations for an individual with intellectual disability may be likened to an attitude that "it is quicker (easier) to just do it myself" and not offering the person the opportunity to perform. Lessened expectations can also emerge from a belief that "they can't do that; it's too hard" and therefore not affording them the opportunity to learn, or "I've tried to teach him but he can't do it," thus preventing the possibility of success for the person with intellectual disability. Necessary active supports are employed to facilitate learning and task performances.

The concepts underlying active supports were well-described in an article by Saunders and Spradlin (1991). It focused on the influence of supported routines (i.e. active supports) on participants' underactivity, low levels of staff involvement with residents, and assistance provided to the residents to actively engage in enjoyable, functional daily routines. Active support is conceptually like the partial participation described by Brown et al. (1979), where the person with intellectual disability performs part of an activity with adaptations or assistance from another person to complete the activity. While the primary aim of active supports is to increase engagement in purposeful and meaningful daily activity, challenging behavior may also be reduced, as engagement in positive activities often reduces the frustration and behavioral sequelae that result (Emerson, Hatton, Robertson, Henderson, & Cooper, 1999; Larson & Lakin, 2012). Using active supports to increase engagement and more independent performance requires increased availability and more effective staff assistance. Occupational therapy practitioners may be especially helpful in educating staff on specific, helpful ways to provide active support to individuals as they learn and practice necessary and desired tasks. When staff learn the best types of cues, directions, supports, and assistance for each specific individual, the persons with intellectual disability will improve their skills, performance, and confidence. Generalization of task performance may also be fostered.

Therefore, the responsibility for occupational therapy practitioners is to evaluate each person's occupational performance, then educate and train caregivers to provide supports that do not involve doing *for* or doing *to* the person who needs assistance. Co-occupational performance, or doing with, is the recommended approach for assisting individuals to learn and perform the tasks they need, want, and must do in their home settings.

"Co-occupations consist of shared physicality, shared emotionality, and shared intentionality" (Pickens & Pizur-Barnekow, 2009, p. 151). *Shared physicality* refers to the motor behavior of two or more persons, while helping or contributing to the occupational performance. Both people are physically involved in doing the occupation. *Shared emotionality* refers to the interactions or responsiveness of each person to others' emotional tone or state within the occupational context. *Shared intentionality* refers to the person's mutual understanding or purpose of the occupation.

An example of shared physicality, emotionality, and intentionality can help clarify the depth and breadth of co-occupation. Cindy (a woman with intellectual disability) and Rose (staff) are working together to make a birthday cake for that evening's celebration of another resident, Betty. Rose carries the stand mixer to the counter, turns on the oven to preheat while Cindy gathers the large mixing bowl and cake mix on the counter. Rose gathers the eggs from the refrigerator and oil from the cupboard while Cindy opens the cake mix box. Cindy excitedly tells Rose that surprising the "birthday girl" will be fun, to which Rose agrees and says, "Chocolate cake is Betty's favorite type of cake." Cindy pours the cake mix into the bowl, and Rose offers Cindy one of the eggs to crack open, as she adds her egg to the mix. Rose measures and adds the oil and inserts the mixer paddle while Cindy finishes adding her egg. Rose asks, "Do you want to turn the mixer on today?" Cindy is eager and Rose helps her adjust the speed just high enough so the mix does not splatter. The women alternate tasks until the cake is mixed, poured into two cake pans, and placed in the oven. The timer is set by Rose, and Cindy brings the used dishes and utensils to the sink. While Rose washes the dishes and Cindy dries, they discuss other plans for the birthday celebration, including presents, decorations for the dining room, and the fact that Betty is a good friend to Cindy. There is anticipation and joy for a fun party, mutual intentionality, and shared physical actions in this simple but meaningful co-occupation.

Shared meaning is embedded in co-occupational experiences and transects the shared dimensions of co-occupations. While the occupations may be simple or complex, co-occupation implies more than the mere assistance by a staff member in performing a task. Co-occupation implies a mutuality, a common experience, and an interconnectedness between two or more individuals. This presupposes an affective or relational foundation for the occupational performance and harkens back to the attitudes and beliefs one holds about the other individual and the task itself. For example, making a cake can also be part of an active support process, but the physical assistance is directed toward helping the other do something well or more independently (i.e., open the cake box, crack the egg, pour the batter). The intentionality involved in active support would be more directed toward the goal of helping Cindy to learn to crack the egg or maintain her attention on the task at hand, and not necessarily as a shared intention or purpose for both parties. Further, with active support, the issue of shared emotionality may not be a factor. A person can assist or support another person without shared emotionality or reciprocal responsivity to the other person. Supporting another can just be part of one's job. In these ways, one can see that the depth and breadth of co-occupation is greater than active support. While both may be part of daily life in the home, co-occupation offers greater collaboration and relationship in the occupational life of another.

Quality of Life

Much has been written about quality of life in the rehabilitation and social sciences literature, and occupational therapy's influence can be significant when considering the quality of life in group home living contexts. *Quality of life* is an overarching term that refers to one's overall, and often subjective, well-being. Bigby, Knox, Beadle-Brown, and Bould (2014) have identified several domains that are foundational to quality of life: emotional well-being, interpersonal relations, material well-being, personal development, physical well-being, self-determination, individual rights, and social inclusion. These domains are interconnected and, together, comprise quality of life.

Emotional well-being encompasses feelings of emotional safety, happiness, a state of satisfaction, and contentment. While emotional well-being and other indicators of quality of life are often assessed using self-report measures, some individuals are not able to self-report their emotional state. The determination of emotional well-being for an individual with intellectual disability requires sensitive observations of arousal level or state, behavior patterns, ease with the presence of and assistance from staff members, engagement and pleasure in activities, and evidence of comfort in their environment.

The domain of *interpersonal relations* includes social interactions that are necessary or chosen, as well as the types and quality of social supports between peers (e.g., other residents) and staff. Interpersonal relations among all members of a home are directly linked to emotional well-being, as well as the emotional tone of the home. Interpersonal relations that are positive, kind, and respectful promote feelings of safety, calmness, respect, and being cared for; whereas, interpersonal relations that are pointed, punitive, or disrespectful will reinforce a divide between individuals. Attitudes such as an us-vs.-them mindset between staff and residents may be noted. Positive interpersonal relations are evident when individuals are supported respectfully, and affection, pleasant interactions, emotional warmth, and concern are demonstrated. More will be said about this in the next section of the chapter.

Another domain pertaining to quality of life is *material well-being*. Examples include having personal possessions that are needed, sufficient, and meaningful, and having the funds to purchase necessary supplies and items. Individuals with intellectual disability should ideally have enough funds to afford essential items, as well as some desired, nonessential items to allow for transportation to access the community, some holiday costs, and some leisure endeavors, such as going into the community for lunch. However, the dire reality for many is that the monthly allotment of funds for individuals is minimal after their monthly income checks are allocated toward rent, food, and other necessities. In many group homes, an individual may receive up to $50 per month to purchase over-the-counter medications, shampoo, new socks, and bus fare. The domain of material well-being also includes an individual's freedom to possess and display items that are important and meaningful to them, such as photographs and personal décor, and to own items to enjoy and perhaps share with others who live in the home. The material well-being domain also pertains to having a range of materials and activities from which to choose for leisure, which increases the probability of engaging occupations for individual or shared enjoyment. Examples include reading materials, art and craft activities, puzzles, availability of music from the radio, CDs or electronic devices, board games, and outdoor spaces to enjoy nature. Choice and supports for engagement should be offered and provided to individuals as appropriate. While quiet times and opportunities for minimal activity are important for restoration, active engagement is more favorable than passive pursuits (e.g., watching television for long periods of time). Further, activities that range from easy to challenging, simple to complex, should be available and offered for individuals' choice. Choice and engagement in purposeful and meaningful activity also contribute to personal development, the next domain related to quality of life.

Personal development is perhaps the most well-understood domain for practitioners who serve adults with intellectual disability, as it refers to supporting the engagement of individuals in activities that expand and enhance their skills, abilities, and interests. The extent to which an individual can make choices and become engaged in a wide range of daily self-care, homemaking, leisure, and productive activities is an important part of an adult's everyday life. Personal development is supported when individuals can try new activities and engage in a range of meaningful occupations. Specific outcomes for personal development may be written as goals into an individualized service plan, yet each day provides a myriad of opportunities for designing and implementing various occupations that foster engagement, enjoyment, and interaction within the home environment. In this way, the domain of personal development conjoins the domains of interpersonal relations and emotional well-being. Consistent with occupational therapy's focus on doing, being, becoming, and belonging (Wilcock, 1999), an individual's personal development is enhanced through engagement in occupation, which fosters satisfaction and emotional health. As individuals with intellectual disability often require active supports to engage in occupations (Mahoney & Roberts, 2009), interpersonal relations are also strengthened.

Physical well-being refers to an individual's health and those lifestyle factors that support safety and effective responses to health care needs. This domain includes simple but essential components of daily life (e.g., ensuring that an individual's food is nutritious and prepared in a way as to be ingested safely; supporting clothing choice to ensure comfort and warmth; maintaining hygienic routines to ensure health and social acceptability), as well as more complex dimensions (e.g., prompt response to pain or illness; access to routine appointments and emergent medical care; maintenance of medication schedules; and support for healthy, yet individualized, lifestyle choices). The physical environment must also be considered, and accommodations made for limited mobility, low vision, accessible and comfortable furniture, and effective tools and utensils for eating, hygiene, and grooming. While safety is paramount, individualized and respectful supports should be provided, without staff being exceedingly risk averse. Physical well-being also includes a component of choice and self-determination. The spaces in an individual's home that express their personality or style, with personal mementos and meaningful items, create an inviting and organized place of belonging. While safety, access, warmth, and provision for the physiological basics are essential, the affective dimension of physical well-being must also be given appropriate attention.

Self-determination, as expanded in Chapter 5, is another domain that underpins quality of life. The exercise of autonomy and choice is an essential way by which one's identity and individualism is seen and honored. Autonomy is important, yet includes aspects of interdependence and relationship with others when living in a community, such as a group home. Individuals support each other by doing necessary and desired activities with, and sometimes for, each other. Individuals should be encouraged and supported to express their choices and preferences and be part of person-centered planning and decisions about their everyday lives as well as their futures. An advocate may be needed to facilitate this understanding and approval process. For many individuals, the use of visual cues or schedules may be important to help them understand and predict their daily activities and appointments, with conscious regard given to their preferences. The extent to which individuals are encouraged and allowed to lead individualized lives and make individual decisions, and to not be treated as just one part of a larger group, provides evidence of self-determination.

Related to self-determination are the individual rights of each person with intellectual disability. The person's rights are essential as the guide to how they are treated and supported. Each person has a right to be treated with dignity and respect in their interactions and actions. Individuals whose quality of life is good are aware of their rights and have strong identities and self-determination.

They recognize their right to make decisions, ask questions, and direct plans and actions that pertain to their daily and future lives. Agencies and group homes often have a human rights committee that oversees behavior and medication plans for each individual, but the domain of rights focuses more on treating an individual with intellectual disability as an adult, with all the rights and privileges afforded adults without disabilities. While many of these rights have been written into legislation, all are underscored by the inherent value and dignity of each individual as a human being.

Finally, *social inclusion* relies on the other domains of quality of life, especially interpersonal relations and refers to being able to participate fully in community settings, organizations, and neighborhood activities without being segregated. Friendships with people within and outside of the home are encouraged. Inclusion in daily life activities, and not just in special outings on weekends, for example, are important. As most group homes are ordinary houses on ordinary streets in residential neighborhoods, where individuals without disabilities live, individuals with and without disabilities are recognized, acknowledged, accepted, and valued, and social inclusion becomes a reality. Further, the ways staff value, respect, and interact with individuals with disabilities as friends, companions, and as equal to themselves, will help to ensure that inclusion in social, community settings can take place. Inclusion is more likely to happen when individuals are valued for their individuality and uniqueness and when accepted and appreciated in both the private and public spaces of their lives (Bigby et al., 2014).

Improved quality of life becomes an important consideration as occupational therapy practitioners intentionally infuse dimensions of each of these domains into their practice, whether through direct interaction with individuals with intellectual disability, consultation and education of staff members, or developing programs and intervention strategies to improve individuals' occupational performance. By enabling occupation in all facets of daily home life, occupational therapy's contributions can be significant and meaningful.

PROVIDING OCCUPATIONAL THERAPY WITHIN THE HOME ENVIRONMENTS

As mentioned earlier in this chapter, approximately 13% of adults with intellectual disability live in supervised residential group home settings (Braddock et al., 2015). The majority of these homes support seven or more residents, with various staff members who cycle in and out of the homes in shifts. The staff-to-resident ratio is greater than 1 staff member to 8 or more residents, which limits available human supports for community outings and opportunities. Direct care staff are often paid a low wage and staff turnover rates are high. A resident may interact with more than 6 paid direct service staff members during a week. It is common for staff to take responsibility for the household tasks, such as cleaning, cooking, shopping, and perhaps laundry, while residents are otherwise occupied in day programs or their work settings outside the homes. While residents are supported to complete certain chores and personal responsibilities, such as doing their own laundry, the bulk of daily life tasks are performed by staff members. Mealtimes typically involve residents eating together with staff and assisting those individuals who require help with cutting their food or feeding themselves; staff may remain close to but positioned away from the dining table and do not simultaneously eat meals with the residents. While many staff may be quite dedicated to the residents and the home in which they work, it may be that other staff consider their responsibilities to be part of "the job."

Occupational therapy practitioners understand the importance of home and individuals' engagement in his or her homes, given the physical, social, and affective dimensions. Occupational therapy is in a unique position to take the lead in creating opportunities for occupational engagement and performance with individuals who have typically not been afforded the experiences to learn and assume responsibility for themselves and their homes. A core commitment of occupational therapy is to enable one's participation in his or her homes, community, and society. Practitioners support individuals to develop their skills and capabilities to perform daily activities in the home and community, and actively address the interaction between the individual and their environment, providing adaptations to promote that person's full participation. Occupational therapy practitioners provide interventions by enabling the development of new skills, modifying the activity or occupation the individual needs and wants to do, or by adapting the environment to create the best person-occupation-environment fit. With their background and training in health care and social sciences, occupational therapy practitioners can contribute to a comprehensive, person-centered approach to individuals' care, and can communicate with other health care and behavioral professionals regarding individuals' functioning and participation.

Occupational therapy can fill an indispensable need through consultation, program development, staff education, as well as the provision of direct services. One constraint, however, is the dearth of occupational therapy positions in organizations that serve adults with intellectual disability. Funding sources for this population typically come from state government initiatives, which vary considerably state to state. Moreover, such service organizations are often not-for-profit, and their funds are typically directed toward immediate, tangible needs, such as housing and food, rather than professional staff. It is, therefore, incumbent upon occupational therapy practitioners to become advocates for this population who have historically been underserved, underfunded, and underappreciated. It is also important to advocate for the profession to be present and committed to providing authentic services to enable individuals with intellectual disability to live their lives fully at home. The strength of the occupational therapy profession's role within home and residential settings for individuals with intellectual disability can be found in efforts directed toward designing and implementing interventions for the individuals related to ADLs, including personal self-care, cooking, homemaking, leisure activities, and community integration. Practitioners can provide educational in-services or programs for caregivers, whether staff, family members, or other professionals, to develop and structure effective ways to engage individuals with intellectual disability to perform daily life tasks in the home and community. What more important role can occupational therapy assume than to support individuals in their homes with all that term implies?

CONCLUSION

This chapter has provided several areas for consideration related to the role, responsibilities, and vision of occupational therapy practitioners who provide services to adults with intellectual disability in their home environments. Such home settings may be institutional, skilled medical, or community environments. Regardless of the setting, the importance of the home to an individual and of living one's life through chosen, relevant, and authentic occupations should be a primary concern of occupational therapy. This author believes that it is an honor to provide services to individuals within their homes—the private spaces in which they reside, play, learn, and take care of themselves and others. As described in the chapter, appropriate supports can and should be provided through a variety of means. Indeed, occupational therapy has much to offer adults with intellectual disability within their home settings.

REFERENCES

Bigby, C., Knox, M., Beadle-Brown, J., & Bould, E. (2014). Identifying good group homes: Qualitative indicators using a quality of life framework. *Intellectual and Developmental Disabilities, 52*, 348-366.

Braddock, D. Hemp, R., Rizzolo, M. C., Tanis, E. S., Haffer, L., & Wu, J. (2015). *The state of the States in intellectual and developmental disabilities: Emerging from the great recession.* Washington, D.C.: American Association on Intellectual and Developmental Disabilities.

Brown, L., Branston-McClean, M. B., Baumgart, D., Vincent, L., Falvey, M., & Schroeder, J. (1979). Using the characteristics of current and subsequent least restrictive environments in the development of curricular content for severely handicapped students. *AAESPH Review, 4*, 407-424. doi: 10.1177/154079697900400408

Emerson, E., Hatton, C., Robertson, J., Henderson, D., & Cooper, J. (1999). A descriptive analysis of the relationships between social context, engagement and stereotypy in residential services for people with severe and complex disabilities. *Journal of Applied Research in Intellectual Disabilities, 12*, 11-29. doi: 10.1111/j.1468-3148.1999.tb00047.x

Hamilton, D., Sutherland, G., & Iacono, T. (2005). Further examination of relationships between life events and psychiatric symptoms in adults with intellectual disability. *Journal of Intellectual Disability Research, 49*, 839-844.

Heller, T., Miller, A. B., & Hsieh, K. (2002). Eight-year follow-up of the impact of environmental characteristics on well-being of adults with developmental disabilities. *Mental Retardation, 40*, 366-378.

Johnson, K. R., & Bagatell, N. (2017). Beyond custodial care: Mediating choice and participation for adults with intellectual disabilities. *Journal of Occupational Science, 24*(4), 546-560.

Larson, S., & Lakin, C. (2012). Behavioral outcomes of moving from institutional to community living for people with intellectual and developmental disabilities: U.S. studies from 1977 to 2010. *Research and Practice for Persons with Severe Disabilities, 37*, 235-246.

Mahoney, W. J., & Roberts, E. (2009). Co-occupation in a day program for adults with developmental disabilities. *Journal of Occupational Science, 16*, 170 179.

McConkey, R., Kelly, F., Mannan, H., & Craig, S. (2011). Moving from family care of residential and supported accommodation: National, longitudinal study of people with intellectual disabilities. *American Journal on Intellectual and Developmental Disabilities, 116*, 305-314.

Moses, K. (1987). The impact of childhood disability: The parent's struggle. *Ways Magazine*, Spring.

Pickens, N .D., & Pizur-Barnekow, K. (2009). Co-occupation: Extending the dialogue. *Journal of Occupational Science, 16*, 151-156. doi: 10.1080/14427591.2009.9686656

Saunders, R. E., & Spradlin, J. J. (1991). A supported routines approach to active treatment for enhancing independence, competence and self-worth. *Behavioral Residential Treatment, 6*, 11-37.

Wehmeyer, M. L., & Bolding, N. (2001). Enhanced self-determination of adults with intellectual disability as an outcome of moving to community-based work or living environments. *Journal of Intellectual Disability Research, 45*, 371-383.

Wilcock, A. A. (1999). Reflections on doing, being, and becoming. *Australian Occupational Therapy Journal, 46*, 1-11.

Woodman, A. C., Mailick, M. R., Anderson, K. A., & Esbensen, A. J. (2014). Residential transitions among adults with intellectual disability across 20 years. *American Journal on Intellectual and Developmental Disabilities, 119*, 496-515.

10

Work Life

Katie Coakley, MOT, OTR/L

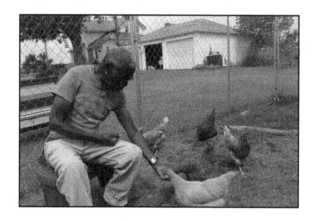

Key Words: Employment First, The philosophy that employment in the general workforce is the first priority and preferred outcome in the provision of publicly funded services for all working-age citizens with disabilities, regardless of level of disability (Association of People Supporting Employment First [APSE], 2015); **sheltered employment,** An approach to employment of individuals with disabilities, which includes adult day care, work activities, and sheltered workshops (Rusch & Braddock, 2004); **supported employment,** Provides an individual with a disability the support he or she needs to work in the community; includes work in small business enterprises, work crews, enclaves within an industry, and individual job placements (Braddock, et al., 2004); **work,** The area of occupational performance that includes activities required in order to participate in paid employment or volunteerism (Larson, 2014)

Bryze, K.
Occupational Therapy for Adults With Intellectual Disability (pp. 109-119).
© 2020 Taylor & Francis Group.

Work is the area of occupation that includes activities required to participate in paid employment or volunteerism (Larson, 2014). It is an integral occupation of adult life. Through work, adults can financially support themselves, interact with members of their communities, feel accomplished and productive, and contribute to society. This is especially true in the United States, where the culture greatly values personal responsibility and independence (Snodgrass & Gupta, 2014).

Productive occupations are an essential component of a balanced life routine. The productive occupations of school and work act to scaffold other dimensions of people's occupational lives from a very young age. Children's productive lives begin early in school, where they learn skills to play, socialize, and gain academic aptitude. School also plays a role in preparing children for future vocational pursuits. From a very young age, children play "work" by dressing up as doctors, police officers, and teachers. They are exposed to the world of work through initiatives like career day and Take Your Child to Work Day. As a part of secondary education, students are further prepared for the future of work, as the focus of school becomes preparation for higher education or post-graduation employment.

The value of work as an occupation is well established in the profession of occupational therapy. *The Occupational Therapy Practice Framework: Domain and Process, Third Edition* identifies work as one of the eight areas of occupation (American Occupational Therapy Association [AOTA], 2014). Work transects other areas of occupation as well. For example, within the occupation of social participation, the workplace is a component of the community, and peers and friends may be a part of one's work environment (AOTA, 2014). Occupational therapy interventions to address challenges in work performance are complex because in order to be successful in the worker role, one must also be able to manage his or her activities of daily living (ADLs)and instrumental activities of daily living (IADLs), and have completed the necessary education and training required for one's work (Wysocki & Neulicht, 2004).

Occupational therapy practitioners have addressed work since the inception of the profession. Eleanor Clark Slagle provided and promoted the value of curative, productive occupations for people with mental illness, as well as return-to-work programs for World War I soldiers. George Barton's Consolation House in New York served as a community-based workshop for the ill and people with disabilities. William Rush Dunton utilized workday planning with psychiatric patients to promote and maintain their work habits (Carrasco, Skees Hermes, & Burgos, 2012).

Work remains an important occupation for practitioners to address with clients today, specifically adults with intellectual disability. Individuals with intellectual disability who are employed report higher quality of life and psychological well-being, engage in social interaction with non-disabled colleagues at work, and report higher levels of autonomy (Jahoda, Kemp, Banks, & Williams, 2008). Employment of adults with intellectual disability in integrated employment settings is also correlated with increased adaptive skills (Stephens, Collins, & Dodder, 2005). These findings suggest that employment leads to significant personal and productive growth for adults with intellectual disability.

Despite these benefits, work remains an inaccessible occupation for many people with disabilities, particularly those with intellectual disability. Current evidence indicates that approximately 34% of adults with intellectual disability in the United States are employed. The percentage of adults with intellectual disability who are competitively employed, meaning they are paid minimum wage and work in the community without support, is far less, at 18% (Siperstein, Parker, & Drascher, 2013). Further, only 13 states report successfully placing at least 60% of individuals utilizing vocational rehabilitation in jobs (Bragdon, 2014). Occupational therapy practitioners are in a unique position to address this issue and support individuals with intellectual disability in shaping their occupational lives as adults and in creating a meaningful work life.

The purpose of this chapter is to empower occupational therapy practitioners who work with this population to provide supports to facilitate the creation of meaningful work lives. This chapter is not an in-depth analysis of employment of adults with intellectual disability. Rather, this chapter will provide an occupational therapy practitioner with a basic understanding of the development of employment services for adults with intellectual disability, current trends, differences between sheltered and supported employment, some barriers to employment for these adults, and how occupational therapy might address work life with a client.

THE HISTORY OF EMPLOYMENT OF ADULTS WITH INTELLECTUAL DISABILITY IN THE UNITED STATES

Employment of adults with intellectual disability has been a recurring challenge in the United States. In the 1960s, family members and advocates for people with disabilities began to organize community-based programs as an alternative to institutionalization (Wysocki & Neulicht, 2004). During this time of limited options, sheltered workshops filled an unmet need by providing an environment where adults with intellectual disability could be safe and occupied during the day, while providing respite for families who chose to care for their loved ones at home instead of in an institution (Dague, 2012). In 1984, the Developmental Disability Act Amendment emphasized employment services for this population as a national priority (Braddock, Rizzolo, & Hemp, 2004). In the 1980s, the movement toward community services and supported employment emerged.

The movement toward community services and community integration of adults with intellectual disability has continued through Employment First, a national movement to promote integrated employment as the priority and preferred outcome of publicly funded services for adults with disabilities, regardless of their level of disability. Employment First is an opportunity to increase the number of adults with intellectual disability who work in integrated settings and to improve the quality of employment experiences for those who are already employed. This effort specifies that employment should pay at least minimum wage and be in integrated settings where most of the workers do not have disabilities (APSE, 2010). The Employment First movement has been adopted by several states; 46 states now have at least some activity toward this end, and 32 states have formal policy action. Tennessee was the first state, in 2003, to have formal policy action in the form of a Statement of Support for Employment First by Tennessee's Division of Mental Retardation Services (APSE, 2015).

APPROACHES TO EMPLOYMENT SERVICES FOR ADULTS WITH INTELLECTUAL DISABILITY

Many adults with intellectual disability who work receive either sheltered or supported employment services. Sheltered employment is most commonly provided in the form of sheltered workshops, which were designed to be both long-term, as well as transitional, placements. Individuals could work in sheltered employment as long as necessary, but the ultimate goal was for individuals to gain the skills necessary for competitive employment and move from the workshops into the community (Wysocki & Neulicht, 2004). The work tasks at these sheltered workshops were and continue to be manual, repetitive work, such as packaging or assembling tasks, contracted by businesses to the sheltered workshop. Employees are often compensated at a piece rate, which is payment for individual work completed given their speed, accuracy, and productivity; piece rate is usually significantly below the minimum wage (Wysocki & Neulicht, 2004).

Sheltered workshops sounded good in theory. Ideally, adults with intellectual disability could work in the sheltered environment for a limited period, gain skills, and go on to work competitively in the community. Unfortunately, this has not been the case. In the mid-1980s, it was determined that a mere 12% of employees at sheltered workshops transitioned to competitive employment each year. Of these individuals who attained competitive employment, only 3% were able to remain in the workforce for longer than 2 years (Bellamy, Rhodes, Bourbeau, & Mank, 1986). One causative factor may have been that the manual and repetitive work opportunities generally offered in sheltered workshops, such as packaging and assembly tasks, do not adequately prepare individuals for competitive employment in dynamic environments with multiple job responsibilities. Another potential reason for such transition failure might be that sheltered workshops are financially incentivized to maintain their client census, as they are paid by the companies who contract work. Financial gains are further increased by paying their employees subminimum wage. Regardless of the reason, sheltered workshops have become a long-term reality and, in turn, have been criticized for promoting the segregation, rather than integration, of adults with intellectual disability (Rusch & Braddock, 2004).

The other type of employment service available to adults with intellectual disability in the United States today is supported employment. Supported employment provides an individual with a disability the support he or she needs to work in the community in small business enterprises, work crews, enclaves within an industry, and individual job placements (Braddock et al., 2004). Supported employment services have increased in popularity since the 1980s. While the percentage of individuals with intellectual disability receiving supported employment services rose, from 9% to 24% between 1988 to 2002, the remaining 76% of this population spent their "work days" in day activity programs, day habilitation programs, or sheltered employment. Despite the value and growth of supported employment, sheltered employment is still the most utilized option (Braddock et al., 2004).

Efforts toward supported employment is beneficial for adults with intellectual disability, in that it is correlated with increased job satisfaction, skills, and interests (Braddock et al., 2004). Adults with intellectual disability working in supported employment, have an increased presence in their communities (Dague, 2012), and their quality of life is greater (Beyer, Brown, Akandi, & Rapley, 2010; Siporin & Lysack, 2004). It is reported that the work in supported employment is more engaging and challenging, provides increased autonomy, and affords more pleasant work environments (Siporin & Lysack, 2004).

BARRIERS TO EMPLOYMENT FOR ADULTS WITH INTELLECTUAL DISABILITY

Despite the benefits of supported and competitive employment, there are barriers to attaining and maintaining the worker role for this population. One such barrier is stigma, or the disapproval of individuals with intellectual disability based on discrimination and judgments made about the members of this population, which cause them to be viewed as less valuable by society. Individuals who are stigmatized face stereotyping and discrimination by other groups (Gormley, 2015). Stigma may be a significant factor leading employers to be hesitant to hire adults with intellectual disability. Stigma is often attributed to a lack of familiarity with intellectual disability, and employers who have experiences interacting with these individuals tend to be more willing to hire them (Duvdevany, Or-Chen, & Fine, 2016).

Another barrier to employment for adults with intellectual disability is a high rate of job separations, including voluntary or forced resignations, such as releasing a person from employment. Job separations have been found to negatively impact quality of life for adults with intellectual disability, with resultant challenges to self-efficacy from job loss and greater risk of boredom (Banks, Jahoda, Dagnan, Kemp, & Williams, 2010). Individuals with intellectual disability have been found to be more likely to separate from jobs than those with other disabilities. Lack of job responsibility and poor social-vocational behavior were the primary reasons cited for job separations (Lagomarcino & Rusch, 1990). There was also a significant relationship between job type and separation; specifically, janitors, maintenance personnel, and food service workers with mild intellectual disability were more likely to separate from these jobs than individuals with other disabilities (Lagomarcino & Rusch, 1990).

The community settings where many people with intellectual disability are employed include office/administration, food service, retail, child and animal care, customer service, manufacturing, and physical labor, such as landscaping or construction (Banks et al., 2010; Siperstein et al., 2013). Many of these work settings afford entry-level jobs with overall higher rates of job turnover (Banks et al., 2010). This serves as a barrier to satisfaction with work for all employees and may especially impact adults with intellectual disability who require more support to be successful in the worker role.

There exists a lack of high-quality, competitive employment options. In the United States, *competitive employment*, defined as independent work in the community that is paid at least the minimum wage, is promoted as the goal for adults with intellectual disability. Unfortunately, of the 18% of adults with intellectual disability engaged in competitive employment, these individuals do not work more than 15 hours per week or receive worker benefits or paid time off. Employees with intellectual disability who had worked in a job for at least 3 years were found to earn higher wages, work more hours, and receive benefits and paid time off at a greater rate (Heyman, Stokes, & Siperstein, 2016). Therefore, the goal for employing adults with intellectual disability should not simply be attaining but sustaining competitive employment.

Policy may also serve as a potential barrier to individuals with intellectual disability in competitive employment. Many adults with intellectual disability receive benefits and income from the federal government in the form of Social Security and/or Supplemental Security Income (SSI). This qualifies them to access health care through Medicare and/or Medicaid and long-term supports, such as residential services. However, Social Security and SSI limits the amount of income an individual can earn before he or she is no longer eligible for benefits, and many individuals will not work or work very few hours to not risk losing their health care and housing support (The Arc, 2015). Initiatives, such as off-setting SSI benefits while continuing Medicare and Medicaid supports, have been implemented in an attempt to address this problem; however, policies still serve as a barrier to many adults with intellectual disability who strive to engage in a fulfilling work life (The Arc, 2015). Additional information specific to policy can be found in Chapter 2.

Another barrier to employment is less self-sufficiency in enacting the worker role. Supported employment ideally provides an employee with intellectual disability with supports to gain the necessary skills and establish a work routine. One such support is that of a job coach, who would work with and support the employee intensively after employment has been attained and who would gradually decrease support as the employee gained independence in his or her worker role. However, research has shown this is not necessarily the case, and job coaches are not consistently reducing their time spent at work sites with supported employees (Cimera, Rusch, & Heal, 1998). Research has also shown that supported employees placed in positions that match their skills and interests require less support from job coaches. The promotion of self-sufficiency in the worker role for adults with intellectual disability is necessary for the long-term, economic viability of publicly funded, supported employment programs (Cimera et al., 1998).

While all adults with intellectual disability experience barriers to attaining and maintaining employment, adults with severe and profound cognitive deficits face even greater challenges. Despite these challenges, these adults have the same occupational needs to participate in productive occupation as part of a satisfying routine. Approximately 25% of people with severe or very severe disabilities in the United States report they are dissatisfied with their lives, compared to around 11% of people without disabilities (Harris Interactive, 2010). For adults with intellectual disability, employment is correlated with increased quality of life. It is imperative to address quality of life by ensuring this population can engage in meaningful work and experience a work life (Jahoda et al., 2008).

Consider the case example of Carol, a woman with profound intellectual disability, blindness, and severe spasticity that limited her range of motion. Carol participated in a developmental training program at the residential facility where she lived. One of her jobs was to crush cans for recycling. The electric can crusher was adapted with a switch that Carol could activate when she was positioned close enough to it. Her developmental training instructor would put the cans into the can crusher and cue her to hit the switch. Although visually impaired, Carol was very motivated by interesting sounds and she received great enjoyment from the can crushing noises. Carol's story is just one example of someone with severe mental and physical limitations benefitting from a work routine with support.

The literature on the work of adults with severe and profound intellectual disability is limited. White and Weiner (2004) found community-based training and least restrictive environments (i.e., students are with non-disabled peers to the greatest extent appropriate for their education) were correlated with young adults attaining employment after a transition program. Mirenda (2014) also found that augmentative and alternative communication was an effective tool to promote individuals with intellectual disability participating in employment. More research must be done to identify interventions to support this population in work.

OCCUPATIONAL THERAPY AND WORK LIFE OF ADULTS WITH INTELLECTUAL DISABILITY

Occupational therapy practitioners can be effective when they address work with their clients who have intellectual disability. The following sections include examples of ways occupational therapy practitioners can address work life using theory, evaluation methods, and varied intervention.

Theory

The profession of occupational therapy utilizes theory to guide its practice. The use of theory enables the practitioner to frame client barriers in terms of occupational performance, identify areas for improvement, and design interventions that are effective, client-centered, and occupational in nature. Similarly, interventions to promote work performance should also be guided by theory. Two theories that might help therapists addressing work life for adults with intellectual disability are occupational adaptation and the Model of Human Occupation (MOHO).

The theory of occupational adaptation describes the integration of two key concepts in occupational therapy: occupation and adaptation. Occupations are the things people need and want to do while adaptation is the way individuals interact with and respond to challenges within their environment. While most theories assume that, as people become more functional they will become more adaptive, this theory assumes that as people become more adaptive their function will increase (Schultz, 2014). The occupational adaptation process results from the interaction between the person and the occupational environment. The individual has an innate desire for mastery, abilities, achievements, and adaptive responses. On the other hand, the occupational environment requires mastery within the physical, social, and cultural contexts, as well as occupational demands placed upon the individual (Schultz, 2014).

One of the criticisms the theory of occupational adaptation has faced is that it is not applicable to individuals with cognitive deficits (Schultz, 2014); however, it actually can be a very useful theory for occupational therapy practitioners addressing work for adults with intellectual disability. Consistent with its proposal that each individual has a desire for mastery and to have an impact on their environment, the occupational adaptation theory implies that this is achieved when individuals create a meaningful work life, as work provides the opportunity to feel productive and contribute to society (Snodgrass & Gupta, 2014). Occupational therapists can support individuals with intellectual disability in the workplace by helping them develop adaptive responses for success in the workplace. Utilizing a visual checklist is one example of an adaptation.

The MOHO presents a very holistic view of the person. Within the person construct, there is a complex interaction among one's volition, habits, routines, roles, and mental and physical performance capacities (Forsyth et al., 2014). It is important for occupational therapy practitioners who work with adults with intellectual disability to consider all these aspects of a person, the impact of the environment, and the occupational demands of the tasks. Further, MOHO conceptualizes occupational engagement as an interaction between one's occupational identity and one's occupational competence (Forsyth et al., 2014). Occupational identity is one's sense of who they have been, are, and wish to become, based on their history of occupational participation. When one's occupational identity and participation match, this leads to high occupational adaptation. In other words, the person is doing the things he or she needs and wants to do and living a meaningful life (Forsyth et al., 2014).

One of the most important roles of adult life is that of worker. Adults who do not work or fill their time with other productive occupations, such as school or volunteering, often experience disruption in their habits and routines. This can negatively impact volition because the individual may not feel as capable as others who are able to work. Occupational therapy practitioners can use the MOHO to articulate why work is such an important occupation to address with adults with intellectual disability. This model is also useful for guiding evaluation and intervention because the therapist will need to assess all the aspects of volition, habituation, and performance capacity, as they all impact how the person will perform at work.

Evaluation Methods

When occupational therapists address work life with adults with intellectual disability, there are several occupational therapy assessments that can be used to identify strengths and barriers to work performance. In keeping with the holistic nature of occupational therapy, it is important to assess the person's habits and routines, values and interests, and performance skills to best support them in the worker role. It is also extremely important to assess the impact of the work environment and task demands, as adaptation of these will be critical to support the success of adults with intellectual disability in the worker role. See assessments in Table 10-1.

Varied Intervention

In the realm of employment services for adults with intellectual disability, vocational rehabilitation professionals, including job coaches, are the primary providers. They are the experts in employment services for this population. Employment for adults with intellectual disability is not a practice area where occupational therapy practitioners are prevalent; however, occupational therapy practitioners possess significant expertise to contribute to employment service teams for adults with intellectual disability in collaboration with vocational rehabilitation professionals. These include the ability to identify matches and mismatches among the person, environment, and occupation; knowledge of adaptive equipment and adaptation strategies; understanding the ways in which habits, routines, and roles intersect with increased independence; and assessments to evaluate occupational performance and competency in the worker role.

The literature demonstrates that when occupational therapy practitioners work as part of employment service teams, they can contribute to the improvement of work performance by identifying strengths and areas of concern, assessing job responsibilities and the work environment, and adapting the work environment and/or job responsibilities to ensure the success of the supported employee in the worker role (Arikawa, Goto, & Mineno, 2013; Dean, Dunn, & Tomcheck, 2015). Occupational therapists can also use their understanding of habits, routines, and roles to facilitate success in aspects of employment, such as job interviews, arriving to work on time, and dressing appropriately (Delahunt, Lowery, & Rudkoski, 2015). Finally, practitioners can add value by assisting with return to work after injury or illness and adapting to this population's ever-changing needs across the life span (AOTA, 2015). In addition to these individual interventions, occupational therapy practitioners can facilitate the employment of adults with intellectual disability by working with potential employers in order to promote employment of people with disabilities (Sabata & Endicott, 2007).

Occupational therapy practitioners can promote employment of adults with intellectual disability even if not directly working with this population. As mentioned previously, one of the major barriers to the population attaining employment is stigma, stemming from a lack of employers who are familiar with individuals with intellectual disability (Gormley, 2015). Therefore, occupational therapy

TABLE 10-1. ASSESSMENTS

ASSESSMENT	AUTHOR	DESCRIPTION
Assessment of Communication and Interaction Skills (ACIS)	Forsyth, Salamy, Simon, & Kielhofner, 1998	The ACIS is an observational assessment that gathers data on communication and interaction skills. Three domains, physicality, information exchange, and relations, are used to describe different aspects of communication and interaction. The ACIS gathers data on skill as it is exhibited during performance in an occupational form and/or within a social group.
Assessment of Motor and Process Skills (AMPS)	Fisher & Jones, 2010	The AMPS is a standardized assessment tool that measures the quality of an individual's occupational performance in a variety of ADL and IADL tasks. The rater scores the effectiveness of the universal motor and process performance skills. This assessment may be applied to work if the work tasks are IADLs (e.g., cleaning bathrooms). Raters must be trained in AMPS administration procedures and calibrated as valid and reliable AMPS raters.
Assessment of Work Performance	Sanqvist, Lee, & Kielhofner, 2010	The Assessment of Work Performance is an observational assessment that provides information about a client's work performance by assessing three skill domains: motor, process, and communication/interaction skills.
Evaluation of Social Interaction (ESI)	Fisher & Griswold, 2015	The ESI is a standardized, highly reliable, and sensitive assessment tool that measures the quality of an individual's social interaction in a natural exchange with typical social partners. The rater scores the effectiveness of the universal social interaction performance skills. This assessment may be applied to work if there are concerns about social participation in the context of work. Raters must be trained in ESI administration procedures and calibrated as valid and reliable ESI raters.
Occupational Self-Assessment (OSA)	Baron, Kielhofner, Iyenger, Goldhammer, & Wolenski, 2006	The OSA is an evaluation tool that allows the client to rate their performance in a variety of occupations and the importance of these occupations. This information can then be used to establishing client-centered occupational therapy goals. This assessment can be modified as a card sort with symbols and words to be more accessible and interactive for clients.

(continued)

efforts to engage in advocacy and promote community integration of individuals with intellectual disability are in service of promoting work opportunities for this population.

Occupational therapy practitioners working in transition services for high school students with intellectual disability are able to be very effective in promoting work as an outcome for students after graduation. As adults with intellectual disability move into adulthood, there is a delicate balance between the need for independence by the young adult with intellectual disability, with the reality of interdependence to support functional performance in daily life. The literature demonstrates the key to finding this balance is planning, to ensure appropriate placement in the services that can maximize the desired independence, such as residential and employment services (Crotty, 2016). Occupational therapy practitioners can contribute significantly to this effort by identifying the strengths and areas of concern for the transitioning students and strategies to maximize students' performance, including but not limited to cues,

TABLE 10-1. ASSESSMENTS (CONTINUED)		
ASSESSMENT	AUTHOR	DESCRIPTION
Vocational Fit Assessment (VFA)	Persch, Gugiu, Onate, & Cleary, 2015	The VFA is a tool that job seekers and employers can use to compare individuals' skills to job demands. The VFA consists of two electronic surveys: the VFA-Worker and VFA-Job. Based on the data from the surveys, job matching reports are generated. Job matching reports identify strengths, needs, pros, cons, and areas for intervention if the job seeker were to pursue a certain job. The reports can be used to guide work placement and job training. For more information and resources, visit www.VocFit.com
Volitional Questionnaire (VQ)	de las Heras, Geist, Kielhofner, & Li, 2007	The VQ is an observational assessment that provides insight into a person's inner motives and information about how the environment affects volition by systematically capturing how a person reacts to and acts within his or her environment. The VQ provides the occupational therapist with insight into a person's inner motives and the effect of the environment on the person's participation in meaningful occupations. This assessment could be used to identify different work tasks and environments that may be more motivating for clients.
Work Environment Impact Scale	Moore-Corner, Kielhofner, & Olson, 1998	The Work Environment Impact Scale is an assessment that allows the client and therapist to identify aspects of the work environment that inhibit or facilitate work performance.
Worker Role Interview	Braveman et al., 2005	The Worker Role Interview is a semi-structured interview to assess the psychosocial and environmental components of the initial rehabilitation assessment process for the injured worker or the worker with a long-term disability and poor or limited work history.

environmental supports, and routines. The literature also demonstrates that job-related social skills, which are necessary for individuals to be successful in the worker role, were inadequately taught in special education (Chu & Zhang, 2015). Occupational therapy practitioners working in the school system, specifically in transition services, can articulate the benefits of teaching job-related social skills in order to promote employment as an outcome for young adults with intellectual disability post-graduation, and help create opportunities for students to practice applying these job-related social skills to daily life.

CONCLUSION

This chapter has defined work as an occupation and its importance to adult life, briefly described the history of employment of adults with intellectual disability in the United States, and explained different approaches to employment services for these adults. This chapter has also outlined some of the major barriers to adults with intellectual disability who want to work, and ways occupational therapy practitioners can support adults with intellectual disability in the creation of a meaningful work life. Although employment services for adults with intellectual disability is not an area where occupational therapy is very prevalent, it is an area where great impact can be made. By supporting adults with intellectual disability in work, several outcomes of occupational therapy services are promoted, including satisfying routine, quality of life, self-efficacy, and participation in the community. It is imperative that occupational therapists working with adults with intellectual disability consider the value of work and support their clients in this productive, meaningful, and integral occupation of adult life.

REFERENCES

American Occupational Therapy Association. (2014). Occupational therapy practice framework: Domain and process, 3rd edition. *American Journal of Occupational Therapy, 68*(Suppl. 1), S1-S48.

American Occupational Therapy Association. (2015), The role of occupational therapy in facilitating employment of individuals with developmental disabilities. Retrieved from https://www.aota.org/media/Corporate/Files/AboutOT/Professionals/WhatIsOT/WI/Facts/Workers%20with%20DD%20fact%20sheet.pdf

Arikawa, M., Goto, H., & Mineno, K. (2013). Job support by occupational therapists for people with developmental disabilities: Two case studies. *Work, 45*(2), 245-251. doi: 10.3233/WOR-131590

The Arc. (2015). National policy matters: Social Security and SSI for people with I/DD and their families. Retrieved from http://www.thearc.org/document.doc?id=5269

Association of People Supporting Employment First. (2010). APSE statement on Employment First. Retrieved from http://apse.org/employment-first/statement/

Association of People Supporting Employment First. (2015). Employment First map. Retrieved from http://www.apse.org/wp-content/uploads/2014/01/activity.html

Banks, P., Jahoda, A., Dagnan, D., Kemp, J., & Williams, V. (2010). Supported employment for people with intellectual disability: The effects of job breakdown on psychological well-being. *Journal of Applied Research in Intellectual Disabilities, 23*, 344-354. doi: 10.1111/j.1468-3148.2009.00541.x

Baron, K., Kielhofner, G., Iyenger, A., Godhammer, V., & Wolenski, J. (2006). *Occupational Self Assessment (OSA)* (V. 2.2). Chicago, IL: MOHO Clearinghouse.

Bellamy, G. T., Rhodes, L. E., Bourbeau, P. E., & Mank, D. M. (1986). Mental retardation services in sheltered workshops and day activity programs: Consumer benefits and policy alternatives. In F. R. Rusch (Ed.), *Competitive employment issues and strategies*. Baltimore, MD: Paul H. Brookes Publishing Company.

Beyer, S., Brown, T., Akandi, R., & Rapley, M. (2010). A comparison of quality of life outcomes for people with intellectual disabilities in supported employment, day services and employment enterprises. *Journal of Applied Research in Intellectual Disabilities, 23*, 290-295. doi: 10.1111/j.1468-3148.2009.00534.x

Braddock, D., Rizzolo, M., & Hemp, R. (2004). Most employment services growth in developmental disabilities during 1988-2002 was in segregated settings. *Mental Retardation, 42*(4), 317-320.

Bragdon, T. (2014). *The case for inclusion*. Washington, D.C.: United Cerebral Palsy.

Braveman, B., Robson, M., Velozo, C., Kielhofner, G., Forsyth, K., & Kerschbaum, J. (2005). *The Worker Role Interview (WRI)* (V. 10.0). Chicago, IL: MOHO Clearinghouse.

Carrasco, R. C., Skees Hermes, S., & Burgos, B. B. (2012). Supported and alternative employment: Developmental disabilities and work. In B. Braveman & J. J. Page (Ed.), *Work: Promoting participation and productivity through occupational therapy* (pp. 118-138). Philadelphia, PA: F. A. Davis Company.

Chu, Y. A., & Zhang, L. C. (2015). Are our special education students ready for work? An investigation of the teaching of job-related social skills in Northern Taiwan. *International Journal of Disability, Development and Education, 62*(6), 628-643. doi: 10.1080/1034912X.2015.1077936

Cimera, R., Rusch, F. R., & Heal, L. W. (1998). Supported employee independence from the presence of job coaches at work sites. *Journal of Vocational Rehabilitation, 10*, 51-63. doi: 10.1016/S1052-2263(97)10020-4

Crotty, G. (2016). People with intellectual disabilities moving into adulthood. *Learning Disability Practice, 19*(5), 32-37.

Dague, B. (2012). Sheltered employment, sheltered lives: Family perspectives of conversion to community-based employment. *Journal of Vocational Rehabilitation, 37*, 1-11. doi: 10.3233/JVR-2012-0595

de las Heras, C. G., Geist, R., Kielhofner, G., & Li, Y. (2007). *Volitional Questionnaire* (V. 4.1). Chicago, IL: MOHO Clearinghouse.

Dean, E., Dunn, W., & Tomchek, S. (2015). Role of occupational therapy in promoting self-determination through consumer directed supports. *Occupational Therapy in Health Care, 29*(1), 86-95. doi: 10.3109/07380577.2014.958887

Delahunt, J. Z., Lowery, L. A., & Rudkoski, T. (2015). Resources and examples of employment for adults with developmental disabilities. *Developmental Disabilities Special Interest Section Quarterly, 38*(3), 1-4.

Duvdevany, I., Or-Chen, K., & Fine, M. (2016). Employers' willingness to hire a person with intellectual disability in light of the regulations for adjusted minimum wages. *Journal of Vocational Rehabilitation, 44*, 33-41. doi: 10.3233/JVR-150778

Fisher, A. G., & Griswold, L. A. (2015). *Evaluation of Social Interaction,* (3rd ed. rev.). Fort Collins, CO: Three Star Press.

Fisher, A. G., & Jones, K. B. (2010). *Assessment of Motor and Process Skill: Development, standardization, and administration Manual* (Vol. 1, 7th ed.), Fort Collins, CO: Three Star Press.

Forsyth, K., Salamy, M., Simon, S., & Kielhofner, G. (1998). *The Assessment of Communication and Interaction Skills (ACIS)* (V. 4). Chicago, IL: University of Illinois.

Forsyth, K., Taylor, R. R., Kramer, J. M., Prior, S., Richie, L., Whitehead, J., ... Melton, J. (2014). The Model of Human Occupation. In B. A. Boyt Schell, G. Gillen, M. E. Scaffa, & E. S. Cohn (Eds.), *Willard & Spackman's occupational therapy* (12th ed., pp. 505-526). Baltimore, MD: Lippincott Williams & Wilkins.

Gormley, M. (2015). Workplace stigma toward employees with intellectual disability: A descriptive study. *Journal of Vocational Rehabilitation, 43,* 249-258. doi: 10.3233/JVR-150773

Harris Interactive. (2010). *The ADA, 20 years later: Kessler Foundation/National Organization on Disability 2010 survey of Americans with disabilities.* New York, NY: Author.

Heyman, M., Stokes, J. E., & Siperstein, G. N. (2016). Not all jobs are the same: Predictors of job quality for adults with intellectual disabilities. *Journal of Vocational Rehabilitation, 44,* 299-306. doi: 10.3233/JVR-160800

Jahoda A., Kemp J., Banks P., & Williams V. (2008) Feelings about work: A review of the socio-emotional impact of supported employment on people with intellectual disabilities. *Journal of Applied Research in Intellectual Disabilities 21,* 1-18. doi: 10.1111/j.1468-3148.2007.00365.x

Lagomarcino, T. R., & Rusch, F. R. (1990). An analysis of the reasons for job separations in relation to disability, placement, job type, and length of employment. In F. R. Rusch (Ed.), *Research in secondary special education and transitional employment.* Retrieved from https://eric.ed.gov/?id=ED331228f

Larson, B. (2014). Evaluation of education and work. In K. Jacobs, N. McRae, & K. Sladky (Ed.), *Occupational therapy essentials for clinical competence* (2nd ed.; pp. 231-240). Thorofare, NJ: SLACK Incorporated.

Mirenda, P. (2014). Revisiting the mosaic of supports required for including people with severe intellectual or developmental disabilities in their communities. *Augmentative and Alternative Communication, 30*(1), 19-27. doi: 10.3109/07434618.2013.875590

Moore-Corner, R., Kielhofner, G., & Olson, L. (1998). *Work Environment Impact Scale (WEIS)* (V. 2.0). Chicago, IL: MOHO Clearinghouse.

Persch, A. C., Gugiu, P. C., Onate, J. A., & Cleary, D. S. (2015). Development and psychometric evaluation of the Vocational Fit Assessment. *American Journal of Occupational Therapy, 69*(6), 6906180080. doi: 10.5014/ajot.2015.019455

Rusch, F. R., & Braddock, D. (2004). Adult day programs versus supported employment (1988-2002): Spending and service practices of intellectual disability and developmental disabilities state agencies. *Research and Practice for Persons with Severe Disabilities, 29*(4), 237-242.

Sabata, D., & Endicott, S. (2007). Workplace changes: Seizing opportunities for persons with disabilities in the workplace. *Work Programs Special Interest Section Quarterly, 21*(2), 1-4.

Sandqvist, J., Lee, J., & Kielhofner, G. (2010). *Assessment of Work Performance (AWP)* (V. 1.0). Chicago, IL: MOHO Clearinghouse.

Schultz, S. W. (2014). Theory of occupational adaptation. In B. A. Boyt Schell, G. Gillen, M. E. Scaffa, & E. S. Cohn (Ed.), *Willard & Spackman's occupational therapy* (12th ed., pp. 527-540). Baltimore, MD: Lippincott Williams & Wilkins.

Sipersterin, G. N., Parker, R. C., & Drascher, M. (2013). National snapshot of adults with intellectual disabilities in the labor force. *Journal of Vocational Rehabilitation, 39,* 157-165. doi: 10.3233/JVR-130658

Siporin, S., & Lysack, C. (2004). Quality of life and supported employment: A case study of three women with developmental disabilities. *American Journal of Occupational Therapy, 58,* 455-465.

Snodgrass, J., & Gupta, J. (2014). Work occupations. In J. Hinojosa & M. Blount (Ed.), *The texture of life* (pp. 318-336). Bethesda, MD: American Occupational Therapy Association.

Stephens, D., Collins, M., & Dodder, R. (2005). A longitudinal study of employment and skill acquisition among individuals with developmental disabilities. *Research in Developmental Disabilities, 26,* 469-486. doi: 10.1016/j.ridd.2003.12.003

White, J., & Weiner, J. S. (2004). Influence of least restrictive environment and community based training on integrated employment outcomes for transitioning students with severe disabilities. *Journal of Vocational Rehabilitation, 21,* 149-156.

Wysocki, D. J., & Neulicht, A. T. (2004). Work is occupation: What can I do as an occupational therapy practitioner? In M. Ross & S. Bachner (Ed.), *Adults with developmental disabilities: Current approaches in occupational therapy* (pp. 291-328). Bethesda, MD: AOTA Press.

11

Leisure Life

Anne F. Kiraly-Alvarez, OTD, OTR/L, SCSS

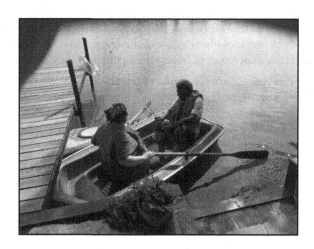

Key Words: leisure, leisure education, leisure exploration, leisure participation, quality of life, self-determination, social participation

Bryze, K.
Occupational Therapy for Adults With Intellectual Disability (pp. 121-136).
© 2020 Taylor & Francis Group.

Many argue that participating in leisure is a fundamental human right (Dattilo, 2013; Dattilo & Schleien, 1994; Yalon-Chamovitz & Weiss, 2008). Therefore, it is essential that occupational therapy practitioners address this occupation when working with adults with intellectual disability. The purpose of this chapter is to highlight the benefits of leisure and the current status of leisure participation for adults with intellectual disability and to emphasize the importance of addressing leisure for this population. Barriers and facilitators of leisure participation for adults with intellectual disability, which have been identified in the literature, are summarized for the purposes of understanding implications for occupational therapy evaluation and intervention. Intervention strategies are also reviewed and case examples are presented to demonstrate how occupational therapy practitioners are presently addressing leisure in practice with adults with intellectual disability.

DEFINING LEISURE

There are many definitions of leisure in the literature, but these definitions often fall into categories of observable activities, quantifiable time, or subjective experiences (MacNeil & Anderson, 1999; Suto, 1998). For example, leisure has been defined as "nonobligatory activity that is intrinsically motivated and engaged in during discretionary time, that is, time not committed to obligatory occupations such as work, self-care, or sleep," (Parham & Fazio [1997] as cited in American Occupational Therapy Association [AOTA], 2014, p. S21). AOTA (2014) further divides the occupation of leisure into *leisure exploration,* which includes identifying interests and appropriate leisure activities, and *leisure participation,* which includes planning for and engaging in leisure activities. However, other authors argue the subjective experience of leisure is more important:

> Rather than conceiving of leisure in terms of time or activity, we may more appropriately view it in relation to an individual's emotional and cognitive response to an activity or experience. Thus, we may conceive of leisure as an emotional condition within an individual that flows from a feeling of well-being and self-satisfaction. This condition is characterized by feelings of mastery, achievement, success, personal worth, and pleasure. (MacNeil & Anderson, 1999, p. 127)

For the purpose of this chapter, the following definition of *leisure* will be used, as it encompasses all three categories of existing definitions:

> … [a]vailable free choice time and the individually selected activities that characteristically are not related to work or to other obligatory forms of activity, and which are expected to promote feelings of pleasure, friendship, happiness, spontaneity, fantasy or imagination, creativity, self-expression and self-development. (Badia, Orgaz, Verdugo, & Ullán, 2013, p. 320)

It is important to note that AOTA (2014) defines social participation as an occupation separate from leisure, although many social participation activities may be defined as leisure in the literature and by clients themselves. Because of this, the following definition of *social participation* is provided:

> "The interweaving of occupations to support desired engagement in community and family activities as well as those involving peers and friends" (Gillen & Boyt Schell, 2014, p. 607); involvement in a subset of activities that involve social situations with others (Bedell, 2012) and that support social interdependence (Magasi & Hammel, 2004). Social participation can occur in person or through remote technologies such as telephone calls, computer interaction, and video conferencing. (AOTA, 2014, p. S21)

Regardless of how leisure is defined in the literature, occupational therapy practitioners working with individuals with intellectual disability need to ensure a client-centered approach by striving to understand how their clients define and experience leisure (Suto, 1998). This understanding should begin with a broader appreciation for the importance of leisure participation for the population of individuals with intellectual disability, as well as an understanding of the current status of participation for this population. These topics are presented in the following sections.

Benefits of Leisure

Leisure participation is important for all individuals but particularly for individuals with intellectual disability. Having leisure activities that are meaningful and purposeful is essential, especially for individuals who may not work full time. Research suggests there are many benefits of leisure, including improved quality of life, social-emotional benefits, and improved skills.

Improved Quality of Life

Much research has investigated the impact of leisure on various quality of life aspects. Although some studies do not find direct correlations between leisure participation and objective measures of quality of life for individuals with intellectual disability (Badia, Orgaz, Verdugo, Ullán, & Martínez, 2013), the literature presents many arguments that individuals with intellectual disability who participate in leisure are more likely to experience enhanced quality of life and life satisfaction (Barret & Clements, 1997; Hawkins, 1997; Salkever, 2000).

Participants with intellectual disability who reported a desire for increasing their participation in leisure activities showed increased levels of material, emotional, and physical well-being (Badia, Orgaz, Verdugo, Ullán, & Martínez, 2013). The benefits of participating in leisure include improved mental and physical health, increased physical activity, experiences of enjoyment, development of self-esteem, and enhanced friendships (Mayer & Anderson, 2014; Specht, King, Brown, & Foris, 2002).

Another important aspect of quality of life is *self-determination*, which is viewed as the "right of a collective group to govern themselves as well as individual control over one's life" (Zakrazsek, Hammel, & Scazzero, 2014, p. 155). Leisure empowers self-determination because intrinsically motivated behaviors, such as participation in leisure, result in feelings of autonomy, which in turn promote the perception of control over one's life (MacNeil & Anderson, 1999). This process of empowering self-determination can be viewed as a very important benefit of leisure.

Social-Emotional Benefits

Although social-emotional factors are encompassed within the concept of quality of life, many benefits of leisure identified in the literature focus on specific social and emotional benefits. Many authors highlight the importance of leisure for individuals with intellectual disability as increasing opportunities to network with peers and build friendships (Barret & Clements, 1997; Dattilo, 1994 as cited in MacNeil & Anderson, 1999; Moisey & van de Keere, 2007; Sutton, 1997). In a study by Mayer and Anderson (2014), participants reported enjoying the social aspects of the recreation programs in which they were involved, as well as increased self-confidence and an appreciation of being people first instead of people with disabilities. Sutton (1997) describes how participating in the community with peers contributes to improved mood and motivation.

Some studies report the social-emotional benefits of specific types of leisure activities. For example, Moisey and van de Keere (2007) noted that participating in online computer activities increases entertainment, decreases boredom, and increases self-esteem. Barret and Clements (1997) identified that involvement in the arts promotes positive attitudes and improves emotional health. Overall, leisure participation provides opportunities for individuals with intellectual disability to interact socially with others, experience positive emotions connected to enjoyment, and develop their confidence and feelings of self-worth.

Skill Development

In addition to the many subjective benefits of leisure related to quality of life and social-emotional factors, the literature has also identified that participation in leisure provides opportunities for individuals with intellectual disability to develop a variety of objective, observable skills. Participation in various leisure activities contributes to the development of adaptive skills (Badia, Orgaz, Verdugo, & Ullán, 2013), social skills, and language skills (Sutton, 1997), and ability to better understand and follow social norms and expectations (Mayer & Anderson, 2014). Another study showed that participation in online recreational activities improves learning of computer-related skills, increases independence with using a computer, and improves cognitive functioning (Moisey & van de Keere, 2007). For adults with intellectual disability who express or demonstrate a need for improved motor, process, and social interaction skills, participation in leisure may be a means through which those improvements can be facilitated.

PRESENT STATUS OF LEISURE PARTICIPATION BY ADULTS WITH INTELLECTUAL DISABILITY

Despite the importance of leisure for adults with intellectual disability, research suggests that leisure participation of these individuals is more limited than that of individuals without disabilities (Boyd, 1997). This decreased participation begins in childhood and adolescence, and children with disabilities, such as Down syndrome or autism, also have fewer friends and fewer opportunities to participate in leisure activities and hobbies (Oates, Bebbington, Bourke, Girdler, & Leonard, 2011; Solish, Perry, & Minnes, 2010). The discrepancies in the status of leisure participation for adults with intellectual disability are well documented in the literature, and can be better understood in terms of the infrequency of participation, the decreased amount and variety of activities, the segregated nature of participation, and the limited ability to choose desired leisure activities. These issues of limited participation occur worldwide, including in Canada (Boucher, Dumas, Maltais, & Richards, 2010); Israel (Azaiza, Croitoru, & Rimmerman, 2012); Netherlands (Zijlstra & Vlaskamp, 2005); Spain (Badia, Orgaz, Verdugo, & Ullán, 2013); Sweden (Hallrup, 2012); Taiwan (Wang, 2013); and the United States (Anderson, 2011).

When adults with intellectual disability participate in leisure activities, they frequently engage in social activities (e.g., hanging out, shopping, eating at restaurants), activities at home (e.g., watching TV, resting, listening to music, talking on the phone) (Badia, Orgaz, Verdugo, & Ullán, 2013). Adults with intellectual disability also engage in physical activities such as swimming, bowling, or basketball, although not as frequently as some of the aforementioned activities (Badia, Orgaz, Verdugo, & Ullán, 2013). Despite this participation, adults with intellectual disability do not participate in leisure activities as frequently as adults without disabilities (Azaiza et al., 2012; Badia, Orgaz, Verdugo, & Ullán, 2013; Van Naarden Braun et al., 2006; Verdonschot, de Witte, Reichrath, Buntinx & Curfs, 2009a; Zijlstra & Vlaskamp, 2005). Additionally, adults with intellectual disability participate in significantly fewer leisure activities than their peers (Van Naarden Braun et al., 2006), and those activities are frequently more passive and solitary in nature (Badia, Orgaz, Verdugo, & Ullán, 2013; Zijlstra & Vlaskamp, 2005). Further, when adults with intellectual disability do participate in leisure activities, their participation is often still occurring in segregated settings, such as special recreation programs or within their residential facilities (Badia, Orgaz, Verdugo, & Ullán, 2013; Mayer & Anderson, 2014; Zijlstra & Vlaskamp, 2005). This limited participation was described in one study as "living everyday life in a restricted area" (Hallrup, 2012, p. 1589). Additionally, adults with intellectual disability frequently have limited choices related to their leisure participation. Oftentimes, family members or staff members make the decisions about the leisure activities in which these adults participate (Anderson, 2011; Badia, Orgaz, Verdugo, & Ullán, 2013; Hallrup, 2012). Other times, adults with intellectual disability make the decisions about participation in activities, but their decisions are based on what is encouraged by their support networks. For example, Mayer and Anderson (2014) found that some adults chose to participate in segregated recreation programs because their family members encouraged it, without knowing about the inclusive recreation programs that were available. Because adults with intellectual disability have limited choices about their leisure participation, the activities in which they participate often do not reflect their personal interests (Badia, Orgaz, Verdugo, & Ullán, 2013). Zijlstra and Vlaskamp (2005) describe the result of this issue, "leisure time consists, to a larger degree, of killing time instead of enjoying 'quality time'" (p. 446).

OCCUPATIONAL THERAPY TO SUPPORT LEISURE PARTICIPATION

Presently, fewer occupational therapy practitioners provide services to adults with intellectual disability compared to those who work in other practice settings, such as schools or hospitals. The practitioners who are employed in settings that serve adults with intellectual disability do not often address leisure because of the need to address more urgent needs, such as activities of daily living. In one study by Anderson (2011), less than half of the facilities serving adults with intellectual disability reported their residents receiving occupational therapy services. Of those facilities, it was reported that services focused on eating/feeding, wheelchair fitting, transportation, and self-care (Anderson, 2011). Because leisure participation is so important to the quality of life for individuals with intellectual disability, and because their participation is so limited, occupational therapy practitioners can and should be addressing leisure exploration and participation. These areas can be addressed through both evaluation and intervention.

Occupational Therapy Evaluation of Leisure

In an initial evaluation, it is important to gather information about leisure as part of the client's occupational profile (AOTA, 2014). This may include current types of leisure activities in which the individual participates; what participation looks like for the individual; the frequency of participation in those activities; the reasons behind the person's participation in those activities; how the person chooses those activities; with whom he or she participates; where participation takes place; in which activities the individual participated in the past; activities in which he or she has never participated, but would like to in the future; and any perceived barriers to past, present, or future leisure participation. Occupational therapy practitioners can gather this information from the individuals themselves or from family members, friends, or other professionals who know the individual well. Some of this information may also be gathered during a more formal assessment of occupational performance (AOTA, 2014), which can be done through interviews, observations of performance, and the use of assessment tools.

Dean, Dunn, and Tomchek (2015) argue that occupational therapy practitioners can contribute to consumer-directed services that facilitate the development of self-determination in individuals with developmental disabilities by utilizing strength-based assessment tools. There are many assessment tools that can be used to assess leisure participation. Some of these tools assess leisure participation more directly by focusing on specific aspects of leisure or by referring to specific leisure activities. Other tools provide information indirectly by looking more globally at occupational performance or by investigating underlying skills and abilities that could impact engagement in leisure. Table 11-1 provides a description of some of these available assessments. Throughout the evaluation process, it is important for occupational therapy practitioners to identify the various barriers and facilitators to leisure participation.

TABLE 11-1. SELECTION OF ASSESSMENT TOOLS
FOR EVALUATION OF LEISURE PARTICIPATION

ASSESSMENT TOOL	DESCRIPTION/APPLICABILITY TO ASSESSMENT OF LEISURE FOR ADULTS WITH INTELLECTUAL DISABILITY
Activity Card Sort (Baum & Edwards, 2008)	This interview-based tool measures a client's participation in occupations, including leisure and social activities.
Assessment of Motor and Process Skills (Fisher & Jones, 2010) and Evaluation of Social Interaction (Fisher & Griswold, 2015)	These occupation-based observational tools assess the quality of a client's occupational performance and can be used to identify strengths and challenges that could impact leisure participation.
Canadian Occupational Performance Measure (Law et al., 2005)	This client-centered interview-based tool is an outcome measure of a client's perceptions of his or her occupational performance, which can give insight into an adult's perceptions of his or her leisure participation.
Interest Checklist UK (Heasman & Brewer, 2008)	This tool identifies a client's leisure interests and engagement in the past, present, and future. An adapted, easy read version is also available.
Leisure Assessment Inventory (Hawkins, Ardovino, Rogers, Foose, & Olsen, 2002)	Originally developed for use with adults with intellectual and developmental disabilities, this tool helps to identify the leisure activities in which an individual engages, preferences for leisure, the degree of unmet leisure participation, and constraints to leisure participation.
Leisure Diagnostic Battery (Ellis, Widmer, & Witt, 2008)	This self-report tool measures "perceived freedom in leisure," as well as preferences and barriers to participation in recreation, and can be used with adults with intellectual and developmental disabilities.
Occupational Performance History Interview-II (Kielhofner et al., 2004)	This interview-based tool identifies a client's daily life roles, routines, and environments where occupations are performed, and can provide information on an adult's leisure and social participation.
Supports Intensity Scale (Thompson et al., 2004)	This strengths-based tool helps to identify available and needed supports for adults with intellectual and developmental disabilities to participate in several areas of daily life, including community recreation and social participation.
Volitional Questionnaire (de las Heras, Geist, Kielhofner, & Li, 2007)	This observational tool assesses a client's motivation to participate in occupations in his or her environment and can be used to determine an adult's volition related to leisure. This tool is helpful if an adult has limited verbal or cognitive abilities that could hinder the administration of an interview or self-report tool.

Identification of Barriers to Leisure Participation

Researchers have identified several common barriers to leisure participation for adults with intellectual disability. These barriers include external factors related to physical or social environments and internal factors related to various personal demographics and experiences. Occupational therapy practitioners should be aware of these potential barriers during an evaluation of a client's leisure participation.

Barriers Within the Physical Environment

Many aspects of the physical environment may present as barriers to leisure exploration and leisure participation for adults with intellectual disability. Announcements of leisure opportunities or instructions for how to use leisure materials may not be made available in formats that match the individuals' reading levels. Often, leisure opportunities are offered in locations that are physically inaccessible (Boucher et al., 2010; MacNeil & Anderson, 1999), which could prevent attendance by adults with intellectual disability who have accompanying physical disabilities. Because many adults with intellectual disability are unable to drive or use public transportation independently, the lack of transportation is another issue that impacts leisure participation (MacNeil & Anderson, 1999; Verdonschot, de Witte, Reichrath, Buntinx, & Curfs, 2009b). An individual's presence in a day center or residence for adults with intellectual disability may limit access to leisure because of decreased leisure offerings at those facilities (Badia, Orgaz, Verdugo, & Ullán, 2013). Additionally, the high costs of some leisure activities (Azaiza, Croitoru, & Rimmerman, 2012) or the lack of access to resources or leisure materials (Moisey & van de Keere, 2007) pose additional barriers to leisure participation. Finally, the lack of accommodations and structure in inclusive recreation programs may prevent some adults from participating in certain leisure activities (Mayer & Anderson, 2014). When evaluating leisure participation, it will be important for occupational therapy practitioners to identify all the objects and physical spaces, or lack thereof, that may be barriers to leisure participation.

Barriers Within the Social Environment

Barriers within the social environment often impact leisure participation more than barriers within the physical environment. Negative, biased, or exclusionary attitudes of staff, caregivers, community members, or even the perceptions of such attitudes, have the potential for limiting the participation in leisure for adults with intellectual disability (Badia, Orgaz, Verdugo, & Ullán, 2013; Hallrup, 2012; Moisey & van de Keere, 2007; Verdonschot et al., 2009b). Oftentimes, adults with intellectual disability are dependent on others' decisions to carry out activities. So, if those others do not follow through on those decisions, their participation could be limited (Badia, Orgaz, Verdugo, Ullán, & Martinez, 2011).

The presence or absence of others may also impact leisure participation. For example, Wang (2013) identified that adults who did not have a spouse or a partner were more likely to be socially excluded, which could result in less leisure participation. Hallrup (2012) found that adults living in institutional care settings participated less in leisure because staff members directed routines and put restrictions in place that limited the opportunities for residents to choose their own activities. The presence of accompanying services such as aides were reported as a barrier for participants with highly restricted levels of participation, perhaps because the services were insufficient to meet their needs (Boucher et al., 2010). Given some adults' difficulty with speech or clear communication, communication barriers may also impede leisure participation (MacNeil & Anderson, 1999). Mayer and Anderson (2014) also identified several social barriers to leisure: the lack of social supports to participate in inclusive recreation programs, the support networks only recommending segregated programs in which to participate, and the exclusive nature of segregated recreation programs limiting the ability of participants to interact with friends or family members without disabilities during those activities. While completing an evaluation, occupational therapy practitioners must take into consideration all social factors that could impede leisure participation.

Personal Factors Impacting Leisure Participation

In addition to these external barriers to leisure participation, researchers have identified some personal risk factors or determinants of decreased leisure participation, including age, education, personal thoughts or feelings, and type of disability or degree of functional limitations. Many studies that investigated the relationship between age and leisure participation have concluded that as individuals with intellectual disability age, their leisure participation decreases and they participate in a fewer number and less variety of activities (Amado, Stancliffe, McCarron, & McCallion, 2013; Badia,

Orgaz, Verdugo, & Ullán, 2013; Boucher, Dumas et al., 2010; Zijlstra & Vlaskamp, 2005). It is important to note that many authors have defined older age for this population as younger than what is typically considered older age for the general population. For example, Zijlstra and Vlaskamp (2005) identified that individuals with intellectual disability aged 38 years and over experienced decreased leisure participation compared to younger individuals with intellectual disability. Boyd (1997) explains this decreased involvement in leisure for older adults with intellectual disability is often connected to age-related changes in physical and psychosocial functional skills.

Several studies have also identified that educational experiences, or lack thereof, result in decreased leisure participation for adults with intellectual disability. For example, Badia, Orgaz, Verdugo, and Ullán, (2013) found that individuals who participated in special vs. general education schooling experienced decreased participation. Wang (2013) found that decreased educational levels resulted in an increased risk of social exclusion. A lack of knowledge and skills, specifically due to a lack of pre-retirement education (Sutton, 1997) or leisure education (MacNeil & Anderson, 1999), has also been linked to decreased leisure participation.

Personal thoughts, feelings, and experiences of adults with intellectual disability can also impact their leisure participation. Participants in one study reported decreased participation in leisure activities at home and socially in the community due to a perception of not enough time to participate in these activities (Badia et al., 2011). They also expressed being tired, afraid of being mocked, and feeling incapable, which impacted their participation (Badia et al., 2011).

The type or degree of disability may also impact leisure participation. While some studies have found no difference in levels of leisure participation by individuals with differing levels of intellectual disability (Badia et al., 2011; Foley, Dyke, Bourke, & Leonard, 2012), other studies have found that individuals with more severe disability or decreased functional ability levels do experience increased social exclusion and decreased leisure participation (Amado et al., 2013; Boucher et al., 2010; Oates et al., 2011; Van Naarden Braun, Yeargin-Allsopp, & Lollar, 2006; Wang, 2013).

Even though these external and internal factors are common barriers to leisure participation for individuals with intellectual disability, they may not be prohibitive for all individuals. It is important for occupational therapy practitioners to remember to consider all factors impacting leisure participation for their individual clients. Using the evaluation process to identify the specific barriers in each individual situation is essential.

Identification of Supports to Leisure Participation

In addition to identifying barriers and deficits, occupational therapy practitioners must identify supports for leisure participation. Some of the most commonly identified facilitators or supports for leisure participation include social and environmental supports.

Social Supports

In the literature, one of the most frequently identified facilitators of leisure participation for adults with intellectual disability is the provision or availability of social support. Many studies found that the adults who have greater levels of support from family, peers, or staff members experience increased participation in leisure activities (Amado et al., 2013; Badia et al., 2011; Badia, Orgaz, Verdugo, & Ullán, 2013; Boucher et al., 2010; Peterson et al., 2008; Sutton, 1997; Verdonschot et al., 2009b). The inclusive nature of religious institutions (Van Naarden Braun et al., 2006), positive staff attitudes (Verdonschot et al., 2009b), and participation in employment (Azaiza, Croitoru, & Rimmerman, 2012) are additional social factors that have been found to increase leisure participation and community integration. Authors have concluded that the promotion of friendships and the provision of social supports can help facilitate leisure participation and reduce social exclusion (Dattilo, 2013; Wang, 2013).

The availability of social supports is important for ensuring active engagement in activities and not just physical presence (Mahoney, Roberts, Bryze, & Parker Kent, 2016). Social supports can also help empower individuals to live self-determined lives (Badia et al., 2011). During an evaluation, occupational therapy practitioners must identify whether adults with intellectual disability have access to friends, family, and staff members to support them in their leisure and participation. If so, they also need to identify if the adults with intellectual disability have opportunities to express their preferences and to make their own choices regarding leisure. Practitioners should investigate the extent to which adults with intellectual disability make decisions about the types of activities in which they participate, the locations of those activities, and the other people with whom they engage. Occupational therapy practitioners must also identify if existing social supports are sufficient for promoting their leisure participation or if additional supports are needed.

Physical Environmental Supports

Access to certain environmental factors and the availability of leisure opportunities have also been identified as facilitators to leisure participation for adults with intellectual disability. Verdonschot et al. (2009b) summarized the variety and stimulation within the environment of facilities, as well as smaller residential facilities, have been identified as supports to leisure participation. Environmental accommodations and modifications (MacNeil & Anderson, 1999; Specht et al., 2002), availability of accessible and affordable transportation (Boucher et al., 2010; MacNeil & Anderson, 1999), and assistive technology (Boucher et al., 2010; Dattilo, 2013; Moisey & van de Keere, 2007; Verdonschot, et al., 2009b) are additional factors that can support leisure participation. Verdonschot et al. (2009b) identified that increased opportunities for adults with intellectual disability to make choices, to be autonomous, and to be involved in policy making led to increased leisure participation. Additional environmental supports include offering a variety of options (Haertl, 2014) and using activities that are attractive, reinforcing, and valuable for individuals with intellectual and developmental disabilities (Lotan, Yalon-Chamovitz, & Weiss, 2011).

During an evaluation, occupational therapy practitioners need to identify the environmental supports that are already in place to support leisure participation and determine if additional supports are necessary. As experts in assessing accessibility, occupational therapy practitioners can identify aspects of both the physical and social environments, which facilitate or inhibit participation. Occupational therapy practitioners can also use their activity analysis skills to determine if the activities that are available to the individuals match their interests, values, and abilities.

Occupational Therapy Intervention to Support Leisure Participation

Following a comprehensive evaluation, occupational therapy practitioners can plan and implement a variety of interventions to facilitate the leisure participation of adults with intellectual disability. The goal of enhanced leisure participation can be achieved through both the increase of supports and the reduction of barriers. Peterson et al. (2008) suggest that interventions designed to increase self-efficacy and social supports have the potential to positively impact leisure participation. Many interventions that have been identified in the literature include advocacy, education, and provision of supports during leisure engagement. While it is important to note that occupational therapy practitioners are not the only professionals qualified to address the leisure needs of adults with intellectual disability, there are unique contributions they can make as part of a collaborative team in both traditional and nontraditional settings. These contributions are highlighted next. The case examples at the end of this section describe how occupational therapists use some of these interventions to address leisure with adults with intellectual disability in different settings.

Advocacy

Badia et al. (2011) found that individuals with intellectual disability who did not need to depend on others' decisions in order to participate reported increased leisure participation. Because of these and similar findings, many authors have identified the importance of promoting self-determination in order to increase participation in leisure (Dattilo, 2013; MacNeil & Anderson, 1999). Occupational therapy practitioners can promote self-determination by advocating for opportunities for adults with intellectual disability to choose leisure activities in which to participate, as well as make decisions about other details of their participation, such as timing, social partners, and location. In a study that focused on identifying factors that contribute to successful individualized residential supports, Cocks and Boaden (2011) highlighted that leadership was important: "At least one person with a clear vision or strong ideas is needed to shape the picture of a desirable living arrangement and lifestyle for the person [with disabilities]" (p. 726). An occupational therapy practitioner could be this one person to take the lead and advocate for the needs and wants of their client.

In addition to advocating for individuals, occupational therapy practitioners can contribute to larger advocacy efforts. For example, Moisey and van de Keere (2007) identified the importance of advocating for accessibility of the physical and virtual environments to promote participation in computer-based leisure activities. Haveman, Tillmann, Stöppler, Kvas, and Monninger (2013) and Wang (2013) highlighted the benefits of advocating for policy changes that promote inclusion for all individuals with intellectual disability. Through advocacy, occupational therapy practitioners can help promote leisure exploration and participation for their clients at the individual, group, or population level.

Education

As many adults with intellectual disability lack knowledge of available leisure opportunities, or lack the skills necessary to participate in some leisure activities, many authors propose leisure education as a support to overcome those barriers (Dattilo, 2013; Hoge & Wilhite, 1997; MacNeil & Anderson, 1999; Wang, 2013). Leisure education is defined as "the use of educational strategies to enhance a person's leisure lifestyle; it is designed to develop awareness of recreation activities and resources and for acquiring skills needed for participating in leisure pursuits throughout the life span" (Dattilo, 2012, p. 267). Occupational therapy practitioners can provide this leisure education for their clients by helping them to explore their needs, interests, and abilities related to leisure, to increase their awareness of leisure activities throughout the community, and to learn the skills needed to participate in their desired leisure activities.

In addition to providing education and training to adults with intellectual disability, many authors have also recommended caregiver and staff training to promote leisure participation (Barret & Clements, 1997; Boyd, 1997; Haertl, 2014; Wang, 2013). One study found that a training workshop for staff members to support self-determination of individuals with intellectual disability to increase their community participation increased their confidence in providing those supports (Zakrazsek et al., 2014). Another study found that staff education and policy changes led to increased community presence, participation, integration, inclusion, and increased community-based transitions for individuals with intellectual disability (Thorn, Pittman, Myers, & Slaughter, 2009). Hoge and Wilhite (1997) describe an eight-step process of recreation integration, of which one step involves creating staff awareness and understanding. Occupational therapy practitioners can contribute to this by educating caregivers or staff members on how to provide a variety of activities that match with individuals' interests and abilities and on how to grade or adapt those activities to maximize participation.

Facilitating Leisure Participation Through Coaching, Training, or Adaptations and Modifications

Many studies have investigated various leisure interventions, which involve coaching/prompting, provision of environmental adaptations or modifications or skills training. Table 11-2 provides a summary of the findings from these studies. Based on these outcomes and other recommendations in the literature, there are many implications for occupational therapy practitioners. Most importantly, occupational therapy practitioners can make sure that adults with intellectual disability engage in leisure exploration and leisure participation. During engagement in leisure activities, occupational therapy practitioners can facilitate participation through prompting or training on discrete skills. They can also utilize various evidence-based interventions, such as video-modeling or visual schedules, to promote participation. Dean, Dunn, and Tomchek (2015) describe that coaching

TABLE 11-2. STUDIES ON LEISURE INTERVENTIONS

STUDY	MAJOR FINDINGS
Cannella-Malone et al., 2016	This study found that video prompting was effective for teaching students with significant disabilities how to participate in various leisure activities, including playing games, playing with toys, or doing crafts.
Chan, Lambdin, Graham, Fragale, & Davis, 2014	This study found that an intervention using a picture-based activity schedule was effective for teaching adults with intellectual disability how to play a game on an electronic device.
Dollar, Fredrick, Alberto, & Luke, 2012	This study found that simultaneous prompting was effective for teaching leisure skills (e.g., operating an iPod [Apple], CD player, and DVD player) to adults with severe intellectual disability in their home environments.
Haveman, Tillmann, Stoppler, Kvas, & Monninger, 2013	This study found that a community mobility intervention that included the targeting of individual skills, adaptations to social and physical environments, and policy changes resulted in a significant increase of individuals with intellectual disability using public transportation (i.e., buses) to access leisure activities.
Kagohara et al., 2013	This systematic review identified evidence that video modeling can be used to teach individuals with intellectual disability how to use iPods for leisure activities, such as watching movies, listening to music, or looking at pictures.
Koyama & Wang, 2011	This literature review found that activity schedules can promote independent performance of recreational activities by adults with intellectual disability living in group homes.

(continued)

interventions in context can help promote self-determination of people with intellectual disability. While providing these coaching interventions, occupational therapy practitioners can identify the most appropriate supports and educate other staff members and caregivers on how to implement those supports on a consistent basis to ensure optimal leisure participation for their clients. Occupational therapy practitioners can also implement a variety of environmental modifications, changes in methods of performing activities, and other strategies to support a client's participation in leisure activities.

TABLE 11-2. STUDIES ON LEISURE INTERVENTIONS (CONTINUED)	
STUDY	**MAJOR FINDINGS**
Lotan, Yalon-Chamovitz, & Weiss, 2011	This study found that a virtual reality–based intervention delivered by caregivers who were initially trained by an occupational therapist was effective for promoting activity participation by all adults with mild to moderate intellectual disability and most adults with severe intellectual disability.
Moisey & van de Keere, 2007	This study found that the direct training in information and communication technology increased the recreational opportunities on computers for individuals with intellectual disability.
Tanner, Hand, O'Toole, & Lane, 2015	This systematic review identified moderate to strong evidence of effectiveness of group-based social skills training, activity-based interventions, and computer-based interventions (e.g., virtual reality, video modeling) to improve social skills and moderate evidence of effectiveness of recess interventions, leisure groups, and social stories to improve leisure participation for children and adults with autism spectrum disorder.
Wilson, Reid, & Green, 2006	This study found that direct service staff providing repeated choices of leisure activity and initial prompting if necessary contributed to increased leisure involvement for adults with disabilities in supported independent living.
Yalon-Chamovitz & Weiss, 2008	This study found that adults with intellectual disability and physical disabilities who participate in virtual reality interventions reported feelings of enjoyment and success.

CASE EXAMPLES

Traditional Setting

Betty, MS, OTR/L and Eric, MSOT, OTR/L are employed as occupational therapists at several day habilitation centers through an agency that provides a variety of services and programming for individuals with disabilities. They primarily provide collaborative and consultative services through educating direct care staff members and suggesting strategies to increase participation and improve progress toward the clients' goals. While most client goals are related to activities of daily living and instrumental activities of daily living, some clients have goals to increase their leisure participation by participating in activities, such as walking on a treadmill or using a computer or iPad (Apple) for recreation.

The day centers offer a variety of programs that encourage leisure exploration and participation, including arts and crafts groups, cooking groups, exercise groups, and community outings to volunteer at community organizations, like a YMCA or local library. Betty and Eric often intervene by providing assistive technology or recommending other adaptations or modifications to improve client access to these types of programs and activities. For example, they provide switches to clients so they can control radios or kitchen appliances and they help to develop picture recipes for cooking groups. They also work with staff members on planning activities that incorporate the interests of the clients and that are graded appropriately to meet the needs of all participants. Additionally, they provide agency-wide in-services to educate staff on a variety of topics. One series of in-services focused on activity engagement, during which they focused on teaching strategies for choosing and adapting activities to increase engagement in enjoyable activities and to decrease the amount of down time clients experience. Overall, the occupational therapy services provided by Betty and Eric result in improved functioning and increased participation in leisure activities for the adults with intellectual disability they serve.

Nontraditional Setting

Barbara, MHS, OTR/L is an occupational therapist who works as a program director at a YMCA. The particular YMCA that she works for embraces an inclusive philosophy aimed at making all spaces and programs accessible to any member, regardless of age, ability, or financial status. One of Barbara's responsibilities is to establish programs to meet the needs of members with disabilities. While she also plans programs for children, Barbara collaborates with the adult members of the YMCA who have intellectual disability to ensure she meets their needs and interests. For example, she has established a variety of group classes and activities that are open to all members, but provide extra support for adults with disabilities, including a music therapy group, video game club, healthy living classes, fitness club, and monthly Friday evening social activities. In addition to developing these programs, Barbara trains the YMCA staff members who run the groups and activities to ensure they have the skills they need to best support the participants with disabilities. Another responsibility that she has taken on involves reaching out to residents of local group homes that serve adults with intellectual disability. She educates them on the opportunities to participate at the YMCA and assists them with obtaining memberships. She also encourages members to participate in all the other YMCA classes and programs, such as craft groups and water aerobics classes.

As a result of Barbara's efforts, adults with intellectual disability who are members at the YMCA experience an increased sense of community. Other members without disabilities are more accepting of members with intellectual disability and are less judgmental of some of the behaviors that they may sometimes exhibit. An employee at the YMCA, who is an adult with intellectual disability, reports that he has made good friends by being a member, and he enjoys working out with his friends after work. Another member with intellectual disability reports that a benefit of participating in programs at the YMCA is that he is healthier; he has lost weight and feels stronger since becoming a member. The mother of one of the members with intellectual disability reports that she has noticed that her son has greatly benefitted socially by participating in activities at the YMCA. She reports that he has made growth in initiating social interactions with others and has more opportunities to interact with others, especially others without disabilities. All of these personal accounts highlight the importance of inclusive recreation opportunities and the provision of appropriate supports for adults with intellectual disability, as well as how an occupational therapy practitioner can be vital to these efforts.

CONCLUSION

Because leisure occupations fall within the scope of occupational therapy, practitioners are in a unique role to be able to address the leisure needs of adults with intellectual disability. Through evaluation and intervention, occupational therapy practitioners can make significant contributions to enhancing leisure participation in a variety of community settings. They can help to decrease barriers or minimize the impact of barriers and to increase availability of supports and accessibility of activities. Practitioners can advocate, educate, and promote engagement in leisure activities for adults with a variety of interests and abilities. By promoting leisure participation for adults with intellectual disability, they can help to ensure that their clients will experience optimal quality of life.

References

Amado, A. N., Stancliffe, R. J., McCarron, M., & McCallion, P. (2013). Social inclusion and community participation of individuals with intellectual/developmental disabilities. *Intellectual and Developmental Disabilities, 51*(5), 360-375. doi: 10.1352/1934-9556-51.5.360

American Occupational Therapy Association. (2014). Occupational therapy practice framework: Domain and process, 3rd edition. *American Journal of Occupational Therapy, 68*(Suppl. 1), S1-S48.

Anderson, J. (2011). *Current trends in occupational therapy services for adults with developmental disabilities in small community living settings,* master's thesis, University of Puget Sound. Retrieved from http://soundideas.pugetsound.edu/ms_occ_therapy/13/

Azaiza, F., Croitoru, T., & Rimmerman, A. (2012). Participation in leisure activities of Jewish and Arab adults with intellectual disabilities living in the community. *Journal of Leisure Research, 44,* 379-391.

Badia, M., Orgaz, B. M., Verdugo, M. Á., & Ullán A. M. (2013). Patterns and determinants of leisure participation of youth and adults with developmental disabilities. *Journal of Intellectual Disability Research, 57,* 319-332. doi: 10.1111/j.1365-2788.2012.01539.x

Badia, M., Orgaz, M. B., Verdugo, M. Á., Ullán, A. M., & Martínez, M. (2013). Relationships between leisure participation and quality of life of people with developmental disabilities. *Journal of Applied Research in Intellectual Disabilities, 26,* 533-545. doi: 10.1111/jar.12052

Badia, M., Orgaz, B. M., Verdugo, M. Á., Ullán, A. M., & Martinez, M. M. (2011). Personal factors and perceived barriers to participate in leisure activities for young and adults with developmental disabilities. *Research in Developmental Disabilities, 32,* 2055-2063. doi: 10.1016/j.ridd.2011.08.007

Barret, D. B., & Clements, C. B. (1997). Expressive arts programming for older adults both with and without disabilities: An opportunity for inclusion. In T. Tedrick (Ed.), *Older adults with developmental disabilities and leisure: Issues, policy, and practice* (pp. 53-64). New York, NY: Haworth Press, Inc.

Baum, C. M., & Edwards, D. F. (2008). *Activity Card Sort* (2nd ed.). Bethesda, MD: AOTA Press.

Boucher, N., Dumas, F., Maltais, D. B., & Richards, C. L. (2010). The influence of selected personal and environmental factors on leisure activities in adults with cerebral palsy. *Disability and Rehabilitation, 32,* 1328-1338. doi: 10.3109/09638280903514713

Boyd, R. (1997). Older adults with developmental disabilities: A brief examination of current knowledge. In T. Tedrick (Ed.), *Older adults with developmental disabilities and leisure: Issues, policy, and practice* (pp. 7-28). New York, NY: Haworth Press, Inc.

Cannella-Malone, H. I., Miller, O., Schaefer, J. M., Jimenez, E. D., Page, E. J., & Sabielny, H. (2016). Using video promoting to teach leisure skills to students with significant disabilities. *Exceptional Children, 82,* 463-478. doi: 10.1177/0014402915598778

Chan, J. M., Lambdin, L., Graham, K., Fragale, C., & Davis, T. (2014). A picture-based activity schedule intervention to teach adults with mild intellectual disability to use an iPad during a leisure activity. *Journal of Behavioral Education, 23,* 247-257. doi: 10.1007/s10864-014-9194-8

Cocks, E., & Boaden, R. (2011). A quality framework for personalised residential support for adults with developmental disabilities. *Journal for Intellectual Disability Research, 55,* 720-731. doi: 10.1111/j.1365-2788.2010.01296.x

Dattilo, J. (2012). *Inclusive leisure services* (3rd ed.). State College, PA: Venture Publishing, Inc.

Dattilo, J. (2013). Inclusive leisure and individuals with intellectual disability. *Inclusion, 1*(1), 76-88. doi: 10.1352/2326-6988-1.1.076

Dattilo, J., & Schleien, S. J. (1994). Understanding leisure services for individuals with mental retardation. *Mental Retardation, 32*(1), 53-59.

de las Heras, C. G., Geist, R., Kielhofner, G., & Li, Y. (2007). *A user's manual for the Volitional Questionnaire (VQ)* (V. 4.1). Chicago, IL: MOHO Clearinghouse.

Dean, E. E., Dunn, W., & Tomchek, S. (2015). Role of occupational therapy in promoting self-determination through consumer-directed supports. *Occupational Therapy in Health Care, 29,* 86-95. doi: 10.3109/07380577.2014.958887

Dollar, C. A., Fredrick, L. D., Alberto, P. A., & Luke, J. K. (2012). Using simultaneous prompting to teach independent living and leisure skills to adults with severe intellectual disabilities. *Research in Developmental Disabilities, 33,* 189-195. doi: 10.1016/j.ridd.2011.09.001

Ellis, G. D., Widmer, M. A., & Witt, P. A. (2008). *Leisure diagnostic battery.* State College, PA: Venture Publishing, Inc.

Fisher, A. G., & Griswold, L. A. (2015). *Evaluation of Social Interaction* (3rd ed. rev.). Fort Collins, CO: Three Star Press.

Fisher, A. G., & Jones, K. B. (2010). *Assessment of Motor and Process Skills: Development, standardization, and administration manual* (Vol. 1, 7th ed.). Fort Collins, CO: Three Star Press.

Foley, K-R., Dyke, P., Bourke, J., & Leonard, H. (2012). Young adults with intellectual disability transitioning from school to post-school: A literature review framed within the ICF. *Disability and Rehabilitation, 34,* 1747-1764. doi: 10.3109/09638288.2012.660603

Haertl, K. (2014). Play, leisure, ADLs, and IADLs for adults with intellectual and developmental disabilities. In K. Haertl (Ed.), *Adults with intellectual and developmental disabilities: Strategies for occupational therapy* (pp. 265-284). Bethesda, MD: American Occupational Therapy Association.

Hallrup, L. B. (2012). The meaning of the lived experience of adults with intellectual disabilities in a Swedish institutional care setting: A reflective lifeworld approach. *Journal of Clinical Nursing, 23*, 1583-1592. doi: 10.1111/j.1365-2702.2012.04208.x

Haveman, M., Tillmann, V., Stöppler, R., Kvas, Š., & Monninger, D. (2013). Mobility and public transport use abilities of children and young adults with intellectual disabilities: Results from the 3-year Nordhorn public transportation intervention study. *Journal of Policy and Practice in Intellectual Disabilities, 10*, 289–299. doi: 10.1111/jppi.12059.

Hawkins, B. A. (1997). Health, fitness, and quality of life for older adults with developmental disabilities. In T. Tedrick (Ed.), *Older adults with developmental disabilities and leisure: Issues, policy, and practice* (pp. 29-36). New York, NY: Haworth Press, Inc.

Hawkins, B. A., Ardovino, P., Rogers, N. B., Foose, A., & Olsen, N. (2002). *Leisure assessment inventory*. Ravensdale, WA: Idyll Arbor.

Heasman, D., & Brewer, P. (2008). *Interest Checklist UK* (V. 6.1). London, United Kingdom: South West London and St. George's NHS Trust—Occupational Therapy Service.

Hoge, G., & Wilhite, B. (1997). Integration and leisure education for older adults with developmental disabilities. In T. Tedrick (Ed.), *Older adults with developmental disabilities and leisure: Issues, policy, and practice* (pp. 79-90). New York, NY: Haworth Press, Inc.

Kagohara, D. M., van der Meer, L., Ramdoss, S., O'Reilly, M., Lancioni, G. E., Davis, T. N., ... Sigafoos, J. (2013). Using iPods and iPads in teaching programs for individuals with developmental disabilities: A systematic review. *Research in Developmental Disabilities, 34*, 147-156. doi: 10. 1016/j.ridd.2012.07.027

Kielhofner, G., Mallinson, T., Crawford, C., Nowak, M., Rigby, M., Henry, A., & Walens, D. (2004). *A user's manual for the Occupational Performance History Interview* (V. 2.1). Chicago, IL: MOHO Clearinghouse.

Koyama, T., & Wang, H-T. (2011). Use of activity schedule to promote independent performance of individuals with autism and other intellectual disabilities: A review. *Research in Developmental Disabilities, 32*, 2235-2242. doi: 10.1016/j.ridd.2011.05.003

Law, M., Baptiste, S., Carswell, A., McColl, M. A., Polatajko, H., & Pollock, N. (2005). *Canadian Occupational Performance Measure* (4th ed.). Toronto, ON, Canada: CAOT Publications.

Lotan, M., Yalon-Chamovitz, S., & Weiss, P. L. (2011). Training caregivers to provide virtual reality intervention for adults with severe intellectual and developmental disability. *Journal of Physical Therapy Education, 25*, 15-19.

MacNeil, R. D., & Anderson, S. C. (1999). Leisure and persons with developmental disabilities: Empowering self-determination through inclusion. In P. Retish & S. Reiter (Eds.), *Adults with disabilities: International perspectives in the community* (pp. 125-143). Mahwah, NJ: Lawrence Erlbaum Associates, Inc.

Mahoney, W. J., Roberts, E., Bryze, K., & Parker Kent, J. A. (2016). Occupational engagement and adults with intellectual disabilities. *American Journal of Occupational Therapy, 70*, 7001350030p1-6. doi: 10.5014/ajot.2016.016576

Mayer, W. E., & Anderson, L. S. (2014). Perceptions of people with disabilities and their families about segregated and inclusive recreation involvement. *Therapeutic Recreation Journal, 8*(2), 150-168.

Moisey, S., & van de Keere, R. (2007). Inclusion and the internet: Teaching adults with developmental disabilities to use information and communication technology. *Developmental Disabilities Bulletin, 35*, 72-102.

Oates, A., Bebbington, A., Bourke, J., Girdler, S., & Leonard, H. (2011). Leisure participation for school-aged children with Down syndrome. *Disability and Rehabilitation, 33*, 1880-1889. doi: 10.3109/09638288.2011.553701

Peterson, J. J., Lowe, J. B., Peterson, N. A., Nothwehr, F. K., Janz, K. F., & Lobas, J. G. (2008). Paths to leisure physical activity among adults with intellectual disabilities: Self-efficacy and social support. *American Journal of Health Promotion 23*, 35-42. doi: 10.4278/ajhp.07061153

Salkever, D. S. (2000). Activity status, life satisfaction, and perceived productivity for young adults with developmental disabilities. *Journal of Rehabilitation, 66*, 4-13.

Solish, A., Perry, A., & Minnes, P. (2010). Participation of children with and without disabilities in social, recreational and leisure activities. *Journal of Applied Research in Intellectual Disabilities, 23*, 226-236. doi: 10.1111/j.1468-3148.2009.00525.x

Specht, J., King, G., Brown, E., & Foris, C. (2002). The importance of leisure in the lives of persons with congenital physical disabilities. *American Journal of Occupational Therapy, 56*(4), 436-445.

Suto, M. (1998). Leisure in occupational therapy. *Canadian Journal of Occupational Therapy, 65*, 271-278. doi: 10.1177/000841749806500504

Sutton, E. (1997). Enriching later life experiences for people with developmental disabilities. In T. Tedrick (Ed.), *Older adults with developmental disabilities and leisure: Issues, policy, and practice* (pp. 65-70). New York, NY: Haworth Press, Inc.

Tanner, K., Hand, B. N., O'Toole, G., & Lane, A. E. (2015). Effectiveness of interventions to improve social participation, play, leisure, and restricted and repetitive behaviors in people with autism spectrum disorder: A systematic review. *American Journal of Occupational Therapy, 69*(5), 6905180010. doi: 10.5014/ajot.2015.017

Thompson, J. R., Bryant, B. R., Campbell, E. M., Craig, E. M., Hughes, C. M., Rotholz, D. A., … Wehmeyer, M. L. (2004). *Supports Intensity Scale: User's manual.* Washington, D.C.: American Association on Intellectual and Developmental Disabilities.

Thorn, S. H., Pittman, A., Myers, R. E., & Slaughter, C. (2009). Increasing community integration and inclusion for people with intellectual disabilities. *Research in Developmental Disabilities, 30,* 891-901. doi: 10.1016/j.ridd.2009.01.001.

Van Naarden Braun, K., Yeargin-Allsopp, M., & Lollar, D. (2006). Factors associated with leisure activity among young adults with developmental disabilities. *Research in Developmental Disabilities, 27,* 567-583. doi:10.1016/j.ridd.2005.05.008

Verdonschot, M. M. L., de Witte, L. P., Reichrath, E., Buntinx, W. H. E., & Curfs, L. M. G. (2009a). Community participation of people with an intellectual disability: A review of empirical findings. *Journal of Intellectual Disability Research, 53,* 303-318. doi: 10.1111/j.1365-2788.2008.01144.x

Verdonschot, M. M. L., de Witte, L. P., Reichrath, E., Buntinx, W. H. E., & Curfs, L. M. G. (2009b). Impact of environmental factors on community participation of person with an intellectual disability: A systematic review. *Journal of Intellectual Disability Research, 53,* 54-64. doi: 10.1111/j.1365-2788.2008.01128.x

Wang, Y-T. (2013). Are adults with intellectual disabilities socially excluded? An exploratory study in Taiwan. *Journal of Intellectual Disability Research, 57,* 893-902. doi: 10.1111/j.1365-2788.2012.01574.x.

Wilson, P. G., Reid, D. H., & Green, C. W. (2006). Evaluating and increasing in-home leisure activity among adults with severe disabilities in supported independent living. *Research in Developmental Disabilities, 27,* 93-107. doi:10.1016/j.ridd.2004.11.012

Yalon-Chamovitz, S., & Weiss, P. L. (2008). Virtual reality as a leisure activity for young adults with physical and intellectual disabilities. *Research in Developmental Disabilities, 29,* 273-287. doi:10.1016/j.ridd.2007.05.004

Zakrazsek, A. G., Hammel, J., & Scazzero, J. A. (2014). Supporting people with intellectual and developmental disabilities to participate in their communities through support staff pilot intervention. *Journal of Applied Research in Intellectual Disabilities, 27,* 154-162. doi: 10.1111/jar.12060.

Zijlstra, H. P., & Vlaskamp, C. (2005). Leisure provision for persons with profound intellectual and multiple disabilities: quality time or killing time? *Journal of Applied Research in Intellectual Disabilities, 49,* 434-448. doi: 10.1111/j.1365-2788.2005.00689.x

12

Spiritual Life

Kimberly Bryze, PhD, OTR/L

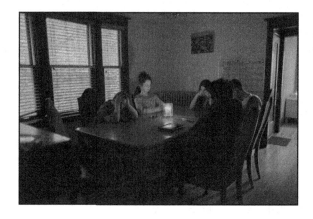

Key Words: becoming, being, beliefs, belonging, doing, L'Arche, spirituality

Bryze, K.
Occupational Therapy for Adults With Intellectual Disability (pp. 137-146).
© 2020 Taylor & Francis Group.

Occupational therapy practitioners assert "people of all ages and abilities require occupation to grow and thrive; in pursuing occupation, humans express the totality of their being, as a mind-body-spirit union," (Hooper & Wood, 2014, p. 38). According to the *Occupational Therapy Practice Framework: Domain and Process, Third Edition* (American Occupational Therapy Association [AOTA], 2014), spirituality, values, and beliefs are important client factors that transect the performance of occupations within relevant contexts. Spirituality is described as "the aspect of humanity that refers to the way individuals seek and express meaning and purpose and the way they experience/perceive their connectedness to the moment, to self, to others, to nature, and to the significant or sacred" (AOTA, 2014, p. S7). Spirituality originates from the Latin word *spiritus*, meaning breath or life. The term "spiritual is generally applied to any human essence connecting us to an unseen world that defies scientific measurement but which we nonetheless believe and feel exists" (Nelson, 2011, p. 17) and refers to direct personal experience, regardless of the social context. Persons with and without disabilities express their spiritual and religious beliefs through such practices as prayer and meditation, consistent with religious traditions, educational programs, and individual choice.

Although the practices and purposes of living a spiritual or religious life may be similar (e.g., seeking peace, practicing gratitude, seeking deeper meaning), spirituality and religion are not necessarily the same. Spirituality reflects the dimension of life in which one seeks the meaning in existence and response to the sacred and relationship with others (George Washington Institute for Spirituality and Health, n.d.). Religion is an organized form of spirituality, centered around certain understandings about God and faith, with associated traditions and practices. Religion may include such activities, practices, or occupations as attending services, meeting as a group for prayer or study, involvement in congregation activities, or reading scripture or religious texts. While spirituality is a personal relationship to the transcendent, religion is community-oriented, codified, and the established aspect of spirituality. One of the questions to be explored in this chapter is "How do individuals with intellectual disability experience spirituality/know God?" While one definitive answer will not be presented, ideas and resources on this topic will be discussed.

Webster (2005) asserts that "knowledge of God must never be reduced to mere propositional judgment or arbitrary logic; it must never be reduced to the proper functioning of neurons and neurotransmitters" (p. 14). Polanyi (1966) describes knowledge as coming through the senses, especially in relationship, and not in the form of logical discourse. Tacit knowledge is based in bodily knowledge that includes cognition and logic, but also the senses, emotion, and relationship with other persons and experiences. This bodily component is vital for understanding spiritual or religious knowledge for persons with intellectual disability (Demmons, 2007). It presupposes that an individual (with or without intellectual disability) knows more than they can express or tell. Such spirituality will not depend on the ability to communicate or express ideas and knowledge with words or logic. Polanyi (1958) suggests there are several forms of knowing, which transcend cognition, including intellectual passions, faith, and doubt. Although persons with intellectual disability lack an intellectual conceptualization or knowledge because of cognitive limitations, there is no reason to assume that they lack a tacit form of knowledge that seeks to discover spiritual truths. Persons with intellectual disability are equally able to experience and know God in this more tacit form, which does not require cognitive consciousness or awareness. Faith steps in where cognitive knowledge is lacking.

While not extensive, there are studies that have addressed spirituality and religion with this population (Harshaw, 2016; Hills, Clapton, & Dorsett, 2016; Watts, 2011), with studies reflecting the practices within service systems, congregations, or the ways in which programs can address the needs of individuals with intellectual disability. Few studies, however, are from the individuals' own perspectives (Demmons, 2007; Liu, Carter, Boehm, Annandale, & Taylor, 2014; Shogren & Rye, 2005). Some researchers have interviewed people with intellectual disability about their beliefs and spiritual lives. Many individuals with intellectual disability view God in personal terms; as a friend, a confidante, someone who is present to talk to, and who understands them (Potter, 2002; Swinton, 2002). They also relate the importance of faith in their lives, the importance of spiritual practices, such as prayer, and the ways in which their faith positively impacts their lives (Liu et al., 2014).

SPIRITUALITY AS OCCUPATION

Engagement in occupation activates and enables the expression of a person's spiritual self in the world (Hasselkus, 2011). *Spirituality* has been referred to as a sense of connection with something greater than the individual that provides meaning for life, or a sense of connection with oneself, others, and beyond, or being attentive to the spirit within. It may be experienced as being or belonging in the moment, at peace, regardless of surrounding circumstances. As stated earlier, spirituality may also refer to how individuals relate to themselves, others, their world, and a higher power, if they believe that one exists. It subsumes the held beliefs (conscious or intuitive) about an individual's relationship to and responsibility for self and others and a source of strength in difficult situations. Spirituality may also include the inquiry "to whom does my life belong?"

Spiritual health is one dimension of wellness, and requires a balance or congruence between one's physical, mental, and social capacities. One's spiritual or inner self contributes to a sense of self, the sense of the reality of who they are. Significant questions are raised about spirituality and the sense of self it implies in questioning what might or might not be accessible to a person with intellectual disability (Gordon, 2009). However, persons with intellectual disability have the right to choose the ways they desire to express their spirituality, and to practice their beliefs and expressions by participating in the faith community of their choice or other spiritual activities. Moreover, they have the right to choose not to participate or express their spiritual or religious beliefs. It is consistent with occupational justice and recommended occupational therapy practice to afford them the opportunity to choose and practice dimensions of spirituality that are meaningful to them.

Chosen activities and occupations may have spiritual significance or meaning as they are integrated into routines and roles (Pentland & McColl, 2011). Spiritual activities can be the certain practices or routines that give meaning to daily life, whether spending time in nature, listening to special music, engaging in an art activity, engaging in wellness practices such as yoga or walking, or sharing time with a favorite person. Certain rituals or routines may, therefore, become "ceremonies of life." A ceremony is an occasion to celebrate a particular event, person, or anniversary. Vanier (2008) writes of celebrating the gifts of others, including individuals with disability, and celebrating them for who they are:

> Every child, every person, needs to know that they are a source of joy; every child, every person, needs to be celebrated. Only when all of our weaknesses are accepted as part of our humanity can our negative, broken self-images be transformed. (p. 26)

A ceremony or celebration of life may be seen in the simple act of making and enjoying a cup of tea with another person. This act may bring a sense of peace and enjoyment in accomplishing the task and the pleasure in being able to do so. One of this author's friends, Neil, found meaning in filling a glass of water daily at a specific time for his roommate, Mark, who needed to take medications at a precise time each afternoon. Thibeault (2011) wrote about the beauty and intensity of rituals that are often linked with grief and loss, and the importance of spiritual rituals to help heal the soul and spirit. Another example of a ceremony of life can be in the story of housemates who were together one evening, shortly after the untimely death of one of their members. The housemates contributed their artistic efforts toward a collage/mural while they remembered and told each other stories of the individual who had recently passed away. The importance of chosen activities and rituals may serve a deeper purpose beyond ready interpretation. Such chosen activities are occupations of the spirit, intentionally engaged in for the development or enhancement of spirituality.

DOING, BEING, BECOMING, BELONGING, AND SPIRITUALITY

Wilcock (1999), an occupational scientist and occupational therapist, published several works centered upon a theoretical framework of occupation that is powerful, yet rarely used as a working model of practice by occupational therapists in the United States. Wilcock (1999) speaks of the need for our profession to understand and embrace occupation as "all the things that people do, the relationship of what they do with who they are as humans, and that through occupation they are in a constant state of becoming different" (p. 2) as the framework commonly referred to as *doing, being, becoming, and belonging*. Indeed, there is a dynamic balance between doing, being, becoming, and belonging; these four elements are interdependent and are central to a healthy physical, mental, and spiritual life. I (the author) assert that these elements can provide occupational therapy practitioners with integral ways to understand and support the spirituality of adults with intellectual disability.

Occupational therapy practitioners are concerned with what people do—their *doing*. People spend their lives doing purposeful, and sometimes meaningful, tasks and activities, even when they are not obligated to do so. They do daily tasks, whether personal self-care, preparing meals, cleaning the home, or working on projects. Some of what they do must be done, and some things are done just because human beings are inherently motivated to learn, grow, and do. What a person does contributes to and helps form who that person is. *Being* is often described with words such as existing, living, or essence. Hegel is attributed with writing that being is the element of the inner life, or "being-within-self" as in being completely developed, or at home with oneself (Inwood, 1992). Being implies a cessation of effort or doing and involves resting and contentment. *Becoming*, however, emerges from doing and being, and denotes a person's potential, growth, and self-actualization (Maslow, 1968). What one does, and how the doing comports with one's being, allows for becoming, or moving closer to self-actualization. Every person is on a path to becoming different, better, stronger, and more whole. Finally, doing, being, and becoming often take place within the physical and psychosocial spaces of *belonging*. Human beings are inherently social, and they establish connections with and find safety and enjoyment within the presence and relationship of others. Initially belonging to one's family expands to belonging to a circle of friends, to a classroom of peers, to a school, and to other groups and communities. What a person does, who they are, and who they are becoming is in relation to their affiliations and friendships, and even more so, to whom they belong.

The concepts of doing, being, belonging, and becoming can be realized by translating them to an understanding of the spiritual life of adults with intellectual disability. Spirituality of people with intellectual disability has long been a neglected area of study, and occupational therapy has not produced much research in this area of inquiry, although faith and spirituality can have an important place in people's lives. By integrating awareness of and an intentional focus on putting spirituality into practice, occupational therapy practitioners can respect the personhood of an individual and their beliefs, values, and experiences. Incorporating valued occupations into occupational therapy interventions, for the meaning the person derives from the activities, is another way of respecting an individual's spiritual self. A sense of wellness, hope, and life purpose may be engendered by focusing on spirituality and is often less obvious than the clinical challenges practitioners typically address.

To provide an example of ways in which doing, being, becoming, and belonging can guide our understanding of the spiritual lives of individuals with intellectual disability, I (the author) will share insights from my experiences in one of the L'Arche communities. L'Arche is an international organization with approximately 150 member communities in more than 35 countries, all united by a common vision and shared mission. In the United States, L'Arche communities are "homes and workplaces where people with and without intellectual disability live and work together as peers; create inclusive communities of faith and friendship; and transform society through relationships that cross social boundaries" (L'Arche, n.d.). While L'Arche was developed according to the Christian tradition, most communities are now interfaith, as they are situated throughout the world. All communities embrace the mission to celebrate the unique value of each person and make known the gifts of those who have disabilities through mutually transforming relationships. People with and without disabilities share life together in faith and friendship. L'Arche communities enact the values and shared life together by engaging in daily practices of personal care and worshipping. Life shared together means that liturgy (i.e., a communal response to and participation in sacred activities) and daily activity become deeply integrated expressions of being human. Some of the practices meet not only spiritual needs but bodily and social needs, such as the need for friendship, care, and recognition, as well.

The doing of daily life in a L'Arche home involves the typical routines of daily living, but daily life tasks are also understood within an intentionality of mindfulness and faith. As stated by Vanier (2012), the founder of L'Arche:

> The community life we live at L'Arche with people who are weak is rooted in simple, material things: cooking meals, spending time together at [the] table, washing the dishes, doing the laundry and the housework, helping meetings to go smoothly, organizing the house so that it is a happy welcoming place: thousands of little things that all take time. It also means looking after the needs of the weaker people: giving them baths, cutting their nails, helping them buy clothes. In the gardens or the workshops, it means doing the best one can with the resources available. These little things can often be seen as insignificant and valueless. However, all these small gestures can become gestures of love that help create a warm atmosphere in which the communion of hearts can grow. (p. 57)

In most homes, preparing and sharing the evening meal has greater meaning than just nourishment for the body; it is a time when the house members, and often friends of the community, live out hospitality, share stories, enjoy each other's company, and communicate with each other. A prayer of blessing is offered before dinner. After dinner, when dishes are cleaned up, the members regather at the table, a candle is lit, and each person offers a prayer, thought, or meditation verbally or silently, as they desire. Such times of prayer and fellowship are built into the fabric of daily life in L'Arche homes. Evidence of doing occupations of faith as part of the spiritual lives of these individuals may include individual and corporate prayer, worship at a church or synagogue, singing together, and participation in traditions throughout the year. Celebrations are held for all members, whether they are core members (i.e., those with intellectual disability) or assistants (i.e., staff). Birthdays, anniversary dates of when they came to L'Arche, and religious, and even secular, holidays are celebrated. One special celebration is held on the Thursday before Easter, when each community enacts the ritual of footwashing, consistent with that which Christ did in service to his disciples. Within the liturgical, as well as daily routines of life, the shared life embodies doing *with*, rather than doing *for*, the other. Such, doing with is the way of life and interfaces with the dimension of being.

One of the inherent tenets of L'Arche communities is the belief that all persons are worthy of respect. In our society, there is an assumption that being a person, or human, requires capabilities of self-representation, agency, memory, and cognitive skill (Reinders, 2008). The fact that these capabilities are diminished for people with intellectual disability places them in vulnerable positions with regard to others' beliefs about their personhood. L'Arche's stance is that individuals with intellectual disability are already persons, are already human, and worthy of care and friendship. They *are*; they have *being* (Vanier, 2010). Individuals with intellectual disability are respected, received, and honored by others. There is mutuality in their relationships, and friendships with those without disabilities. The assistants are friends, not merely caregivers, of those with disability. Such, *being with* bestows the gift on the other that they are more than their stigma, negative social narrative, or biological identity. Therefore, people with intellectual disability become far more than a cared for resident, and instead, they are a person in whom one finds joy, connection, and delight. A person's being is not dependent on the extent to which they can *do*; they are worthy in their own right and are valued as such. Not only does this afford confidence and resting in relationship and trust, but instills hope, encouragement, or inspiration toward growth and greater potential. This is lived out in L'Arche. One example was when Joan learned that her father had just been diagnosed with a serious, progressive disease that would likely be terminal. She was understandably sad and very quiet during the weekly house meeting. When another core member asked her what was wrong, Joan told him and began to cry. The other core members at first were quiet, but soon rose from their seats and came to sit alongside Joan, touching her arms, rubbing her back, allowing her to weep. They seemed to come alongside her to just be with her in her grief.

Doing and being are interrelated and thus influence becoming, of which there are different aspects: becoming "I" or oneself, becoming competent, and becoming a social being in relation to others (Fidler, 1983). Becoming implies potential, growth, and self-actualization. Occupational therapy practitioners often consider becoming in terms of doing (e.g., becoming better at doing …) or as a state of being (e.g., becoming calmer). Becoming can include the assumption of a role and its inherent responsibilities (i.e. becoming a worker and performing a specific job). However, becoming, as aligned to being, is to become what one has the potential to become and to be true to one's essence or own nature. The conception of friendship in L'Arche speaks to this aspect of becoming within relationships, whereby persons accept each other as they are, while becoming what they are meant to be. Through daily routines within an atmosphere of respect, there is support and encouragement toward wholeness and growth. Therefore, becoming is strengthened within the reality of belonging.

Belonging speaks to connection, relationship, and friendship. Belonging is seen in one's position within a family, in assumption of roles and responsibilities, and in the choices a person makes regarding spending time with others. In L'Arche, belonging is noted in the intentionality of daily life, the hospitality shown to those who live in the homes, as well as friends or guests to the community, and in the regular celebrations, open houses, or community nights when they open their doors to others for conversation, fellowship, and connection. The reality of belonging extends beyond immediate, interpersonal connections. Individuals who choose to live in this intentional community are not just choosing a good group home in which to live, but are choosing a lifestyle and value-oriented way of life. Core members are members for life, into and through illness and aging to death. This speaks to the value and stability that comes from belonging, with its resultant security and interconnection.

MAKING SPIRITUALITY A PART OF PRACTICE

An important first step to making spirituality a part of practice is recognizing that the occupational therapy process of evaluation and intervention carries with it certain ethical and moral values. Gaventa (2018) speaks of these values as the spirituality of the therapeutic relationship:

> To understand others "thickly" means professionals need to understand themselves that way as well. To learn and exercise practical wisdom means knowing when to do something as well as how, knowing who it is being done to as well as who is doing it, so that a caring and empowering partnership evolves. It also means being able to talk about the "whys" of a suggested treatment in terms of the core meanings in someone's life. Stated another way, good professional care is an art form, one that is not just about the skilled application of pain on the surface but also about the depth of shared symbols, meaning, and story between the artist and viewer, the professional and the people being served—the spirituality of that relationship. (pp. 189-190)

The occupational therapy process always begins with the therapeutic use of oneself as a practitioner, and establishing rapport within the client-centered context (Fisher, 2009). A person with intellectual disability may be able to provide information about their spiritual beliefs and values directly, although it may also be helpful to learn from a family member or caregiver who knows the person well and can provide insights about them. Seeking information about the person's spiritual practices and religious affiliations may be included in initial interviews or assessment processes as part of the occupational profile. Listening to and engaging the person, learning about who they are, and respecting the essence of the person are crucial qualities in the early phases of the occupational therapy process. Moreover, practitioners must learn to listen differently when understanding the meaning of spiritual practice for people whose personality is at least partially characterized by cognitive impairment. In speaking of the work of Vanier and the L'Arche movement, Reinders (2010) writes:

> Vanier does not think that [cognitive impairment] is a serious problem, because they communicate through their bodily gestures and simple words of love, or of anger. In Vanier's

understanding, their spirituality is very much about communication, which appears from the fact that they celebrate whatever gifts there are to thank God for. The gestures of rejoicing can be shared, if not always in words. (p. 8)

As such, persons with intellectual disability do indeed communicate—in embodied form. Assessments can be an important way to learn about and support individuals with intellectual disability. The FICA Spiritual History Assessment (Borneman, Ferrell, & Puchalski, 2010; Puchalski & Romer, 2000) is a tool that can be used in practice. It is a structured series of questions used to gather spiritual history information about a person, and the name, FICA, is an acronym, with each letter representing a category or type of question. *Faith* (F) and belief questions seek to shed light on the individual's recognition and acknowledgement of spiritual or religious beliefs, or more simply, that which may bring meaning to the person's life. *Importance* (I) questions are aimed toward ways in which the person's spirituality has influenced health, decision-making, and daily life. *Community* (C) inquiries seek to identify whether the individual is connected to a spiritual community or a support system of like-minded individuals. Finally, *Address* (A) in care questions seek ways the individual would like those spiritual and meaningful practices to be integrated into daily routines and care.

In the broadest sense, occupational therapy practitioners assess persons' occupational strengths and needs from a holistic, often quality of life, perspective in which spirituality is one component. A quality of life framework includes certain guiding human or spiritual questions and practices that are fundamental to each person. Although not specific to adults with intellectual disability, a thorough occupational profile, with questions designed to increase awareness of a person's spiritual history, may be used to guide the approach to spiritual assessment. As information is gathered from assessments, observations, and narrative accounts from and about an individual, practitioners will be challenged to explore and implement ways to integrate spirituality into practice.

Practitioners are not called upon to intervene in areas of spirituality, as are chaplains or counselors, yet as has been discussed, spirituality is an important dimension of human life. Identifying the occupations that are meaningful and that bring enjoyment, purpose, and engagement in life to the person is crucial when initiating interventions. The practitioner must be sensitive and open to the meaning an occupation may hold for a person and the positive impact it may have for them. As reported earlier, Neil's act of preparing and offering Mark a glass of water every afternoon held meaning to him beyond the obvious doing something good for Mark, or Neil's tendency to perform tasks within rigid routines and schedules. These explanations are the common and often misleading reasons. When asked about the glass of water for Mark, Neil explained, "'Cuz he's my friend," and "He needs water." The meaning of this faithful, daily task performance was in friendship and a simple way Neil could demonstrate care for Mark.

Meaningful occupations can be used through creative activities, such as decorating a room or the home for holidays, displaying photographs, or exhibiting items from travel. Participation in meaningful occupations helps organize and provides a sense of presence and purpose for individuals. In one home, Andrew looks forward to, and assumes great responsibility for decorating the different rooms for the holidays. Not only does he place Christmas decorations in the kitchen, on the dining room table, the coffee table in the living room, and in his bedroom; he hangs strings of tiny, white lights along the curtain rods in the sitting room, ensures that the red and gold placemats are ready to be used for each night's dinner, and organizes everyone for tree-trimming activities the first day of December. Other meaningful activities might involve exhibiting individual treasures and engaging in conversation about the objects. The process of engaging in storytelling, with few or many words actually spoken, is also one of the ways to bring meaning to shared time.

Certain practices are becoming common in occupational therapy for the purposes of bringing relaxation, organization, and mindfulness. Yoga, deep breathing, and mindfulness reflections are some simple and easily integrated strategies for individual and small group occupational therapy sessions. Such calming or meditative practices may also be evident with individuals who enjoy and find rest when walking in nature, bird watching, gardening, or sitting in a sanctuary or place where they feel safe, protected, and calm.

Participation in spiritual practices can be diverse and varied. Such practices can include the simplicity of practicing acts of kindness, practicing forgiveness and assuming an intentional mindset toward gratitude, and seeking ways to celebrate life and joy. Meditation, journaling, writing, artistic activities, and prayer are also practices that deepen and inform spirituality for many persons. Activities may be individualized or shared with others, depending on the person or persons involved.

IMPLICATIONS FOR OCCUPATIONAL THERAPY

Among the limited studies exploring spirituality of individuals with intellectual disability, several have focused on the experiences of older adults (Bassett, Perry, Repass, Silver, & Welch, 1994; McNair & Swartz, 1997; Minton &. Dodder, 2003). Studies have indicated that the majority of individuals with intellectual disability have been exposed to religious experiences and traditions, and that prayer and attending worship services are common practices (Shogren & Rye, 2005). Spiritual identity, spiritual community involvement, and spiritual expression can hold great importance in the lives of adults with intellectual disability, as they may for adults without disabilities (Liu et al., 2014). Occupational therapy practitioners, with other professionals, do great disservice to this population if they assume they are unable to comprehend concepts of God or a higher power and to need spirituality as part of their lives.

Religious and spiritual beliefs can and do shape a practitioner's views of disability, and, likewise, disability can also shape religious beliefs (Boswell, Knight, Hamer, & McChesney, 2001). One group of researchers (Baglieri, Valle, Connor, & Gallagher, 2011) studied individuals with intellectual disability, some of whom reported seeing design in their disability, while others spoke of their disability as a gift to be shared. However, most of their participants considered themselves to be loved, valued, and understood by God. While only one study, these results do offer another perspective, contrary to prevailing societal and professional views that disability is something that needs to be fixed, solved, or changed. Mark, mentioned previously, also stated, "You don't need to be afraid to have a disability. That's the way that God made you."

Occupational therapy practitioners are called upon to develop the skills needed to deal with individuals' spiritual interests and needs. The willingness to develop these skills may be somewhat dependent on the practitioner's own beliefs and attitudes. Moreover, the way a practitioner uses their knowledge and skills is crucial and can provide hope and energize care, or can lead to fear, frustration, and resistance. Within person-centered approaches and therapeutic use of self, which are two of the foundational constructs of occupational therapy practice, persons with intellectual disability could benefit from encouragement and opportunities to express the beliefs and values that shape their daily lives, relationships, and future. Their thoughts and perspectives about the types of community involvement they desire, including involvement in meaningful spiritual activities and practices in a faith community, and the particular supports they want and need in their lives (e.g., personal, spiritual, instrumental supports), are essential aspects to be actively integrated into occupational therapy practices for individuals with intellectual disability. Practitioners can and should empower their clients to live the lives they want to live. This can be realized by embracing the stance that people with intellectual disability bring their own unique spiritual gifts and benefits to communities, just as people without disabilities do. In this way of occupational therapy practice, the lives of all people are strengthened and enlarged.

REFERENCES

American Occupational Therapy Association. (2014). Occupational therapy practice framework: Domain and process, 3rd edition. *American Journal of Occupational Therapy, 68*(Suppl. 1), S1-S48.

Baglieri, S., Valle, J. W., Connor, D. J., &. Gallagher, D. J. (2011). Disability studies in education: The need for a plurality of perspectives on disability. *Remedial and Special Education, 32*, 267-278.

Bassett, R. L., Perry, K., Repass, R., Silver, E., & Welch, T. (1994). Perceptions of God among persons with mental retardation: A research note. *Journal of Psychology and Theology, 22*, 45-49.

Borneman, T., Ferrell, B., & Puchalski, C. M. (2010). Evaluation of the FICA tool for spiritual assessment. *Journal of Pain and Symptom Management, 40*, 163-173.

Boswell, B. B., Knight, S., Hamer, M., & McChesney, J. (2001). Disability and spirituality: A reciprocal relationship with implications for the rehabilitation process. *Journal of Rehabilitation, 67*, 20-25.

Demmons, T. A. (2007). Tacit and tactile knowledge of God: Toward a theology of revelation for persons with intellectual disabilities. *Journal of Religion, Disability & Health, 11*, 5-21.

Fidler, G. (1983). Doing and becoming: The occupational therapy experience. In: Kielhofner G. (Ed.), *Health through occupation: Theory and practice in occupational therapy*. Philadelphia, PA: F. A. Davis.

Fisher, A. G. (2009). *Occupational therapy intervention process model: A model for planning and implementing top-down, client-centered, and occupation-based interventions*. Fort Collins, CO: Three Star Press.

Gaventa, W. C. (2018). *Disability and spirituality: Recovering wholeness*. Waco, TX: Baylor University Press.

George Washington Institute for Spirituality and Health. (n.d.). About GWish. Retrieved from http://smhs.gwu.edu/gwish

Gordon, J. (2009). Is a sense of self essential to spirituality? *Journal of Religion, Disability & Health, 13*(1), 51-63

Harshaw, J. (2016). Finding accommodation: Spirituality and people with profound intellectual disabilities. *Journal of Disability and Religion, 20*, 140-153.

Hasselkus, B. R. (2011). *The meaning of everyday occupation*. Thorofare, NJ: SLACK Incorporated.

Hills, K., Clapton, J., & Dorsett, P. (2016). Towards an understanding of spirituality in the context of nonverbal autism: A scoping review. *Journal of Disability and Religion, 20*, 265-290.

Inwood, M. (1992). *A Hegel dictionary*. Malden, MA: Wiley-Blackwell.

L'Arche. (n.d.). About L'Arche. Retrieved from https://www.larcheusa.org/who-we-are

Liu, E. X., Carter, E. W., Boehm, T. L., Annandale, N. H., & Taylor, C. E. (2014). In their own words: The place of faith in the lives of young people with autism and intellectual disability. *Intellectual and Developmental Disabilities, 52*(5), 5, 388-404.

Maslow, A. H. (1968). *Toward a psychology of being*. New York, NY: D. Van Nostrand Company.

McNair, J., & Swartz, S. L. (1997). Local church support to individuals with developmental disabilities. *Education and Training in Mental Retardation and Developmental Disabilities, 32*, 304-312.

Minton, C. A., &. Dodder, R. A. (2003). Participation in religious services by people with developmental disabilities. *Mental Retardation, 41*, 430-439.

Nelson, K. (2011). *The spiritual doorway in the brain: A neurologist's search for the God experience*. New York, NY: Penguin Group.

Newberg, A., & Waldman, M. R. (2009). *How God changed your brain: Breakthrough findings from a leading neuroscientist*. New York, NY: Ballantine Books.

Pentland, W., & McColl, M. A. (2011). Occupational choice. In M. A. McColl (Ed.), *Spirituality and occupational therapy*, (2nd ed., pp. 141-149). Ottawa, ON: CAOT Publications.

Polanyi, M. (1958). *Personal knowledge*. London, United Kingdom: Routledge & Kegan Paul

Polanyi, M. (1966). *The tacit dimension*. London, United Kingdom: Doubleday.

Potter, D. (2002). Spirituality and people with learning disabilities, *Tizard Learning Disability Review, 7*, 36-38.

Puchalski, C., & Romer, A. L. (2000). Taking a spiritual history allows clinicians to understand patients more fully. *Journal of Palliative Medicine, 3*(1), 129-137.

Reinders, H. S. (2008). *Receiving the gift of friendship*. Grand Rapids, MI: W. B. Eerdmans.

Reinders, H. S. (2010). *The paradox of disability: Responses to Jean Vanier and L'Arche communities from theology and the sciences*. Grand Rapids, MI: W. B. Eerdmans.

Shogren, K. A., & Rye, M. S. (2005). Religion and individuals with intellectual disabilities: An exploratory study of self-reported perspectives. *Journal of Religion, Disability & Health, 9*, 29-53.

Swinton, J. (2002). Spirituality and the lives of people with learning disabilities, *Tizard Learning Disability Review, 7*, 29-35.

Thibeault, R. (2011). Ritual: Ceremonies of life. In M.A. McColl (Ed.), *Spirituality and occupational therapy* (2nd ed., pp. 233-240). Ottawa, ON, Ca: CAOT Publications.

Vanier, J. (2008). *Becoming human*. Mahwah, NJ: Paulist Press.

Vanier, J. (2010). What have people with learning disabilities taught me? In H. S. Reinders (Ed.), *The paradox of disability* (pp. 19-24). Grand Rapids, MI: W. B. Eerdmans.

Vanier, J. (2012). *The heart of L'Arche: A spirituality for every day*. Toronto, ON, Canada: Novalis.

Watts, G. (2011). Intellectual disability and spiritual development. *Journal of Intellectual & Developmental Disability, 36*, 234-241.

Webster, J. (2005). *Holiness*. Grand Rapids, MI: W. B. Eerdmans.

Wilcock, A. A. (1999). Reflections on doing, being, and becoming. *Australian Occupational Therapy Journal, 46*, 1-11.

13

The Use of Technology to Enhance Participation

Minetta Wallingford, DrOT, OTR/L and Joy M. Hyzny, MS, OTR/L

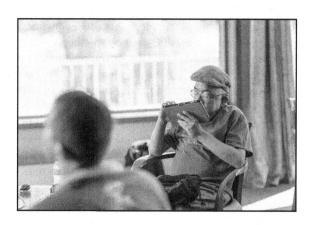

Key Words: assistive technology, mainstream technology, prompts, technology

Bryze, K.
Occupational Therapy for Adults With Intellectual Disability (pp. 147-159).
© 2020 Taylor & Francis Group.

Technology and assistive technology service delivery enhances occupational participation for people with intellectual disability in numerous ways. The professional literature reviewed for this chapter included individuals both with intellectual and also developmental disabilities. Therefore, some of the information discussed may refer to both populations.

Although technology continues to advance at amazing rates, there are limited studies that address the effectiveness of using technology for the intellectual disability population (Wehmeyer et al., 2006). Moreover, there are few peer-reviewed outcome studies and literature pertaining to specific interventions that support evidenced-based practice in occupational therapy for individuals with intellectual disability across occupations and environments over time. This chapter integrates professional literature and current evidence, along with clinical reasoning based on occupational therapy principles, related theories, and relevant assistive technology practice models, to address how technology may be utilized to support occupational participation for individuals with intellectual disability. Given the ever-changing landscape of technology, the authors provide some examples but do not endorse any specific products.

It is easy to be excited by the capabilities of technology, since the general population now has greater access to high-tech devices. Technology can be used to simplify a task, make the task more efficient, or provide the support necessary to decrease the physical or cognitive load to accomplish the task. Technology can transform how individuals with intellectual disability participate during play, leisure, recreation, at home, at work, or while engaging in multiple roles across various occupations.

Definitions of technology and assistive technology have commonly included references to equipment, a device, or a product. The Assistive Technology Act of 1998 defines an *assistive technology device* as "any item, piece of equipment or product system, whether acquired commercially, modified, or customized, that is used to increase, maintain, or improve functional capabilities of individuals with disabilities" (29 U.S.C. 3002, §3). There are many definitions of technology, but for the purpose of this chapter, technology is considered applying knowledge and tools to accomplish a task (Technology, n.d.).

There is often overlap in the various types of technology that are used to address the needs of a person with an intellectual disability. Blackhurst (2001) describes a range of technology categories, from no to high technology. *No tech*, consists of strategies to adapt the method, conditions, or services in the environment to support an individual's participation (Blackhurst, 2011). *Low tech* is often considered easy to utilize and is more readily or commercially available (Blackhurst, 2011). *High tech* includes devices that frequently include electronic components (Blackhurst, 2001). *Mainstream technology* refers to technology that is utilized by consumers that was not developed explicitly for individuals with disabilities (Cook & Polgar, 2015).

The advances in mainstream technology have increased the availability of useful features incorporated into devices that were previously only available in products that were initially designed specifically for people with disabilities (Stow & England, 2016). Consequently, consumers may not necessarily consider assistive technology a specialized area because many tech products, such as portable devices and smartphones, are used as universal tools with multipurpose functionality. This has been an exciting development resulting in some lower-cost applications that mimic the functionality of high-tech devices. However, there are often continuous updates that may require greater knowledge and time investment for those using or supporting individuals with intellectual disability. New updates may lead to unforeseen issues with functionality of certain applications (apps). Yet, technological advances provide many additional options for integrating technology into daily life and may create additional opportunities to support occupational participation for people with intellectual disability.

FUNDING

Occupational therapy practitioners need to consider funding sources early in the occupational therapy service delivery process, particularly when recommending expensive technology solutions that require customization. Occupational therapy services are typically provided within the contexts of where services are provided (e.g. school, work, hospital, home). As a result, there can be special rules or requirements for funding equipment, devices, services, and training based on the setting or service delivery model (Ripat & Booth, 2005). Funding sources include public funding, private insurance, private pay, workman's compensation insurance, crowdfunding, or nonprofit organizations. Some nonprofit organizations may also offer loaner programs or reutilize equipment they provide to consumers. In the United States, public sources may be available at the federal, state, or local level.

Unfortunately, many funding systems or organizations do not consider all the costs, benefits, and other relevant implications as part of their decision-making process. There are important questions for funding agencies to consider when making funding decisions. When providing assistive technology or making decisions on funding, it is important to consider whether using technology will lead to fewer resources required for caregiving and if this is preferable for the user (Ripat & Booth, 2005). Quality of life factors, such as increasing autonomy or social participation, are also essential considerations. Many of these quality of life benefits are often overlooked, yet important to consider for individuals with intellectual disability who may experience occupational deprivation. Participation in meaningful occupations can impact physical, psychological, and emotional well-being for people with intellectual disability and the people who support them. Ultimately, the allocation of funding for services and technology elicits many questions regarding what is valued by society and where to invest resources.

ASSISTIVE TECHNOLOGY SERVICE DELIVERY

Occupational therapy best practice develops from theoretical models for guiding the critical reasoning, evaluation processes, and intervention practices for enabling occupation in a person's daily life. When occupational therapy practitioners are involved in assistive technology service delivery, such models may come from occupational therapy or from the assistive technology practices. The University of Wisconsin–Milwaukee has compiled a thorough taxonomy of models applicable to assistive technology (Assistive Technology Outcomes Measurement System [ATOMS], n.d.). Assistive technology models include the Human-Activity-Assistive Technology Model (Cook & Polgar, 2015), the Matching Person and Technology Model by Sherer (Institute for Matching the Person and Assistive Technology, 2007), and the Student, Environment, the Tasks, and the Tools Model by Zabala (Zabala, 2005). These models overlap with essential shared characteristics that include the person, environment, and tool or technology that supports participation in tasks, activities, or occupations (ATOMS, n.d.).

The inter-relationship between these factors is particularly important for individuals with intellectual disability, as assistive technology is often used across multiple contexts. High quality assistive technology service delivery requires an in-depth understanding of the person, his or her interests and abilities, and the environments where he or she engages in occupational tasks. The American Occupational Therapy Association *Occupational Therapy Practice Framework: Domain and Process, Third Edition* (2014) serves as a guide to current occupational therapy practice and service delivery. The occupational therapy process and components of the *Framework* comport with many assistive technology models in that they emphasize:

- Understanding of the person's past, current, and future abilities and needs that assistive technology might address
- The person's interests, values, and skills

- Environmental supports and barriers to participation
- Collaboration in the development of the individual's assistive technology goals
- Clinical reasoning of intervention approaches based on understanding how assistive technology can enhance participation
- Relevant assistive technology service delivery outcomes

SPECIAL CONSIDERATIONS IN ASSISTIVE TECHNOLOGY SERVICE DELIVERY FOR INDIVIDUALS WITH INTELLECTUAL DISABILITY

There are several factors influencing assistive technology service delivery that must be considered for individuals with intellectual disability. Occupational therapy practitioners are often part of a team who work together to develop, implement, and achieve individual client or organizational goals. The team members may include caregivers, family, personal care assistants, speech-language pathologists, physical therapists, orientation and mobility specialists, equipment vendors, resident service coordinators, case managers, and others. The use of technology and its integration varies across environments and settings. For example, research indicates that considerations such as time, resources, training, organizational culture, staff perceptions, and knowledge of technology may impact how information and communication technology is used and valued in different environments that serve people with intellectual disability (Parsons, Daniels, Porter, & Robertson, 2008). Therefore, it is imperative to consider the impact of various contexts and environments on the individual's current and future occupational participation. For assistive technology to be an effective intervention, it must be integrated into the individual's daily occupations and across the environments in which the person participates (Hammel, 2000). It may require training the individual and the team, not only on using the equipment, but also on maintaining it (Hammel, 2000). This may include cleaning the screen of an augmentative and alternative communication (AAC) device, charging a wheelchair battery, updating the operating system or apps, and knowing who to contact for technical support or repairs.

There are many methods for introducing technology to individuals with intellectual disability when they have not used it previously. Whenever possible, it is best to utilize strategies that are engaging and do not increase the cognitive demand, such as errorless learning activities. This is especially important for individuals with intellectual disability, who may have difficulty changing routines and incorporating new information. It may be beneficial to begin with a device or strategy that is familiar to the individual, easy to implement, and not too overwhelming. The individual should practice incorporating the technology across environments and in various situations (Hammel, 2000). It is also essential to provide hands-on training to caregivers to increase familiarity with the technology, so they can model the assistive technology tool or strategy to facilitate successful use. This can enable the caregiver to empower the individuals they support. The importance of appropriate training and matching the person with the right technology, to participate in occupations across environments cannot be overemphasized.

Instructional methods that may be relevant to individuals with intellectual disability include demonstration or hands-on exploration to apply the information. This may involve repetitive practice, simulations, or participation in occupations to generalize the skills or methods across other environments or tasks. A multisensory (e.g., auditory, visual, kinesthetic, tactile) approach may be beneficial to learning tasks and using tools. Modifications may include changing the rate and speed of directions, repeating directions, using simple words, gestural or tactile cues, or visuals (e.g., photos, pictures, diagrams, social stories, words, symbols, emojis). Visual directions, visual schedules, and charts can support sequencing tasks and routines. These methods may be applied to enhance occupational participation across multiple environments (e.g., work, education, volunteer, home, community). However, even a skilled occupational therapy practitioner can have difficulty finding the exact technology match for the individual's skills, abilities, and unique interests due to the challenges and limitations in current practice. These include the capabilities and complexity of current technology, cost of equipment, access to assistive technology, and limitations in the systems that support the individual. According to Lauer, Longenecker Rust, & Smith (n.d.), assistive technology device abandonment rates vary from "8% to 75%" (p. 2). Even though technology has many benefits usage rates differ for a variety of reasons including device function, service issues, or improvement in the individual user's functional abilities (Lauer, et al., n.d.).

Successful adoption of assistive technology involves the skills of the therapist during the assessment process to ensure appropriate feature match. Other considerations include device trials, training, funding options, and environmental supports. It is essential that individuals with intellectual disability and caregivers invest time to learn and implement the assistive technology into a daily routine. An individual's current and future abilities, as well as their values and response to technology, are also important considerations that may contribute to success and satisfaction in technology adoption (Ripat & Booth, 2005). Ideally, the individual and their team collaborate during the entire assistive technology service delivery process, including decisions regarding features, costs, and understanding maintenance of equipment. This is extremely critical, because technology may require both a financial and time investment for the individual and/or caregiver to learn to optimally use the technology in their daily lives (Ripat & Booth, 2005). Successful assistive technology adoption may require advocating for funding or working with family, agencies, or caregivers across environments to ensure that follow up, follow through, and carry over occurs. Research supports the benefits of collaborating with the consumers of assistive technology and the individuals who support them in order to facilitate effective assistive technology integration and environmental interventions for adults with intellectual disability as they age (Mirza & Hammel, 2009).

USING ASSISTIVE TECHNOLOGY TO SUPPORT OCCUPATIONAL ENGAGEMENT

The performance of occupations (e.g., activities of daily living [ADLs], instrumental activities of daily living [IADLs]) is influenced by both physical and cognitive abilities, as well as supports and training. Some people with mild intellectual disability may be independent with basic ADLs and other occupations, while others may require varying levels of supports, depending on the severity of the intellectual disability, individual client factors, and performance skills. Adaptive equipment, durable medical equipment, and assistive technology is often used by individuals with intellectual disability to support participation, particularly when there are physical challenges. Since individuals with intellectual disability have cognitive challenges, the occupational therapy practitioner must thoroughly understand the occupational demands, the individual's habits, routines, motor and process skills, interests, and temperament. They must also consider the relevant environments and contexts and the features of technology for effective assistive technology intervention.

It is also important to support occupational routines (e.g., grooming, ADLs, IADLs, work). Routines can be facilitated through prompts, visual schedules, organizational systems, and various applications or devices. It is essential to utilize the correct amount of supports and to decrease supports as appropriate to foster independence and participation. For example, an individual may be able to initiate brushing his or her teeth independently but require a prompt or other support to remember to put the toothpaste back where it belongs. An occupational therapy practitioner may need to provide a variety of supports to ensure that an individual organizes the environment and performs all of the steps in a task appropriately.

Recent research indicates that service providers who work with individuals with intellectual disability, identified a variety of devices, such as wheelchairs, walkers, computers, applications, AAC, and adapted eating utensils, as valued supports (Bryant, Seok, Ok, & Bryant, 2012). Moreover, a systemic review on the effectiveness of assistive technology, to support cognitive function, revealed that prompting or reminding technology can support participation in activities ranging from personal care to social participation (Gillespie, Best, & O'Neill, 2012). Since a variety of technology solutions are often used across multiple environments to support different occupations, there is often overlap in the technology that is used, depending on the individual's occupational needs, demands, and the environment. Further examples of technology that may support individuals with intellectual disability in their occupations are presented in the following sections.

Personal Device Care

Personal devices that may support people with intellectual disability across occupations include hearing aids, eyeglasses, orthotics, prosthetics, medical devices, or other types of mainstream technology and adaptive equipment. Since some of these devices are essential to daily function, training on how to care for and maintain the devices is imperative. Individuals with intellectual disability may care for the devices on their own or with support from systems or other individuals. For example, a visual schedule that involves step-by-step directions for device care and maintenance may help support this important routine. It is also vital to train individuals on how to problem solve potential issues and provide them with visuals or other resources to support this process (Hammel, 2000).

Grooming, Hygiene, Toileting, Showering, and Bathing

Occupational therapy practitioners are typically familiar with adaptive equipment to support ADLs for physical challenges, but they also need to keep in mind the cognitive challenges of using this equipment for people with intellectual disability. Items to support grooming and hygiene may include cylinder foam, built-up handles, and universal cuffs, used with personal care items to support decreased grip for a variety of occupations, such as shaving, oral care, and combing hair. Mainstream tech may be particularly useful for individuals with intellectual disability. For example, an electronic toothbrush can also act as a timer to ensure proper brushing time; a curling iron with an automatic shut-off may provide a needed safety feature.

Toilet safety frames, raised toilet seats, and bedside commodes can be used to assist with transfers during toileting. Bath mitts, long-handled sponges, grab bars, shower chairs, roll-in shower chairs, bath benches, shower hoses, non-skid mats, and barrier free showers are a few types of equipment or adaptations that may support bathing and showering. Providing lighting or high-contrast tape to designate the lip of a walk-in shower may assist with safety while showering. However, if an occupational therapy practitioner recommends equipment to support the individual with intellectual disability, it is important to make sure an individual can safely and effectively use the equipment during the actual occupation (e.g., showering, bathing). It is also imperative to identify the supports (e.g., physical assistance, verbal prompts, visual prompts) that are needed to safely carry out the occupation in his or her daily or weekly routines.

Dressing

Dressing sticks, reachers, sock aids, elastic or Velcro tie shoes, adapted clothing, and adapted dressing techniques can be used to assist with dressing; however, training an individual in the use of assistive technology and adapted dressing methods requires consideration of the organization and sequence of the task. Individuals with intellectual disability may benefit from visual or organizational supports that may include tactile supports, visual instructions, charts, diagrams, color codes, tags, labels, or organizing items to support daily and weekly routines.

Swallowing, Eating, and Feeding

Eating can provide pleasure, nutritional support, and a means for socialization for individuals with intellectual disability. Positioning can be an important consideration for eating and swallowing for some individuals. Occupational therapy practitioners may need to adapt utensils, eating surfaces, or provide seating supports, such as seat belts, chest straps, wedges, or footrests to allow for better positioning. A Swedish sling, mobile arm supports, wheelchair trays, different mounting devices, or seating systems may assist with positioning and supporting extremities to enhance self-feeding. Other technology to increase participation in feeding for individuals with intellectual disability includes built-up utensils, divider plates, cup holders (Bryant et al., 2012), universal cuffs, plate guards, self-feeding devices, or different kinds of cups or glasses.

Although there is a great deal of technology and positioning equipment available to support eating, it is also imperative to consider the social context of eating when recommending assistive technology for individuals with intellectual disability by asking several questions:

- How much training is required to use the equipment?
- How will the equipment impact the social experience of the individual and others at the table?
- Does the individual want to use the equipment?
- Is the equipment aesthetically acceptable?
- Will the adaptive equipment increase independence and participation in eating?
- Will it decrease reliance on another person for feeding?

Functional Mobility and Community Mobility

Functional mobility can be assisted in various ways. People with intellectual disability may use various types of canes, walkers, scooters, wheelchairs, power wheelchairs, or other devices. Bed rails or hospital beds that raise and lower may assist with transfers out of bed. Lift chairs are sometimes used as both a bed and a chair and can assist individuals who are having difficulty with transfers from sit to stand. If a person requires any mobility device, it is important to consider the person's current and future needs. This is especially critical when considering a wheelchair or a scooter, as insurance may only replace equipment every several years. For individuals with intellectual disability, it is imperative to consider the cognitive demands, as well as the other implications, of using any functional mobility device. When recommending power mobility, it is also vital to think through the potential need for an integrated system, which allows components from the wheelchair to communicate with other technology to perform additional tasks, such as controlling aspects of the environment. This can include turning on lights, playing music, and accessing a personal computer. Other considerations may include a wheelchair tray and the need to identify locations for mounting switches and other devices.

Enhancing functional mobility requires consideration of the environment and contexts that the person participates in as part of his or her daily life. When a person starts using a mobility device, it is essential to utilize it in all applicable environments. People with intellectual disability may need guided practice and reminders to support the safe use of the devices. For example, when they first start using a walker, they may need repeated practice or other supports to remember to reach for the arm of a chair when sitting down. They may have difficulty opening a heavy door or it may bump them when using a walker or wheelchair. Options to address this can include door holders, automatic door openers, and door openers or closers that adjust the time or pressure required. In some cases, home modifications may be necessary to enhance mobility and accessibility (Sanford & Fagan, 2004). Ramps, elevators, and levers vs. knobs on doors (Sanford & Fagan, 2004), adapted bathrooms, wide doorways, and height accessible light switches are some design features or adaptations that may enhance accessibility and mobility. A low tech option to increase safety in functional mobility may involve applying colored tape or paint to contrast thresholds and stairs.

Positioning is extremely important for individuals with intellectual disability who may have physical impairments or mobility concerns. An individual might perform the majority of his or her daily occupations from a wheelchair, so proper seating and positioning is essential to enhancing occupational performance, preventing skin breakdown, and addressing concerns that occur with decreased mobility. Many major medical centers, hospitals, clinics, and schools have seating and mobility clinics with experienced therapists and personnel who conduct evaluations, recommend equipment, and provide training. It is essential to work with reputable therapists, contractors, providers, and companies who are current with the latest technology and products when considering home modifications, seating, positioning, or the need for a manual wheelchair or power mobility. Transporting power wheelchairs or scooters, and providing required maintenance are also a consideration in functional and community mobility.

Community mobility can be supported by tech options, such as maps, landmark identification, written and visual directions, GPS devices, public and private transportation, transportation websites, and related apps. Technology to support orientation and mobility in the home and community are continuing to evolve, and effectiveness is being explored (Gillespie et al., 2012; Lancioni et al., 2009; Mengue-Topio, Courbois, Farran & Sockeel, 2011). Individuals with intellectual disability who have low vision or use mobility devices such as wheelchairs, scooters or walkers may find even more challenges with accessing the community at large. Accessibility is still a concern in many communities; however, there are several websites and organizations, such as centers for independent living, regional Americans with Disabilities Act centers, and the National Council on Independent Living that may have information on accessible options.

Communication and Social Participation

Several technology options and methods can support communication for individuals with intellectual disability across various occupations. No-tech options for prompts include gestures, pointing, or sign language. Expressive communication may be supported by asking questions, offering choices, or demonstrating actions. Low-tech methods include emphasizing core vocabulary (i.e., common words that can be used in multiple contexts), as well as fringe vocabulary (i.e., words that are relevant to a particular context) through the use of objects, pictures, photos, or icons, along with printed words, to reinforce the visual supports. Other AAC options may include picture-based communication boards or more complex options, such as speech generating devices.

Effective AAC implementation entails a collaborative team process focused on matching the most appropriate options and features to the individual to facilitate optimal utilization across environments. Occupational therapy practitioners can contribute to successful evaluation, intervention, device selection, and implementation. They can assist with access selection, positioning, and mounting strategies to promote maximal efficiency when using a device across multiple environments. This information assists the team in better understanding the amount of vocabulary, the size of the pictures or icons, as well as their location on the device. It is important for staff working with individuals with intellectual disability to undergo training with the AAC device or system to facilitate effective implementation (Sutherland et al., 2014).

Mainstream tech used for communication include computers, tablets, cell- or smartphones, and landline telephones. There are some feature-packed apps to enhance written communication, which are available for both phones and tablets. At this time, there are apps that support communication by including word and picture supports, color coding, and sentence structure.

Electronic communication has also greatly expanded the ability to socialize with others in various environments and across social networks. Some of these options include email, video chat, and social networking platforms. Research on the experiences of adults with intellectual disability who were using Facebook revealed that participants viewed it positively and mostly interacted with family and others they already see in- person (Shpigelman & Gill, 2014). Engaging in social networks to share photos and other exchanges may provide additional opportunities for socializing with others and enhance the quality of life for individuals with intellectual disability.

Meal Preparation, Home Management, and Financial Management

Technology to support meal preparation includes electronic can openers, rocker knives, adapted or built-up utensils, or items that stabilize objects when cutting or stirring. Individuals with intellectual disability may benefit from visual recipes and instructions to assist with organizing and sequencing steps for meal preparation. Tactile cues, symbols, pictures, or other visuals can be attached to appliances to provide cues for use. Appliances may be activated through various switches, environmental control units, or mobile technology. Meal items can be transported via rolling carts and walker or wheelchairs trays.

Other home management tasks may be assisted by environmental control systems, smart technology, reaching devices, organization systems, and visual schedules. Additional supports for daily living tasks may include picture, auditory and tactile prompts, and prompts via electronic devices (Mechling, 2007). Smart technologies, assistive care systems, personal robots, and virtual technologies continue to develop and may support individuals with cognitive disabilities (Braddock, Rizzoli, Thompson, & Bell, 2004). Mainstream technology has evolved so that voice-controlled devices (i.e., smart speakers) may be used to obtain information, set timers, and control lights and thermostats.

Individuals with intellectual disability may benefit from large key calculators, use of debit cards with a specified dollar amount, and other systems for managing money. Shopping may be supported by shopping lists, picture lists, and organizational systems for locating items either online or in stores. Computer programs, applications, or websites may support financial management through options such as automatic bill payment. However, the use of financial management applications and systems may require step-by-step training and should be geared to a person's abilities and needs.

Health and Safety, Relaxation, and Sleep

Health and safety technology supports include medication reminders, secured dispensers, devices that monitor vital signs, and safety monitors and systems (Sanford & Fagan, 2004). Health management and maintenance routines for individuals with intellectual disability may be supported by exercise videos, devices with alarms or reminders, or health and fitness apps. As with any other technology, for a routine to be established it is important that individuals with intellectual disability take an active interest in using the equipment or systems and that appropriate supports and training be provided.

Health and safety for individuals with intellectual disability may be impacted by changes in vision and hearing as a normal part of aging. Technology to support visual changes may include glasses, lenses that filter light, magnifiers, visuals, large print books, large signage, tactile cues, and lighting. Additionally, reducing glare, providing contrast, and reducing the environment's visual clutter (e.g., patterns) may be advantageous (Whittaker, Sheiman, & Sokol-McKay, 2016). Auditory supports include hearing aids, acoustic supports, visual signage, and phones or other devices that display text or vibrate.

There are also sleep and relaxation apps that include exercises for deep breathing, sleep journals, and soothing sounds if sleep routines are a concern for the individual with intellectual disability; however, there is limited evidence on the overall effectiveness of the use of behavioral health applications at this time (Wiederhold, 2015). Other technology to support sleep includes ear plugs or earphones to decrease sounds or eye masks to decrease light. In addition, there are a several kinds of beds, mattresses, mattress toppers, and pillows that may support positioning and comfort or help prevent deformities and pressure sores.

Education and Work

Adults with intellectual disability may participate in formal or informal education, hands-on exploratory learning, paid or supported employment, or volunteering. A meta-analysis on the use of technology (e.g., computers, audio prompting devices, video training devices) indicated positive benefits to support employment interests, pursuits, and work-related tasks for individuals with intellectual and developmental disabilities (Wehmeyer et al., 2006).

Technology that offers speech to text, word prediction, and accessibility options may be particularly useful to support education or work for individuals with intellectual disability. Tablets, computers, and even cell phones can help individuals who have some foundational keyboarding skills and struggle with print or cursive writing. Computer programs, applications, and access tools and strategies may be especially applicable to the education or work environment, depending on the occupational demands.

To determine the most appropriate applications and devices, it is necessary to identify the features that the person and task require. This involves a thorough understanding of the individual's skills and abilities, including the ability to access various devices. For example:

- How much prompting does the individual require?
- Do they require a picture or video support to complete the particular occupational task?
- Do they require auditory feedback?
- Do they respond better when seeing a video of each work task component, or do they respond better with a subtle visual cue in a checklist?
- Do they require support from another person to search the internet or to use other devices and applications effectively?

All of these questions are necessary to consider because the answers will guide the occupational therapy practitioners and team members to select the features that the technology must integrate to assist the individual.

Play and Leisure

Computer technology, smart phones, environmental control devices, and switch interfaces may assist with play and leisure for individuals with intellectual disability. There are numerous games, music, and videos that can be accessed using a switch. The use of a switch interface and switch may be required for online games if the individual has difficulty manipulating a computer mouse. Some battery-operated games can be accessed by using a battery interrupter and connecting a switch to the interrupter.

Touch screens are a common way to directly access the online activities on tablet devices if a wireless connection is available. Other assistive technology products to promote access on tablets may include keyguards, touch-screen gloves, an adapted stylus, and joysticks. Nevertheless, some switch interfaces are designed to work with the built-in operating system, while others may only be compatible to a specific device. Other leisure options for individuals with intellectual disability may include participation in games, sports, arts, or crafts. Games or sports can be modified by adapting equipment, changing the rules, context, or some of the materials. Adaptive scissors, large markers, digital art software or apps, and other media may be used in art projects or other activities to support individuals with intellectual disability in leisure participation.

CASE EXAMPLE

Jan is a 72-year-old adult with intellectual disability who lives in a group home in Chicago, Illinois and attends a senior community center daily. Jan has her lunch at the center and participates in many activities. She enjoys eating and socializing at the center, using the computer, and participating in arts and craft activities. Jan is an avid baseball fan, who cheers for her favorite north-side team. She knows several of the team members' names and likes to watch them on TV. Occasionally, the center will get complimentary tickets and take Jan to the game.

Jan has osteoarthritis in her knees and started using a rolling walker last month after losing her balance and falling. Previously, Jan required only minimal prompting from support staff to perform most of her ADL routines (e.g., dressing, grooming, bathing in a walk-in shower, laundry). The group home has some adaptive bathroom and shower equipment that Jan has not needed in the past. However, the recent fall has impacted her ADL and IADL performance.

Jan is assigned various tasks at her group home. The staff prints out recipes for residents to use when making dinner. Jan requires some verbal prompting to remember the next step in the recipe and how to set the table. Jan also requires minimal prompting to sequence the steps needed to do her laundry. Prior to the fall, Jan was able to physically perform tasks, such as washing lettuce, putting items in bowls, clearing dishes, and loading and unloading the dishwasher. However, the tasks were not always performed efficiently (e.g., carries one utensil to dishwasher at a time) or completely (e.g., leaves items on the table, forgets to finish task).

Since Jan fell, she has had difficulty with reaching to load the dishwasher and the washer and dryer. She occasionally drops items, and it is challenging for her to safely bend down to pick them up. Her balance impacts her ability to reach higher and lower shelves to obtain items that she frequently uses in the kitchen. She currently requires minimal physical assistance with getting up from a low chair. This is most problematic at the end of the day. Jan recently fell when she got up from her low bed to go to the bathroom and no one found her until the morning. Jan now appears to have a fear of falling and is not participating in many of the activities that she did in the past.

CONCLUSION

Advances in technology continue to occur at an increasingly faster rate. These advances may provide occupational therapy practitioners with more tools and opportunities to support occupational participation for individuals with intellectual disability; however, these continuing changes may also require that individuals with intellectual disability learn new technology and systems. Therefore, occupational therapy practitioners stay up-to-date with the latest technology and make sure that new innovations are a better match for these individuals. Moreover, further research is needed to examine the effectiveness of technology use on occupational participation outcomes for individuals with intellectual disability. It is an exciting time for occupational therapy practice, as these continued advances in mainstream technology may make devices and other technology more affordable and available for those individuals who need them the most.

ACKNOWLEDGMENTS

We would like to acknowledge Evan Rockefeller, Meredith Kaulbach, and Thomas Mercier for sharing their time and expertise regarding assistive technology service delivery for individuals with intellectual disability.

REFERENCES

American Occupational Therapy Association. (2014). Occupational therapy practice framework: Domain and process, 3rd edition. *American Journal of Occupational Therapy, 68*(Suppl. 1), S1-S48.

Assistive Technology Act of 1998, 29 U. S. C. 3002, §3. (1998). Retrieved from www.congress.gov/105/plaws/publ394/PLAW-105publ394.pdf

Assistive Technology Outcomes Measurement System. (n.d.). *ATOMS project: Models and taxonomies relating to assistive technology resource.* Retrieved from www.r2d2.uwm.edu/atoms/archive/technicalreports/fieldscans/fs7/tr-fs-taxonomiesmodels-resource.html

Blackhurst, E. A. (2001). What is assistive technology? National Assistive Technology Research Institute. Retrieved from http://natri.uky.edu/resources/fundamentals/defined.html#continuum

Braddock, D., Rizzolo, M. C., Thompson, M., & Bell, R. (2004). Emerging technologies and cognitive disability. *Journal of Special Education Technology, 19*(4), 49-56. doi: 10.1177/016264340401900406

Bryant, B. R., Seok, S., Ok, M., & Bryant, D. P. (2012). Individuals with intellectual and/or developmental disabilities use of assistive technology devices in support provision. *Journal of Special Education Technology, 27*(2), 41-57. doi: 10.1177/016264341202700205

Cook, A. M., & Polgar, J. M. (2015). Principles of assistive technology: Introducing the human activity assistive technology model. In A. M. Cook & J. M. Polgar (Eds.) *Assistive technologies: Principles and practice* (4th ed., pp. 1-15). St. Louis, MO: Elsevier Health Sciences.

Gillespie, A., Best, C., & O'Neill, B. (2012). Cognitive function and assistive technology for cognition: A systematic review. *Journal of the International Neuropsychological Society, 18*, 1-19. doi: 10.1017/S1355617711001548

Hammel, J. (2000). Assistive technology and environmental intervention (AT-EI) impact on the activity and life roles of aging adults with developmental disabilities: Findings and implications for practice. *Physical & Occupational Therapy in Geriatrics, 18*(1), 37-58., doi: 10.1080/J148v18n01_04

Institute for Matching the Person and Assistive Technology. (2007). Matching person & assistive technology model and assessment process. Retrieved from https://sites.google.com/view/matchingpersontechnology/products

Lancioni, G. E., O'Reilly, M. F., Singh, N. N., Sigafoos, J., Campodonico, F., & Oliva, D. (2009). A wheelchair user with visual and intellectual disabilities managing simple orientation technology for indoor travel. *Journal of Visual Impairment and Blindness, 103*(5), 308-313.

Lauer, A., Longenecker Rust, K., & Smith, R. O. (n.d.). ATOMS project technical report—Factors in assistive technology device abandonment: Replacing "abandonment" with "discontinuance." Assistive Technology Outcomes Measurement System. Retrieved from www.r2d2.uwm.edu/atoms/archive/technicalreports/tr-discontinuance.html

Mechling, L. C. (2007). Assistive technology as a self-management tool for prompting students with intellectual disabilities to initiate and complete daily tasks: A literature review. *Education and Training in Developmental Disabilities, 42*(3), 252-269.

Mengue-Topio, H., Courbois, Y., Farran, E. K., & Sockeel, P. (2011). Route learning and shortcut performance in adults with intellectual disability: A study with virtual environments. *Research in Development Disabilities, 32*, 345-352. doi: 10.1016/j.ridd.2010.10.014

Mirza, M., & Hammel, J. (2009). Consumer-directed goal planning in the delivery of assistive technology services for people who are ageing with intellectual disabilities. *Journal of Applied Research in Intellectual Disabilities, 22*(5), 445-457. doi: 10.1111/j.1468-3148.2009.00495.x

Parsons, S., Daniels, H., Porter, J., & Robertson, C. (2008). Resources, staff beliefs and organizational culture: Factors in the use of information and communication technology for adults with intellectual disabilities. *Journal of Applied Research in Intellectual Disabilities, 21*, 19-33. doi: 10.1111/j.1468-3148.2007.00361.x

Ripat, J., & Booth, A. (2005). Characteristics of assistive technology service delivery models: Stakeholder perspectives and preferences. *Disability and Rehabilitation, 27*(24), 1461-1470. doi: 10.1080/09638280500264535

Sanford, J. A., & Fagan, L. A. (2004). Assistive technology to facilitate occupational performance in the home. *Technology Special Interest Section Quarterly*, 1-4.

Shpigelman, C. N., & Gill, C. J. (2014). How do adults with intellectual disabilities use Facebook? *Disability and Society*, *29*(10), 1601-1616. doi: 10.1111/jcc4.12059

Stow, J., & England, S. (2016). The rise of inclusive mainstream technology: Implications for occupational therapists. *British Journal of Occupational Therapy*, *79*(8), 457-458. doi: 10.1177/0308022616657110

Sutherland, D., van der Meer, L., Sigafoos, J., Mirfin-Veitch, B., Milner, P., O'Reilly, M. F., ... Lancioni, G. E. (2014). Survey of AAC needs for adults with intellectual disability in New Zealand. *Journal of Developmental and Physical Disabilities* *26*, 115-122. doi: 10.1007/s10882-013-9347-z

Technology. (n.d.). Merriam-Webster Online. Retrieved from http://www.merriam-webster.com/dictionary/technology

Wehmeyer, M. L., Palmer, S., Smith, S., Parent, W., Davies, D., & Stock, S. (2006). Technology use by people with intellectual and developmental disabilities to support employment activities: A single-subject design meta analysis. *Journal of Vocational Rehabilitation*, *24*, 81-86.

Wiederhold, B. K. (2015). Behavioral health apps abundant, but evidence-based research nearly nonexistent. *Cyberpsychology, Behavior and Social Networking*, *18*(6), 309-310. doi: 10.1089/cyber.2015.29001.bkw

Whittaker, S. G., Scheiman, M., & Sokol-McKay, D.A. (2016). Environmental modification. In S. G. Whittaker, M. Scheiman, & D. A. Sokol-McKay. (Eds.), *Low vision rehabilitation: A practical guide for occupational therapist.* (2nd ed., pp. 203-218). Thorofare, NJ: SLACK Incorporated.

Zabala, J. S. (2005). Using the SETT framework to level the learning field for students with disabilities. Retrieved from www.joyzabala.com/Documents.html

14

Peer Mentoring and Support

Alisa Jordan Sheth, PhD, OTR/L; Jenna Heffron, PhD, OTR/L; and Joy Hammel, PhD, OTR/L, FAOTA

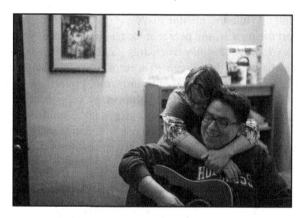

Key Words: community participation, health behaviors, peer mentoring, person-environment-occupation-performance model, Photovoice, post-secondary education, self-advocacy

Bryze, K.
Occupational Therapy for Adults With Intellectual Disability (pp. 161-171).
© 2020 Taylor & Francis Group.

The concept of the mentor dates back to ancient Greek mythology, although it has increasingly been formally conceptualized, utilized, and studied in the United States in recent decades. While there are many available definitions of mentoring, they typically involve a relationship where a person with certain experiences or skill-sets provides advice, teaching, or help to a less-experienced person. Since the 1970s, mentoring has gained increasing utilization and study as a strategy to improve career outcomes, such as job satisfaction and promotion opportunities, across a wide variety of fields (Allen, Eby, Poteet, Lentz, & Lima, 2004). It is also a common intervention utilized with youth, particularly those identified as at-risk for negative outcomes, such as limited academic achievement or criminal behavior, and is seen throughout secondary and post-secondary educational programs (National Mentoring Partnership, 2016). Mentoring for youth and in professional settings often involves not only an experience gap but also an age gap, serving to provide exposure to new opportunities, coaching, role modeling, and affirmation (Allen et al., 2004). However, mentoring can be applied to many populations and settings beyond traditional youth and employment programs. Since its rise to popularity in various aspects of vocational and educational domains, different variations of traditional methods have emerged. For those in the occupational therapy field, structured mentoring programs are often developed for students (Jacobs, Doyle, & Ryan, 2015; Milner & Bossers, 2004), for faculty (Falzarano & Zipp, 2012; Provident, 2006), and as a means for ongoing professional development for practitioners (Cusick, Johnson, & Bissett, 2010; Le Maistre, Boudreau, & Paré, 2006).

One such variation, peer mentoring, has developed as a mutual support model where people are typically closer in experience level or age and are able to provide each other with guidance (Ensher, Thomas, & Murphy, 2001). While the mentor may have slightly more experience and training in how to successfully assist the mentee, the peer mentor relationship is designed to provide opportunities for growth and development for all participants (Gillman, 2006). Peer mentors and mentees typically share common characteristics, circumstances, or interests. The potential power of shared or similar experiences between peers differs significantly from professional/client relationships, and this model has increasingly been implemented within many support and resource programs for people with disabilities, often based on diagnostic or experiential similarities. The growing body of research, detailing the use of peer mentoring strategies with adults with intellectual disability, will be explored, including the theoretical background underpinning these programs and applications to occupational therapy.

THEORETICAL BACKGROUND

Peer mentoring, and its use with people with intellectual disability, draws from a variety of theoretical backgrounds and frames of reference. One major influence is social cognitive theory (Bandura, 1986), which emphasizes the importance of the social environment for learning and acquiring knowledge. Modeling, imitating, and observing others, such as peer mentors, are strategies important to personal or social processes. Social cognitive theory can be related to health-promotion and occupational therapy. As individuals observe and learn from each other, such "socially mediated pathways" (Bandura, 2004, p. 151) help to connect individuals to varied networks and communities of information, support, and navigation that can meet their unique and individualized needs. These influences can affect people's perceived self-efficacy and significantly impact learning and change. Higher levels of self-efficacy can lead to goal achievement; successful knowledge translation can lead to behavior change and to more positive experiences.

Building on social cognitive theory's emphasis on self-efficacy, empowerment theory is also influential in the development of peer mentoring in occupational therapy interventions. While the concept can have a variety of definitions and operate on individual, community, and systemic levels, empowerment is a process focused on individuals gaining and exerting control over their lives through awareness and participation (Zimmerman & Warschausky, 1998). As rehabilitation sciences and related fields have transitioned over recent decades to be more client- and consumer-oriented, empowerment theory has become more commonly used as a guide for practice. As such, professionals are regarded less as experts and more as collaborators with service recipients in order to achieve goals and promote self-determination and self-advocacy. The knowledge and experiences of people with disabilities is seen as important to acknowledge, cultivate, and share, aligning it squarely with the use of peer mentors. These beliefs align with those of occupational therapy as it envisions "our goals will be our clients' goals, based on their needs and values" (Law, 1991, p. 176). Occupational therapy practitioners' use of empowerment theory will guide clients to utilize their strengths and address environmental barriers to maximize meaningful engagement and performance (Redick, McClain, & Brown, 2000). Peer mentoring can be seen as one intervention element to encourage empowerment within occupational therapy services.

Incorporating many tenants of empowerment theory, but specifically conceptualized with people with intellectual disability in mind, the Mutual Support Model (Keyes & Brandon, 2012) is another frame of reference influential to the use of peer mentoring in interventions. The model specifically discusses the importance of peer mentoring as a way to educate and capitalize on the strengths and needs of different members of groups or communities of people with intellectual disability. Concepts common to other models and theories related to peer mentoring include accessing supports and addressing barriers through collaboration and encouragement. The Mutual Support Model also illuminates some elements that may be more unique to the experience of people with intellectual disability, such as the importance of accessible communication and the interactions between people with and without disabilities. The Mutual Support Model also incorporates the social model of disability, which examines the impact of physical and attitudinal barriers in society on people with physical or cognitive impairments, and emphasizes the role that social environments have on creating disability (Oliver, 1990). The model views supports among people with intellectual disability and those without disabilities (i.e., non-disabled allies) as essential to addressing these barriers and working towards more inclusion and increased participation within communities and society.

A common thread among these theories, frameworks, and models informing peer mentoring, is the interaction between the individual and the social elements within the larger environment. As such, the person-environment-occupation (Law et al., 1996) and person-environment-occupation-performance models (Christiansen, Baum, & Bass, 2014) can help inform occupational therapy professionals who utilize peer mentoring in their practice. The interactions between the person and the physical, cultural, economic, political, and social environments are vital. These interactions also incorporate the role of the occupation, or specific tasks, and activities that are meaningful to a person, and all of these elements combine to impact a person or community's functioning or performance. This performance is also seen as a way that individuals connect and are part of their larger environments, leading to multiple pathways of influence and connectedness. Therefore, the interactions between the people with intellectual disability and their peers, within the larger social environment, are seen as powerful forces upon occupational performance.

PEER MENTORING AND ADULTS WITH INTELLECTUAL DISABILITY

Peer mentoring has increasingly been incorporated into various interventions for adults with intellectual disability, including those related to community participation, post-secondary education, and health behaviors. Table 14-1 highlights recent research from diverse fields and covers various content areas that specifically identify and utilize peer mentoring as an intervention element for adults with intellectual disability.

As noted in Table 14-1, peer mentoring can develop from a variety of sources. For example, some programs, specific to post-secondary education, utilized students without intellectual disability, typically those studying health science or educational fields, as the mentors (Jones & Goble, 2012; O'Brien et al., 2009; Shields, Taylor, & Dodd, 2008; Stanish & Temple, 2012). Another program used older adults without disabilities, who were involved in community organizations or volunteering

TABLE 14-1. EXAMPLES OF PROGRAMS USING PEER MENTORING FOR ADULTS WITH INTELLECTUAL DISABILITY						
NAME	**FOCUS**	**TARGET POPULATION**	**SETTING**	**PEER MENTORS**	**PEER MENTOR TRAINING**	**ROLE OF PEER MENTORS**
Active Mentoring Program (Chng, Stancliffe, Wilson, & Anderson, 2013; Wilson et al., 2013)	Transitioning into retirement; active aging	Adults with intellectual disability working in segregated supported employment (i.e., sheltered workshops) but close to retiring	Local community senior centers or groups	Staff, volunteers, or group members without disabilities at the senior centers/groups	Disability interaction training and interactive support training	Providing basic and task-specific support throughout group activities
Certificate in Contemporary Living (O'Brien et al., 2009)	Post-secondary university education	Young adults with intellectual disability	University campus	Occupational therapy and speech-language students	Not specified	Taking classes with students; supporting participation
Team Up For Fitness (Stanish & Temple, 2012)	Community-based exercise	Young adults with intellectual disability	Local YMCA gyms	Young adults without intellectual disability	Formal training in providing support	Engaging in exercise program with participants with intellectual disability, offering encouragement, monitoring for safety, teaching technique
Going Walkabout Together Through the Suburbs (Lloyd, 2009)	Community-based living support	Community-dwelling adults with intellectual disability and/or mental illness	Various community meetings and workshops	Adults with intellectual disability and/or mental illness participating in a community project including workshops on service-user experiences and perspectives	No formal training	Sharing personal stories related to community living and navigating service systems, providing support and feedback for others

(continued)

TABLE 14-1. EXAMPLES OF PROGRAMS USING PEER MENTORING FOR ADULTS WITH INTELLECTUAL DISABILITY (CONTINUED)

NAME	FOCUS	TARGET POPULATION	SETTING	PEER MENTORS	PEER MENTOR TRAINING	ROLE OF PEER MENTORS
Peer to Peer: Health Messages Program (Marks, Sisirak, Medlen, & Magallanes, 2012)	Health behaviors, physical activity, nutrition, etc.	Adults with intellectual disability	Community-based organizations for people with intellectual disability	Undergraduate students without intellectual disability majoring in general and special education	Orientation and ongoing assignments as part of service-learning course	Attending classes, campus events, and studying with students with intellectual disability; providing accommodations
Peer-Mentored Preparation (Eiseman et al., 2014)	Disaster preparedness	Community-dwelling adults with intellectual disability	Community-based organizations	Community-dwelling adults with intellectual disability	Formal training on program content, mentoring, leadership, and motivation	Ensuring participation in program activities, leading small group exercises, facilitating activities, acting as role models
Strength Training (Shields et al., 2008)	Progressive resistance training	Young adults with Down syndrome	Local, community gyms	Physical therapy students	Formal training on progressive resistance training program and supporting participants; ongoing monitors	Completing a log book of training session, providing teaching and motivation as needed
Inclusive Individual Support Model (Jones & Goble, 2012)	Post-secondary education	Young adults with intellectual disability	University campus	Undergraduate students without intellectual disability, majoring in general and special education	Orientation and ongoing assignments as part of service-learning course	Attending classes, campus events, and studying with students with intellectual disability; providing accommodations

opportunities, to assist with the inclusion of adults with intellectual disability who were in the process of transitioning from sheltered workshops into retirement (Wilson et al., 2013). While in these instances the peer mentors did not share a common disability category with the mentees, they did share similarities, such as occupational role or similarity in age or position in their season of life.

Other interventions utilized peer mentors with intellectual disability, often in a co-leader role with a professional without intellectual disability (Eisenman et al., 2014; Factor et al., 2010; Marks et al., 2012). Often, these mentors had also participated in the program as a mentee and had transitioned to serve as facilitators of small-group activities, provide individual assistance as needed, encourage member participation, and provide modeling or demonstration. In other program models, mentoring was provided by peers with varied disabilities who had a shared experience, such as living with a disability in the community or being a service consumer (Lloyd, 2009). The amount and type of training for peer mentors with intellectual disability varied depending on expectations of the mentor-mentee relationship and the previous knowledge or experience of the mentors.

The use of peer mentoring, regardless of who served as the mentors, has been shown to have many benefits for adults with intellectual disability. Mentorship assists in improving social inclusion and interaction opportunities for the mentees with intellectual disability, as well as increased access through individualized supports or adaptations, to encourage meaningful engagement in a variety of contexts and environments (O'Brien et al., 2009; Jones & Goble, 2012; Wilson et al., 2013). Mentorship also promotes increased participation in activities for adults with intellectual disability, particularly in promoting health-related behaviors, such as engagement in exercise or nutrition programs, rather than programs that do not provide these tailored supports (Marks et al., 2012; Shields et al., 2008). The provision of modeling and supports can be powerful tools to create more inclusive programs that promote self-expression and opportunities to learn from others, instead of those programs that rely solely on professional or authority-driven supports (Lloyd, 2009; Stanish & Temple, 2012). Participation in these programs can also prompt adults with intellectual disability to become interested in becoming mentors and advocates, not only for themselves, but for others with intellectual disability as well (O'Brien et al., 2009). The positive impact of peer mentoring for adults with intellectual disability actively reflects its theoretical background in behavior change, self-efficacy, and empowerment.

Mentors also benefit from participation in these interventions. Those without intellectual disability report more inclusive attitudes and behaviors toward peers with disabilities, as well as overall transformed views on disability (Jones & Goble, 2012; Wilson et al., 2009). Positive attitudinal changes toward disability have also been observed beyond the mentor-mentee dyad, with impacts felt throughout the larger social environments of these programs (O'Brien et al., 2009). Mentoring can be a particularly valuable experience for those studying to work with people with disabilities in the future, by giving opportunities to gain experience in making adaptations, implementing person-centered planning, effectively communicating with those with various abilities, and promoting self-advocacy (Jones & Goble, 2012). Mentors have also described perceived improvements in their leadership and collaboration skills (Wilson et al., 2013). The benefits of mentoring are shared by all involved in the relationship, not just those directly receiving services.

While the literature on peer mentoring does not specifically include occupational therapy, there are wide-reaching implications for occupational therapy professionals working with adults with intellectual disability. Given the established use of peer mentoring programs for adults pursuing post-secondary education, occupational therapy professionals working with students transitioning out of high schools to college could be instrumental in assisting their clients in accessing these programs, as well as consulting with universities and peer mentors without disabilities to provide supports to help those with intellectual disability participate in meaningful occupations related to the college student role. In post-secondary environments, involving occupational therapy students in peer-mentoring programs may provide valuable experiences in working with adults with intellectual disability and developing skills that may help them professionally, such as effective communication and activity adaptation. These experiences can also encourage students to interact with people with intellectual disability in non-clinical contexts and provide meaningful insight into the experiences of people with intellectual disability, including discrimination and other social barriers, which will help inform their practice in the future.

Occupational therapy professionals providing educational groups related to health behaviors, social interaction, community living skills, or other occupations, should consider the use of peer mentors who have disabilities in their programming. While groups may not start with peer mentors, group leaders can identify members who may be able to assume more leadership roles in subsequent groups to support group members in accessing intervention content and achieving goals.

CASE EXAMPLE

Photovoice Peer-Mentoring Program Overview

A team of researchers at the University of Illinois at Chicago used peer mentoring and Photovoice to understand supports and barriers to community participation for adults with intellectual disability (Heffron, Spassiani, Angell, & Hammel, 2018; Spassiani, Hammel, & Heffron, 2016). Peer mentors with intellectual disability supported participants throughout the research, and additional peer-mentoring relationships emerged during the Photovoice intervention and supported community participation.

Participants

Study participants were 30 years of age or older, residing in community-based settings in or around Chicago, and had diagnoses of mild to moderate intellectual disability. All participants provided informed consent and authorized the use of their photographs and Photovoice books for research and teaching purposes.

Method

Participants identified participation goals and worked with a peer mentor and an access specialist to choose, plan, and go on community outings related to these goals. While on community outings, participants (once again with peer mentor and access specialist support) conducted in-context audits by taking photographs of supports and barriers they considered to be influencing or interfering with their ability to participate in the community. After the outings, participants discussed how their photos represented supports and/or barriers to community participation for them. This process of using photography to document, reflect on, and critically discuss community issues is called *Photovoice* (Wang & Burris, 1997). Photovoice has been shown to support people with intellectual disability's engagement in action and advocacy, improve therapist-client relationships and understandings of community's strengths and needs, and support individual empowerment (Catalani & Minkler, 2010). In this research, Photovoice was coupled with peer mentoring, as a method for supporting active engagement in the research process and meaningful participation in the community.

Outcomes

During the community outings, it became clear that peer support and mentoring were facilitating participants' community participation. For example, participants worked together to strategize and problem solve their participation, as evidenced by linking arms while navigating through a crowd, helping each other purchase library cards, order food, and use public transportation. Further, the Photovoice process itself became a way for participants to support and mentor one another. Participants who had more experience using disposable cameras helped others who were newer to photography, and after the outings participants discussed their photographs together, pointing out helpful supports and advising each other about barriers they encountered. Both during and upon completion of the study, several participants reported an interest in participating in continued peer mentoring relationships, such as with groups like People First. Participants found meaning in both mentoring and being mentored by their peers, while choosing, planning, and going on community outings and Photovoice further facilitated these mentoring relationships. Further, the combination of peer mentoring and Photovoice resulted in an improved understanding of supports and barriers to community participation from the perspectives of people with intellectual disability.

Implications for Occupational Therapy

Occupational therapy practitioners are experts in evaluating and facilitating the person-environment fit, making them well equipped to support meaningful community participation for people with intellectual disability (Ideishi, D'Amico, & Jirikowic, 2013). Occupational therapy practitioners can further support client participation and carryover of skills into daily life by incorporating the experiential expertise of peer mentors into practice. Peer mentors can provide clients with firsthand accounts of environmental supports and barriers that practitioners might not be familiar with. In this way, the client, peer mentor, and occupational therapy practitioner can each contribute their own unique expertise to problem solve actual or potential participation concerns. This sharing of knowledge and lived experiences can enhance clients' ability to problem solve and participate in context.

Peer mentors can be recruited from support groups, centers for independent living, and other disability service agencies. They may also be former clients a practitioner knows to be knowledgeable and experienced in areas relevant to the client's situation. When choosing peer mentors, practitioners should consider age, personality, communication style, and other factors to ensure a good mentor-mentee fit. Peer mentors should be trained to facilitate client problem solving without being overly directive. Photovoice can be used to facilitate mentor-mentee relationships and to identify and negotiate participation barriers and supports. In addition to incorporating peer mentors into practice, occupational therapy practitioners can also refer clients to peer mentors outside of a clinical context. In either case, peer mentors can be a valuable resource for clients and can complement or enhance the usefulness of occupational therapy interventions to more fully support participation for people with intellectual disability.

INFORMAL PEER MENTORING AND SUPPORT

It is important to note that peer mentoring can also occur in more informal contexts. Self-advocacy groups for adults with intellectual disability, such as People First (2016) and Self-Advocates Becoming Empowered (2019), were created by and for people with intellectual disability to foster opportunities to exert more control over their lives, through understanding their rights and communicating choices and decisions. While many groups do have non-disabled allies and professional support, ideally, the primary control remains with the members, who set agendas and run the meetings, with emphasis on working together interdependently and using community building to achieve group goals. Examination of these groups highlight the natural opportunities for members to establish mentoring support for each other, such as reading materials aloud for those with limited literacy and encouraging each other to participate or take on more leadership roles within the group (Garcia-Iriarte, Kramer, Kramer, & Hammel, 2009). Participation in these groups has also been illustrated to help build confidence for adults with intellectual disability through educating members on their rights to receive support, as well as fostering their ability to provide support to others (Williams & Porter, 2015).

As one member of People First of California reported:

> When I first went to a [People First] support group, I felt scared to talk in front of the group with all these people. I heard other people talking and not being judged I felt safe, and WOW, I felt my voice coming out. Now, I have so much passion … and people can't shut me up! (People First of California Member, 2010)

On a more community and societal level, engaging in peer support, such as that of People First, Self-Advocates Becoming Empowered, or other self-advocacy groups, is believed to empower adults with intellectual disability to challenge larger attitudinal barriers they face, such as discrimination (Keyes & Brandon, 2012). While many of these groups may not utilize formal peer mentoring approaches, the benefits of opportunities to give and receive support from others with intellectual disability are numerous. Occupational therapy professionals should consider assisting their clients in connecting with these community resources or incorporating elements of mutual support into their services as much as possible.

For adults with intellectual disability, it is important to note that siblings are a critical source of informal support and mentoring. This can be particularly vital as people with intellectual disability get older and their traditional caregiving networks (e.g., parents) become less able to maintain previous levels of support, as they experience their own increasing support needs as they age (Kramer, Hall, & Heller, 2013). Siblings are often the family members who assume caregiving roles, but the relationship has been found to operate reciprocally, as all family members assume increased responsibilities within the family unit, while non-disabled siblings help to access community resources and networks (Kramer et al., 2013). Organizations such as the Sibling Leadership Network (SLN, 2016) provide advocacy opportunities for siblings of adults with intellectual disability, and encourage collaboration between siblings with and without disabilities, to address causes and concerns important to this population. Identifying and working with an individual's networks of support is essential to providing client-centered and effective services.

CONCLUSION

Although there is little research on peer mentoring for adults with intellectual disability within occupational therapy literature, other sources suggest that this is a beneficial component to interventions addressing a wide range of occupational areas, from education to health behaviors to community participation. Formal peer mentoring, either using mentors with or without disabilities, where mentors are trained to provide supports depending on the context and needs of the mentee, has been shown to have multiple positive outcomes for all participants, regardless of role. Based in varied theoretical frameworks, peer mentoring for adults with intellectual disability encourages behavior change, skill building, self-efficacy, empowerment, and improved occupational performance. Accessing informal networks of support, such as self-advocacy groups and sibling networks, can also be important to adults with intellectual disability and critical for ensuring their participation in meaningful occupations. Peer mentoring and support can be a powerful tool for occupational therapy practitioners to use when working with this population, whether in structured group environments or referrals to community resources.

REFERENCES

Allen, T. D., Eby, L. T., Poteet, M. L., Lentz, E., & Lima, L. (2004). Career benefits associated with mentoring for proteges: A meta-analysis. *Journal of Applied Psychology, 89*, 127-136.

Bandura, A. (1986). *Social foundations of thought and action: A social cognitive theory.* Upper Saddle River, NJ. Prentice Hall, Inc.

Bandura, A. (2004). Health promotion by social cognitive means. *Health Education & Behavior, 31*, 143-164.

Catalani, C., & Minkler, M. (2010). Photovoice: A review of the literature in health and public health. *Health Education & Behavior, 37*, 424-451.

Chng, J. P. L., Stancliffe, R. J., Wilson, N. J., & Anderson, K. (2013). Engagement in retirement: An evaluation of the effect of active mentoring on engagement of older adults with intellectual disability in mainstream community groups. *Journal of Intellectual Disability Research, 57*, 1130-1142.

Christiansen, C. H., Baum, C. M., & Bass, J. D. (2014). *Occupational therapy: Performance, participation, and well-being* (4th ed.). Thorofare, NJ: SLACK Incorporated.

Cusick, A., Johnson, L., & Bissett, M. (2010). Continuing professional development for occupational therapy emergency department services. *Australian Occupational Therapy Journal, 57*, 380-385.

Ensher, E. A., Thomas, C., & Murphy, S. E. (2001). Comparison of traditional, step-ahead, and peer mentoring on protégés' support, satisfaction, and perceptions of career success: A social exchange perspective. *Journal of Business and Psychology, 15*, 419-438.

Eisenman, D. P., Bazzano, A., Koniak-Griffin, D., Tseng, C. H., Lewis, M. A., Lamb, K., & Lehrer, D. (2014). Peer-mentored preparedness (PM-Prep): A new disaster preparedness program for adults living independently in the community. *Intellectual and Developmental Disabilities, 52*, 49-59.

Factor, A, DeBrine, E., Caldwell, J., Arnold, K., Nelis, T., & Heller, T. (2010). *The future is now: A future planning training curriculum for families and their adult relatives with developmental disabilities* (3rd ed. rev.). Chicago, IL: University of Illinois at Chicago.

Falzarano, M., & Zipp, G. P. (2012). Perceptions of mentoring of full-time occupational therapy faculty in the United States. *Occupational Therapy International, 19*, 117-126.

Garcia-Iriarte, E., Kramer, J. C., Kramer, J. M., & Hammel, J. (2009). 'Who did what?': A participatory action research project to increase group capacity for advocacy. *Journal of Applied Research in Intellectual Disabilities, 22*, 10-22

Gilman, D. (2006). *The power of peer mentoring.* Waisman Center, University of Wisconsin–Madison. Retrieved from http://www2.waisman.wisc.edu/hrtw/PPM.pdf

Heffron, J. L., Spassiani, N. A., Angell, A. M., & Hammel, J. (2018). Using Photovoice as a participatory method to identify and strategize community participation with people with intellectual and developmental disabilities. *Scandinavian Journal of Occupational Therapy, 25*(5), 382-395. doi: 10.1080/11038128.2018.1502350.

Ideishi, R., D'Amico, M., & Jirikowic, T. (2013). *AOTA fact sheet: Supporting community integration and participation for individuals with intellectual disabilities.* Bethesda, MD: American Occupational Therapy Association.

Jacobs, K., Doyle, N., & Ryan, C. (2015). The nature, perception, and impact of e-mentoring on post-professional occupational therapy doctoral students. *Occupational Therapy in Health Care, 29*, 201-213.

Jones, M. M., & Goble, Z. (2012). Creating effective mentoring partnerships for students with intellectual disabilities on campus. *Journal of Policy and Practice in Intellectual Disabilities, 9*, 270-278.

Keyes, S. E., & Brandon, T. (2012). Mutual support: A model of participatory support by and for people with learning difficulties. *British Journal of Learning Disabilities, 40*, 222-228.

Kramer, J., Hall, A., & Heller, T. (2013). Reciprocity and social capital in sibling relationships of people with disabilities. *Intellectual and Developmental Disabilities, 51*, 482-495.

Law, M. (1991). The environment: A focus for occupational therapy. *Canadian Journal of Occupational Therapy, 58*, 171-179.

Law, M., Cooper, B., Strong, S., Stewart, D., Rigby, P., & Letts, L. (1996). The person-environment-occupation model: A transactive approach to occupational performance. *Canadian Journal of Occupational Therapy, 63*, 9-23.

Le Maistre, C., Boudreau, S., & Paré, A. (2006). Mentor or evaluator? Assisting and assessing newcomers to the professions. *Journal of Workplace Learning, 18*, 344-354.

Lloyd, R. (2009). How the all fruits salad creates sweeter futures in rural and remote mental health. *Australasian Psychiatry, 17*(Suppl. 1), S142-S145.

Marks, B., Sisirak, J., Medlen, J. & Magallanes, E. (2012). *Peer to peer health messages program: Becoming a healthy lifestyle coach.* Chicago, IL: Rehabilitation Research and Training Center on Aging with Developmental Disabilities.

Milner, T., & Bossers, A. (2004). Evaluation of the mentor-mentee relationship in an occupational therapy mentorship programme. *Occupational Therapy International, 11*, 96-111.

National Mentoring Partnership. (2016). Mentoring impact. Retrieved from http://www.mentoring.org/why-mentoring/mentoring-impact

Oliver, M. (1990). *The politics of disablement*. Basingstoke, United Kingdom: Macmillan.

People First (2016). What is people first? Retrieved from www.peoplefirst.org

People First of California. (2010). Peer to peer get-together guide. Retrieved from https://static1.squarespace.com/static/5823ce091b631b02ca6b6f60/t/5823fd8e8419c2fcb11bcd03/1478753687113/PFCA+Peer+to+Peer+Book.pdf

Provident, I. M. (2006). Outcomes of selected cases from the American Occupational Therapy Foundation's curriculum mentoring project. *American Journal of Occupational Therapy, 60*, 563-576.

O'Brien, P., Shevlin, M., O'Keefe, M., Fitzgerald, S., Curtis, S., & Kenny, M. (2009). Opening up a whole new world for students with intellectual disabilities within a third level setting. *British Journal of Learning Disabilities, 37*(4), 285-292.

Redick, A. G., McClain, L., & Brown, C. (2000). Consumer empowerment through occupational therapy: The Americans with Disabilities Act Title III. *American Journal of Occupational Therapy, 54*, 207-213.

Self-Advocates Becoming Empowered. (2019). About SABE. Retrieved from www.sabeusa.org/meet-sabe

Shields, N., Taylor, N. F., & Dodd, K. J. (2008). Effects of a community-based progressive resistance training program on muscle performance and physical function in adults with Down syndrome: A randomized controlled trial. *Archives of Physical Medicine and Rehabilitation, 89*, 1215-1220.

Sibling Leadership Network. (2016). Our mission and core values. Retrieved from http://siblingleadership.org/about

Spassiani, N., Hammel, J., & Heffron, J. (2016). Using Photovoice to increase awareness of barriers and supports to community participation as identified by adults with I/DD living in the community. Manuscript in preparation.

Stanish, H. I., & Temple, V. A. (2012). Efficacy of a peer-guided exercise programme for adolescents with intellectual disability. *Journal of Applied Research in Intellectual Disabilities, 25*, 319-328.

Wang, C. C., & Burris, M. (1997). Photovoice: Concept, methodology, and use for participatory needs assessment. *Health Education & Behavior, 24*, 369-387.

Williams, V., & Porter, S. (2015). The meaning of 'choice and control' for people with intellectual disabilities who are planning their social care and support. *Journal of Applied Research in Intellectual Disabilities*. doi:10.1111/jar.12222

Wilson, N. J., Bigby, C., Stancliffe, R. J., Balandin, S., Craig, D., & Anderson, K. (2013). Mentors' experiences of using the active mentoring model to support older adults with intellectual disability to participate in community groups. *Journal of Intellectual and Developmental Disability, 38*, 344-355.

Zimmerman, M. A., & Warschausky, S. (1998). Empowerment theory for rehabilitation research: Conceptual and methodological issues. *Rehabilitation Psychology, 43*, 3-16.

15

Person-Centered Planning

Susan M. Cahill, PhD, OTR/L, FAOTA

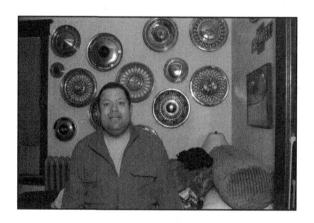

Key Words: facilitator, person-centered planning, supported decision making

Bryze, K.
Occupational Therapy for Adults With Intellectual Disability (pp. 173-181).
© 2020 Taylor & Francis Group.

As services for individuals with intellectual disability have moved into the community, the need for transition plans that support community engagement has become critical (Martin, Grandia, Ouellette-Kuntz, & Cobigo, 2015). Transition out of high school and into post-secondary life can prove challenging for many individuals, and developing plans to support successful transitions can help mediate the experience for both the individual with intellectual disability and his or her family members (Kim & Turnbull, 2004). The concept of person-centered planning emerged in the 1980s and is now widely used to support the transitions of individuals with intellectual disability (Claes, Van Hove, Vandevelde, van Loon, & Schalock, 2010).

Different from traditional planning models, where professionals plan for the individual with intellectual disability (Martin et al., 2015), person-centered planning models are used to actively engage the individual with intellectual disability in the planning process (Claes et al., 2010; Martin et al., 2015). Person-centered planning is focused on the development of collaborative goals and individualized plans that promote community presence and participation, positive friendships, and life skill development (Claes et al., 2010). Person-centered planning is future oriented and grounded in the hopes and dreams of the individual with intellectual disability and his or her family (O'Brien & O'Brien, 2000).

Individuals with intellectual disability may benefit from person-centered planning during the transition between high school and post-secondary life. This chapter defines person-centered planning, provides a review of three popular person-centered planning models, and includes implications for practice. In addition, the case of Jacob is used to illustrate how one person-centered planning model was used by an occupational therapist working for a community agency that supports individuals with intellectual disability.

PERSON-CENTERED PLANNING MODELS

There are several different person-centered planning models that can be used by teams to help individuals with intellectual disability plan for transitions. While there are nuances to all of the models, they generally focus on documenting an individual's interests, strengths, fears, and goals; outlining the individual's past history; identifying the individual's current and potential social networks; and describing the steps that are needed to assist the individual in achieving his or her goals (Hagner, 2010). The planning process typically involves the individual with intellectual disability, family members, caregivers, and other allies (e.g., friends, community members, service providers). The meetings can be held in the family's home, at school, or in a community setting. The meetings are often run by a facilitator (i.e., an individual who will guide the process, but who will not participate directly by sharing his or her personal vision for the individual or offering solutions). The facilitator often generates a written document that archives the process and outlines any future action steps. In some instances, this document can take the form of flip-chart paper (Hagner, 2010) or in other cases, a more narrative form. Three of the most common models will be discussed here. All of the models are future focused, based on the strengths and interests of the person with intellectual disability, and geared at providing the necessary supports, so that he or she can be an actively engaged community member.

Personal Futures Planning

Personal Futures Planning (PFP) is a process that uses pictorial images and words to graphically depict who the person with intellectual disability is now and who that person would like to become, his or her ideas about the future, and the actions that are needed to move towards achievement of future goals (Mount, 2000). The PFP process is conducted with the person with intellectual disability, as well as individuals who have been identified as potential allies or supports. Everyone participating in the PFP process is encouraged to consider the client and his or her goals within the context of what Mount (2000) calls *windows for change*. These windows for change help to describe the important people, places, and resources that can lead to the person with intellectual disability achieving his or her future goals. After the plan is developed, the individual with intellectual disability, and a smaller group of allies, get together somewhat frequently and revisit the plan to discuss challenges to implementation, identify additional resources, and revise the initial plan (Mount & O'Brien, 2002).

Essential Lifestyle Planning

Essential Lifestyle Planning (ELP) focuses on the individual's daily life and what is important to him or her (Smull & Sanderson, 2005). The ELP process can also be used to identify what the individual perceives as health or safety risks, and these perspectives are then balanced with perspectives of the individual's allies, family members, or caregivers (Smull & Sanderson, 2005). The product of the ELP process is a written document that includes four sections: an administrative section, the person's section, the support section, and the action section. The administrative section describes who the plan is for and how it was created. The person's section outlines his or her priorities, or what is perceived to be personally most important. The support section summarizes what is needed to keep the individual safe and healthy and, when possible, who can implement such strategies. Finally, the action section includes a list of questions or concerns that still need to be addressed, as well as what aspects of the individual's life can be maintained and which need to be changed to keep the individual safe and healthy.

Planning Alternative Tomorrows with Hope and the McGill Action Planning System

Planning Alternative Tomorrows with Hope (PATH) and the McGill Action Planning System (MAPS; O'Brien, Pearpoint, & Kahn, 2010) are two complimentary group processes that are used by teams to help individuals with intellectual disability move toward attainable goals. The PATH process is based on the individual's vision for himself or herself. This future vision is presented in pictures and images and is often based on the individual's hopes and dreams related to where he or she hopes to reside, how the individual hopes to spend time (e.g., at work, at vocational school, or on vacation), and with whom the individual wants to share his or her life (i.e., social connections) (Armstrong & Dorsett, 2015; O'Brien et al., 2010). The MAPS process is often used in conjunction with PATH and is used to clarify the unique gifts that are possessed by the individual with intellectual disability and leads the team to consider how to best capitalize on these gifts to provide opportunities for further growth and life satisfaction.

PERSON-CENTERED PLANNING MODELS IN PRACTICE

The person-centered planning process can be initiated by an individual with intellectual disability, his or her family members, or members of his or her team. Regardless of how the process gets started, the individual with intellectual disability must always be present and actively participate to the extent that he or she is able (Martin et al., 2015). Efforts should be taken to ensure the person with intellectual disability also understands the purpose of the meeting (Dumas, De La Garza, Seay, & Becker, 2002).

Unlike some other meetings, person-centered planning meetings are generally attended by participants on a voluntary basis (Hanger, 2010). These meetings are time intensive, and teams working in traditional systems are sometimes challenged to engage in authentic, person-centered planning due to beliefs that individuals with intellectual disability are unable to make their own decisions (Claes et al., 2010). However, teams that can dedicate adequate time to the person-planning process and value supported-decision making will have successful outcomes.

The concept of supported decision making is closely tied to self-determination and has been shown to improve post-secondary outcomes for people with disabilities in the United States (Blanck & Martinis, 2015). Supported decision making is used by most adults when making informed decisions. The process generally involves asking knowledgeable and trusted friends and family for advice before taking action (Blanck & Martinis, 2015). All the person-centered planning models encourage supported decision making, and the team may select a certain model over another based on their familiarity with the models, their access to resources, or their precise focus.

Once the person-centered planning model has been determined, a facilitator needs to be selected. A good facilitator should value person-centered planning and be committed to the process. In addition, the facilitator should have a true desire to support the individual with intellectual disability, be willing to assist with inviting other allies, create a welcoming environment that supports participation for all group members and have well-developed group facilitation skills (Amado & McBride, 2001). A good facilitator is "non-judgmental, a good listener, self-confident, flexible, genuine, and hospitable" (Amado & McBride, 2001, p. 17).

The role of the facilitator is to expedite the person-centered planning process. To do this, the facilitator must always keep the individual with intellectual disability and his or her concerns and priorities in the foreground. In addition, the facilitator resolves conflicts as they arise, works to build consensus related to needed resources and action items, and helps to construct a network of allies for the individual with intellectual disability (Amado & McBride, 2001).

In some cases, the facilitator will help the individual with intellectual disability and his or her family determine who will be invited to the person-centered planning meeting and assist with the production of invitations. Encouraging involvement of the individual with intellectual disability at all stages in the person-centered planning process, starting with guest list formation and production of invitations, will help to ensure that the process is truly person-directed (Eisenman, Chamberlin, & McGahee-Kovac, 2005). The facilitator might also enter into an inquiry process with the individual with intellectual disability to determine his or her perspectives on personal strengths, challenges, dreams, wishes, and nightmares (Amado & McBride, 2001; Eisenman et al., 2005). The facilitator would then collaborate with the individual to document this information, so it could later be shared with the team. Many of the person-centered planning resources provide worksheets and other graphic organizers to capture this information. In addition, the facilitator may assist the individual with intellectual disability in selecting an alternative format, such as a Microsoft PowerPoint presentation or a video.

The facilitator leads the planning meetings and takes notes, typically on a flip chart, to document the process (Hagner, 2010). During the meeting, the facilitator's most important function is to ensure that the perspectives of the individual with intellectual disability are honored. In addition, the facilitator will set the pace of the meeting, encourage the group to stay on task, and create an atmosphere where all members' opinions can be expressed freely (Amado & McBride, 2001). After the meeting has concluded, the facilitator will disseminate the planning document and follow up with team members regarding their action steps (Amado & McBride, 2001). If needed, the facilitator will also schedule and lead follow-up meetings.

Occupational therapy practitioners can engage in person-centered planning meetings as participants or facilitators. Occupational therapy practitioners may be effective facilitators because they possess an understanding of the demands that an individual with intellectual disability may face during the school-to-adult-life transition, including living away from parents, getting and maintaining employment, and the need to advocate for oneself (Juan & Swinth, 2010). The literature suggests that individuals with severe communication difficulties and challenging behaviors are often excluded from the planning process (Claes et al., 2010; Mansell & Beadle-Brown, 2004). However, occupational therapy practitioners can use multiple strategies to encourage the engagement of individuals with intellectual disability in the person-centered planning process. Further, occupational therapy practitioners can assist teams in framing a client's behaviors, such as expressing positive affect and showing focused attention, as engagement (Mahoney, Roberts, Bryze, & Parker Kent, 2016).

Case Example

Jacob is a 21-year-old, young adult who is getting ready to exit the public-school system. Jacob currently lives with his mom and dad in a suburban neighborhood, approximately 40 minutes outside of a large metropolitan city in the Midwestern United States. Jacob has three older sisters and a large, extended family. In general, Jacob and his family have been pleased with the education and services that Jacob received in school and feel satisfied with his transition plan. Jacob's transition plan was focused on his obtaining gainful employment, taking public transportation, and visiting a local health club. Jacob has achieved his transition goals and has been working as a bagger at local grocery store for over 1 year.

One of Jacob's cousins, Adam, recently moved out of his family's home and into an apartment in the city with two roommates. Jacob and his family visited Adam 2 weeks ago and ever since, Jacob has been telling his mom that he wants to get an apartment. Jacob's parents are in their 60s and starting to think seriously about where Jacob will live as they age.

Jacob's mom contacted a local community support agency that provides services to adults with intellectual disability and is connected with a person-centered planning facilitator. The person-centered planning facilitator, Diane, has a background in vocational education and is a licensed occupational therapist. Diane agrees to meet with Jacob and his parents to discuss person-centered planning. After learning more about the person-centered planning process, the family agrees it is the right choice for them. Diane determines that the PATH model (O'Brien et al., 2010) will be used to guide Jacob's person-centered planning process.

Forming the Team

Diane interviews Jacob and his parents to determine who Jacob would like to invite to his meeting. Diane explains that everyone invited to the meeting should be considered by Jacob as a confidant and a person willing to support him in reaching his goals. Diane, Jacob, and his parents talk about Jacob's daily routines and who he encounters daily. The group also looks through photo albums and discusses the pros and cons of inviting Jacob's particular family members and friends. At the close of the conversation, Jacob has decided to invite his oldest sister, his teacher, his job coach, both of his parents, and his cousin, Adam.

Diane shows Jacob a few sample meeting invitations, ranging from handmade cards to emails. Jacob decides that he would like to invite guests with handwritten invitations, but is worried that he will not be able to complete them soon enough to give people adequate time for the meeting. Diane designs a handwritten invitation template for Jacob to fill in and photocopies it at the community agency. Jacob and his mom address the invitations and take them to the post office to be mailed.

Setting Up the Environment

Jacob asked to have this meeting take place in his family's home. Jacob's parents were ultimately supportive of this decision, but had asked Jacob to consider a meeting room at the local library. Jacob chose the family's home because he wanted to have snacks at the meeting. Diane and Jacob discussed the snack options. Initially, Jacob was hoping to provide guests with pizza, pasta, salad, and breadsticks. Diane provided Jacob guidance on how these meetings typically flowed and encouraged him to select finger foods that could easily be eaten in the family's living room, away from a dining table. Jacob decided to offer cheese pizza cut into small squares. He deferred to his mom for beverage items and other snacks and she selected water, soft drinks, and vegetables and dip.

To further prepare for the meeting, Jacob, Diane, and Jacob's dad brought in a few folding chairs from the garage and arranged the living room furniture in a semicircle. They also set up a place for Diane that included a flip chart on an easel and different colored markers. Next to the flip chart, was another easel, which would hold a vision board (i.e., pictures that symbolize what Jacob wants for his future) that would later be created by Jacob, with his mom's support.

On the day of the person-centered planning meeting, Jacob greeted his guests and showed them to their seats. He also offered them refreshments. Diane provided each of the participants with small notebooks and pencils, so they could also take notes if desired. After brief introductions, Diane explained the person-centered planning process and objectives. She also informed all of the guests that they were invited here directly by Jacob because they were people he trusted and hoped would support him in reaching his goals.

The North Star (The Dream)

Diane led the group through the first step of the PATHS process. The step is referred to as the *North Star*, or the *Dream* (O'Brien et al., 2010). During this discussion, Diane asked Jacob what goals he wants to realize and what he is excited about. Jacob was a little nervous to speak in front of the group and referring to his vision board allowed him to participate in this step. After Jacob had shared his perspectives, Diane summarized Jacob's North Star:

> Jacob wants to be able to live in an apartment with friends, like Adam. He wants to take the bus or train to go to the library, try new restaurants, and attend baseball games. Jacob wants to do this with friends or family members but would also do it by himself. Jacob doesn't want to have to wait for someone to take him on outings. He wants to go on his own schedule. Jacob also wants to work in a bakery and learn how to make bread. Jacob might want to get married someday, but right now he just wants to meet girls that like the same movies, so that they can maybe go on a date.

The Goal

After reviewing Jacob's North Star, Diane suggested that the group keep in mind Jacob's perspectives and set a time frame (e.g., 6 months from now) and talk about what Jacob's day-to-day life would look like if he was making progress toward these goals. Diane encouraged the group to remember to frame these ideas positively. For example, Jacob's mom said that Jacob would be doing his laundry and Jacob's job coach said that he would be sending out applications to local bakeries. Diane then guided the group to develop some goals for Jacob.

> Jacob decided to set his goals for 1 year from the day of the meeting. Jacob said that in 1 year's time he would be doing his own laundry, getting up for work on his own, packing his lunch, and working at a bakery. Jacob also said that he would have gone to three baseball games with family members and that he would have gone to the movies, at least once, with just friends.

The Now

In the next part of the process, Diane brings everyone back from thinking about the future, to thinking about present day. Diane encourages Jacob and the rest of the group to brainstorm words and phrases that describe Jacob's current reality. The team says things like *reliant on others, bagger, safe, bus rider, hardworking,* and *fun to be around.* Diane draws a picture of an arrow on the flip chart. She writes the words that describe Jacob's Now on the left side and his North Star and his goals on the right side. Diane tells the group that this picture represents the path that Jacob will take to reach his goals in the next 6 months.

Enrolling Supports

The group took a short break before starting the next phase in the PATH process. When they regrouped, Diane asked Jacob, "Who can help you to achieve your goals?" This question was answered by Jacob and served as the backdrop to a larger discussion related to the people and resources that would be needed to help Jacob reach for his dreams. During this discussion, Jacob and his team discussed additional people, besides those who were present, would need to be included in the action plan for Jacob to meet his targeted goals. Jacob and his parents identified that his other two sisters, who also lived at home, could be a resource for Jacob related to doing laundry, getting up on time for work, and packing his lunch. Jacob and his job coach identified Jacob's current boss and a pastry chef at a local technical college, as supports for helping Jacob to obtain a job in a bakery. Jacob identified his cousin Adam for support with going to baseball games and two other cousins for going to the movies. Jacob also considered joining an adult recreation program at the park district to potentially meet new friends.

Getting Stronger

During this phase of the meeting, Diane stressed the amount of work it would take on everyone's part, especially Jacob's, to get him to the point of realizing his goals. Diane then encouraged all of the group members to speak about *"what it would take"* to be able to support each other through this process. Jacob and the people who attended his person-centered planning meeting came up with the following list:

- Engaging in regular communication between Jacob, his parents, and the other members of the group on the action steps.
- Providing Jacob and his family with opportunities to learn about the transition from living in one's family, to a home, to an apartment with friends, from other adults with intellectual disability who have made the transition.
- Providing Jacob with opportunities to try things out in a way that is safe but also allows for him to learn from his mistakes.
- Providing Jacob with opportunities to learn about the different jobs at a bakery and what he is interested in doing.

Action Planning

Diane then directed the group to think about what would need to happen within the next 3 months to reach his goals. Once these action steps were prioritized, she asked them to think about what needed to happen in the next 30 days. Diane asked Jacob and the members of his person-centered planning team to consider exactly what they would do, when they will do it, and where their actions would take place. Each group member spent some time writing down the steps that they would personally be responsible for in their notebooks. Then, they tore off their pages and turned them into Diane. Diane summarized the responses on the flip chart. One of the examples of the action steps that would be taken by group members comes from Jacob's cousin, Adam. Adam was going to help Jacob get to three baseball games in the city. The steps Adam wrote down with Jacob's input follow.

Three Months

- Take the train from the city to the stop near Jacob's house to look for potential challenges and safety considerations that might arise when Jacob rides alone.
- Take the train with Jacob from his train stop to the city. Help Jacob to identify challenges and safety considerations. We might have to do this a few times.
- Program my phone number into Jacob's phone. Teach Jacob how to text me when he is three stops from the city, so that I can meet him at the station.
- Get matching team shirts.

One Month

- Get team schedule.
- Get train schedule.
- Determine which games are a possibility based on the train schedule.
- Determine which games I can go to because of my work schedule.
- Contact Jacob and my aunt to see if the games that work for me also work for him.
- Buy tickets for the games that fit our schedules.

First Step

After all the action steps were compiled, Diane asked the group members which of the steps in the 1 month time period they were ready to do now. She asked them to be specific about when they would accomplish this step and to check in with each other at specific time intervals to promote accountability.

Adam shared that he would get the team schedule and the train schedule by the end of the weekend. Adam said he would email his uncle (Jacob's dad) to check in once he completed these two tasks.

Closing the Meeting

After the meetings' participants went around the room speaking about their commitments, Diane asked each of them to reflect on the person-centered planning process and to share their thoughts.

Some of the participants said words like hopeful and excited. Adam said, "I think this will help Jacob really be the man he wants to be." Jacob said, "I'm ready!"

CONCLUSION

Person-centered planning models can be used with persons with different types of medical conditions and disabilities, but are thought to be particularly beneficial when working with individuals with intellectual disability. Through person-centered planning, individuals with intellectual disability and their allies can practice supported decision making (Blanck & Martinis, 2015), which is particularly important as individuals transition out of high school into post-secondary life (Kim & Turnbull, 2004). This process allows individuals with disabilities to actively engage in the planning process, rather than having professionals and family members plan for them (Claes et al., 2010; Martin et al., 2015).

REFERENCES

Amado, A., & McBride, M. (2001). *A manual for person-centered planning facilitators.* Institute on Community Integration UAP, University of Minnesota. Retrieved from http://rtc.umn.edu/docs/pcpmanual1.pdf

Armstrong, M. L., & Dorsett, P. (2015). Panning for gold: The personal journey of mental health wellness and its relationships with Planning Alternatives Tomorrows with Hope (PATH). *Journal of Social Inclusion, 6*(2), 36-50.

Blanck, P., & Martinis, J. G. (2015). "The right to make choices": The National Resource Center on Supported Decision-Making. *Inclusion, 3*(1), 24-33.

Claes, C., Van Hove, G., Vandevelde, S., van Loon, J., & Schalock, R. (2010). Person-centered planning: Analysis of research and effectiveness. *Intellectual and Developmental Disabilities, 48*(6), 432-453.

Dumas, S., De La Garza, D., Seay, P., & Becker, H. (2002). I don't know how they made it happen, but they did. In S. Holburn & P. Vietze (Eds.), *Person-centered planning: Research, practice, and future directions* (pp. 223-246). Baltimore, MD: Brookes.

Eisenman, L., Chamberline, M., & McGahee-Kovac, M. (2005). A teacher inquiry group on student-led IEPs: Starting small to make a difference. *Teacher Education and Special Education, 28*(3-4), 195-206.

Hagner, D. (2010). The role of naturalistic assessment in vocational rehabilitation. *Journal of Rehabilitation, 76*(1), 28-34.

Juan, H., & Swinth, Y. (2010). As students become adults: The role of occupational therapy in the transition process. *Journal of Occupational Therapy, Schools, & Early Intervention, 3*(3), 255-267.

Kim, K., & Turnbull, A. (2004). Transition to adulthood for students with severe intellectual disabilities: Shifting toward person-family interdependent planning. *Research and Practice for Persons With Severe Disabilities, 29*(1), 53-57.

Mahoney, W. J., Roberts, E., Bryze, K., & Parker Kent, J. A. (2016). Occupational engagement and adults with intellectual disabilities. *American Journal of Occupational Therapy, 70,* 7001350030p1-6. doi: 10.5014/ajot.2016.016576

Mansell, J., & Beadle-Brown, J. (2004). Person-centered planning or person-centered action? A response to commentaries. *Journal of Applied Research in Intellectual Disabilities, 17,* 31-35.

Martin, L., Grandia, P., Ouellette-Kunz, H., & Cobigo, V. (2015). From framework to practice: Person-directed planning in the real world. *Journal of Applied Research in Intellectual Disabilities, 29*(6), 552-565.

Mount, B. (2000). *Person-centered planning: Finding directions for change using personal futures planning.* Amenia, NY: Capacity Works.

Mount, B., & O'Brien, C. L. (2002). *Building new worlds: A sourcebook for students with disabilities in transition from high school to adult life.* Amenia, NY: Capacity Works.

O'Brien, C. L., & O'Brien, J. (2000). The origins of person-centered planning: A community of practice perspective. ERIC. Retrieved from http://eric.ed.gov/?id=ED456599

O'Brien, J., Pearpoint, J., & Kahn, L. (2010). *The PATH and MAPS handbook—Person-centred ways to build community.* Toronto, ON, Canada: Inclusion Press.

Smull, M., & Sanderson, H. (2005). *Essential lifestyle planning for everyone.* Stockport, United Kingdom: HSA Press.

16

Preventative and Primary Care for Persons With Intellectual Disability

Monika Robinson, DrOT, OTR/L and Daniel Stumpf, OTR/L

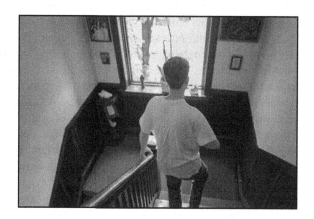

Key Words: chronic disease management, health promotion, interprofessional collaboration, occupational justice, primary care, tiered prevention

Bryze, K.
Occupational Therapy for Adults With Intellectual Disability (pp. 183-204).
© 2020 Taylor & Francis Group.

Individuals with intellectual disability face unique health challenges. Compared to the general population, people with intellectual disability are more likely to live with multiple medical morbidities that co-occur in patterns, such as mental health/neurologic, cardiovascular/metabolic, and liver/lung/joint/eye patterns (Hermans & Evenhuis, 2014; Perry et al., 2014). Higher incidences of hypothyroidism, obesity, epilepsy, dementia, asthma, type 2 diabetes, arthritis, periodontal infection, epilepsy, cardiovascular disease, and mental illness, as well as behavioral, visual, and hearing problems are associated with individuals with intellectual disability (Hermans & Evenhuis, 2014; Oguni, 2013). It is also well documented that there are higher incidences of multiple psychosocial health issues for people with diagnoses of intellectual disability compared to the general population, such as anxiety, depression, behavioral problems, anger control issues, suicidal tendencies, self-talk, loneliness, sleep problems, and stress (Melville et al., 2008; Merrick, Merrick, Lunsky, & Kandel, 2006; Scott & Havercamp, 2014).

People with intellectual disability are also at a higher risk for developing secondary conditions, which go undiagnosed or untreated, and experience, on average, 5.4 chronic health conditions (Lennox, Van Driel, & van Dooren, 2015). They are often undiagnosed or underdiagnosed due to numerous contributing factors, ranging from genetic pre-dispositions, poor access to preventative health services, limited health literacy, sedentary lifestyles, and frequent administration of prescriptive psychotropic drugs (Krahn & Fox, 2014; Perry et al., 2014). Consequently, compared to the general population, people with a diagnosis of intellectual disability have higher rates of emergency department visits, hospitalizations, hospital readmissions, and increased duration of stay (Axmon, Karlsson, & Ahlstrom, 2016; Ervin, Hennen, Merrick, & Morad, 2014).

The medical and social models of health often marginalize this population and do not promote primary care service participation for people with intellectual disability. The inability to meet the health care needs and provide prevention services for avoidable health conditions constitutes the existence of health inequities for this population (Lennox et al., 2015; Weise, Pollack, Britt, & Trollor, 2016). These health inequities lead to poorer health outcomes, which negatively affect quality of life and the capacity for social inclusion and participation. As a result, life expectancies are lower than the general population by approximately 20 years, noting an average life expectancy from the late 50s to mid-60s (Lauer & McCallion, 2015; Lennox et al., 2015). While the overall life span for individuals with a diagnosis of intellectual disability is reduced compared to the general population, advancements in medicine have prolonged their life expectancy compared to previous decades.

As occupational therapy practitioners, we view individuals as occupational beings and advocate for participation and inclusion by addressing their occupational needs for meaningful engagement and enhanced quality of life. As occupational scientists, we realize that social inclusion and participation are related to occupation and that the performance of occupation is inseparable from the surrounding social or community issues (Cutchin & Dickie, 2012). Consequently, exclusion of people with intellectual disability from mainstream health care services, such as primary care interventions, results in poorer health outcomes and reduced participation in meaningful activities.

This population exhibits limited function in areas of self-care, communication, and literacy that restricts their ability to establish good health and their access to health care services compared to non-disabled individuals (Ouellette-Kuntz, 2005). The limited affordance of good health and reduced participation, which is outside of the control of individuals with intellectual disability, could be considered an occupational injustice. Occupational injustice is present when people's choice and ability to engage in meaningful occupations is reduced, resulting in occupational deprivation and marginalization (Channon, 2014; Townsend & Wilcock, 2004). The inability to receive basic health care services, the lack of opportunity to make or act on health care decisions, imposed sedentary lifestyles, and reduced engagement in occupations, illustrate some of the many contextual conditions surrounding the individual with intellectual disability. These contextual factors may confine the occupational opportunities and limit health care options that could otherwise treat and prevent the onset of secondary conditions within the primary care setting (Channon, 2014).

Occupational therapy's role, in addressing the basic health care needs of people with intellectual disability in a primary care setting, has the potential to address some of these occupational injustices. The provision of necessary services, within the primary clinic by occupational therapy practitioners, could detect the often-overlooked lack of meaningful engagement in occupation and poor health habits and routines, which constrain optimal health and wellness. Occupational therapy practitioners are able to provide the needed education for caregivers to enhance supports for a healthier lifestyle and access to preventive health care services.

Occupational therapy practitioners are uniquely situated to address the specific needs of individuals with intellectual disability in the primary care setting by:

- Understanding the associated medical conditions and how they may challenge occupational performance
- Assisting with the management of multiple chronic conditions that increase with aging, especially the high rates of dementia for this population
- Identifying or adapting the environmental supports that typically consists of in-person supports and residential or supported living contexts

The lens of occupational therapy is unique, in that it focuses on creating the goodness of fit between the person, occupation, and environment.

The profession's client-centered, holistic approach is congruent with the principles of self-determination, a much needed policy for individuals with intellectual disability (American Association on Intellectual and Developmental Disabilities [AAIDD], 2008). According to the AAIDD (2008), self-determination focuses on the ability of individuals to actively participate in decision making to allow for "… opportunities and experiences that enable them to exert control in their lives and to advocate on their own behalf," thereby reducing the risk for occupational marginalization. Occupational therapy practitioners can help support the primary care team to instill practices that are geared toward self-determination for the person with intellectual disability and improve overall client care, helping to make services more inclusive, comprehensive, and valuable for users. All of these examples are efforts that promote occupational justice and reduce health inequities.

The role of occupational therapy within the primary care setting is an emerging area of practice. The transformative evolution of primary care models highlights collaborative team approaches, which supply coordinated and integrated patient-centered care. The occupational therapy profession is called upon to expand and establish distinct roles that assist in achieving better outcomes for populations with complex conditions, such as individuals with intellectual disability within these new primary care models. This chapter will review (1) overview of the types of primary care models and services, (2) meeting primary care needs for individuals with intellectual disability, and (3) occupational therapy's role in primary care for health promotion and prevention.

OVERVIEW OF THE TYPES OF PRIMARY CARE MODELS AND SERVICES

Primary care is a "… setting that provides entry into the health care system for new needs and problems, provides person-focused (rather than condition-oriented) care, and offers services for all except rare conditions" (World Health Organization [WHO], 2015). Primary care, as defined by the Patient Protection and Affordable Care Act (ACA), highlights the importance of providing health care services in collaboration with the patient and family within the community context (ACA, 2010). The goals are for early identification, prevention, and treatment of conditions to improve overall health and increase the life span. Primary care physicians are physicians who are often the first point of contact for clients, and provide continuing care, regardless of clients' diagnoses or conditions. Primary care physicians are often supported by nurse practitioners and physician assistants, and act as gatekeepers to the entire health care system, including the potential to advocate for patients to access a variety of services (American Academy of Family Physicians, 2016).

Primary Care Models

As stated earlier in Chapter 2, "Health Policy and Funding for Adults With Intellectual Disability: Past, Present, and Future Directions," the ACA greatly impacted the landscape and delivery of primary care services. The health care reform strategies emphasize health promotion to encompass health of populations and deliver high-quality care based on value, not volume, of services (U.S. Department of Health and Human Services, 2010). As of January 2017, the Comprehensive Primary Care Plus (CPC+) Model, under the Centers for Medicare & Medicaid Services (CMS), began a 5-year, multi-payer initiative to improve primary care in the United States (CMS, 2017). The CPC+ model is part of the innovative payment model initiative that is centered on five functions (CMS, 2017):

1. Access and continuity
2. Care management
3. Comprehensiveness and coordination
4. Patient and caregiver engagement
5. Planned care and population health

This model has direct implications for the population with intellectual disability and occupational therapy practice, as it affects the extent to which access and support is available for the necessary services in the primary care clinic, including those provided through occupational therapy.

CMS payment reforms have changed the landscape of primary care services to focus on coordinating the care of populations through patient-centered medical homes (PCMHs) and accountable care organizations (ACOs), using cost containment and value-based care for populations under one organization. Focusing on population outcomes via cost management and shared financial risk agreements between CMS and health care organizations forces service delivery re-design that creates new processes and roles for health care providers. The ACO, PCMH, and newly introduced CPC+ care models continue to emphasize the importance of primary care services as the first point of contact; however, they have also introduced new team members, such as care coordinators, new types of interventions, such as transitional care, and new uses for health risk assessments to provide risk-stratification of patients who require more frequent follow-up appointments. The effectiveness of all these efforts, as determined by cost-savings and patient outcome measures for ACOs and PCMH primary care settings, continues to be determined (Patient-Centered Primary Care Collaborative, 2017). Results of such efforts creates new occupational therapy roles and opportunities for the profession to address the gaps in services for individuals with intellectual disability within primary care.

An identified barrier to achieving better outcomes for individuals with complex medical conditions and comorbidities was lack of time for care coordination, and lack of resources or community supports to effectively deal with the negative social determinants of health (Rabin, 2014; Rich et al., 2012). These aforementioned barriers (i.e., the need for additional time for care coordination during an office visit) exist for individuals with intellectual disability in the primary care setting. The newer CPC+ model payment reform attempts to consider the additional time needed to follow up and coordinate care for high-risk populations, such as individuals with intellectual disability (CMS, 2017).

MEETING PRIMARY CARE NEEDS FOR PEOPLE WITH INTELLECTUAL DISABILITY

The primary care clinic may be the first place that people with intellectual disability seek out health care; however, research shows that this population does not readily utilize this setting for regular annual exams or preventive care but tends to enter through costlier, acute care settings (Ervin et al., 2014). Factors that limit the effective provision of primary care services to people with intellectual disability include, but are not limited to communication problems, client anxiety, poor self-reporting skills, transportation issues, poor self-advocacy, inadequate health promotion, lack of access to quality health care service, and physician time constraints (Krahn, Hammond, & Turner, 2006; Perry et al., 2014; Scott & Havercamp, 2014). According to a recent review (Krahn & Fox, 2014), core recommendations for improved health outcomes through primary care services for people with intellectual disability were (1) promote early identification, inclusion, and self-determination, (2) prevent and/or manage the onset of health conditions, (3) empower caregivers and family members to meet the needs of persons with intellectual disability, and (4) promote healthy behaviors.

SUPPORTS AND BARRIERS IN PRIMARY CARE SERVICES FOR THE POPULATION WITH A DIAGNOSIS OF INTELLECTUAL DISABILITY

Recognition is given to the existence of newer primary care models that are specifically designed for people with intellectual disability (Sullivan, et al., 2011; Surrey Place Center, 2011; Vanderbilt Kennedy Center, 2014; Woodbury-Smith, 2016). These newer primary care models for individuals with intellectual disability strive to overcome the numerous typical barriers for this population to receive necessary primary care services. Examples to improve care are the use of an intellectual disability tool kit for primary care providers that suggests more frequent and tailored health screenings, behavior checklists, tailored office procedures specific to the population, communication strategies, and educational information for practitioners, as well as other resources for families and caregivers.

These newer primary care models address specific barriers to good health care for individuals with intellectual disability, who often have limited health literacy, social and financial constraints restricting follow through on suggested treatment guidelines, sensory sensitivities, reliance on others to communicate health needs limiting self-determination and control, and incomplete care from untrained health professionals, who lack an understanding of their specific needs (Sullivan et al., 2011). The updated primary care model guidelines designed for people with intellectual disability are to provide general, physical, behavioral, and mental health recommendations, especially for those conditions not typically found on a routine exam. The early detection and treatment of pain and distress, and avoidance of inappropriate long-term use of antipsychotic medications for behavioral management is targeted for individuals with intellectual disability (Sullivan et al., 2011).

Although these primary care model guidelines exist for individuals with intellectual disability, they are not widely instituted nor available to a majority of these individuals and primary care providers. As a result, there are continued gaps and barriers in accessing adequate primary care services for this population, as well as a lack of essential supports for the primary care team to attend to the specialized needs of these individuals (Lennox et al., 2015). Occupational therapy in primary care can ameliorate the prevalent and common barriers for individuals with intellectual disability to specifically address such areas as sensory sensitivities through sensory regulation in the clinic environment, coordination of care amongst the interprofessional team and communication with the client's social supports regarding methods to enhance the client's occupational performance. The outcomes of such efforts could facilitate the awareness of the primary clinic team to understand how the client's occupational performance influences their medical condition and strategies to meet their special needs. Becoming familiar with occupational therapy's role and function in primary care is fundamental to understanding how occupational therapy services benefit this population.

OCCUPATIONAL THERAPY AND PRIMARY CARE FOR HEALTH PROMOTION AND PREVENTION

The core concepts of primary care are harmonious to the practice of occupational therapy, in that it is a holistic, integrated team approach that focuses on supporting healthy lifestyles for individuals within their communities (American Occupational Therapy Association [AOTA], 2014b; Killian, Fisher, & Muir, 2015). The occupational therapy practitioner's knowledge of the behavioral and physical health of humans, through the use of occupation-based interventions, focuses on a holistic and top-down approach that addresses client roles, values, and occupations within the primary care clinic (AOTA, 2014a; Dahl-Poplizio, Manson, Muir, & Rogers, 2016; Lamb & Metzler, 2014; Muir, 2012; Roberts, Famer, Lamb, Muir, & Siebert, 2014).

Occupational therapy practitioners are actively involved in prevention and health promotion efforts for all types of individuals in various settings (Donnelly et al., 2013; Lamb & Metzler, 2014). These interventions ultimately focus on enhancing health, well-being, and participation (AOTA, 2014a). The primary care setting lends itself to these efforts, as the purpose of primary care is to *promote* early identification, engage in disability prevention, and provide treatment (Muir, 2012). McColl et al. (2009) suggested six delivery models for occupational therapy services to be implemented in primary care for individuals with chronic conditions (e.g., those with diagnosis of intellectual disability):

1. Traditional clinic model
2. Chronic disease management
3. Outreach
4. Community-based rehabilitation
5. Shared care
6. Case management

Most likely, the selection of the type of delivery model is determined by the process and structures within the organization, dictated by reimbursement methods, geographical/physical space, allocation of staff resources, and types of ancillary services available within the medical organization.

OCCUPATIONAL THERAPY FOR INDIVIDUALS DIAGNOSED WITH INTELLECTUAL DISABILITY IN PRIMARY CARE

Occupational therapy practitioners are able to add value and efficiency to the services delivered in a primary care setting (Rexe, Lammi, & von Zweck, 2013). As an example, time constraints in the primary care setting often limit the physician's intervention to addressing the acute condition, disease process, or patient's complaints during the visit (Altshuler, Margolius, Bodenheimer, & Grumbach, 2012). To address these situations, the occupational therapy practitioner sees the client following the physician's visit, and as a result, is able to shift the focus from the disease process to health factors, collaborating with the client on strategies to engage in occupations that improve their health through their daily routines and habits (AOTA, 2014a; Dahl-Poplizio et al., 2016; Donnelly, Brenchley, Crawford, & Letts, 2014; Muir, 2012).

Another obstacle encountered because of time constraints, obliges the primary care practitioner to refer out or schedule additional follow-up care services in order to meet the specific needs of individuals with multiple chronic conditions (Altschuler, Margolius, Brodenheimer, & Grumbach, 2012), as could be pertinent to individuals with intellectual disability. Occupational therapy practitioners are equipped to potentially assist individuals to manage multiple comorbidities in a primary care clinic providing same day services (Leland, Fogelberg, Halle, & Mroz, 2017). One example is that of OPTIMAL, a self-management support program tailored by occupational therapy practitioners using occupations for improved activity participation, self-efficacy, and quality of life for individuals with multiple comorbidities (Garvey, Connolly, Boland, & Smith, 2015). Another example of a self-management program for individuals with chronic diseases, which occupational therapy could facilitate, is performed in a group workshop format called the Chronic Disease Self-Management Program (Stanford Medicine, 2017).

Additionally, occupational therapy practitioners could fulfill some of the initial acute needs that physicians feel they do not need to address and therefore, would defer to the occupational therapy practitioner, enabling higher levels of cost containment, especially as reimbursement is based on high-quality care and value (Dahl-Poplizio et al., 2016). These are some of the ways in which occupational therapy practitioners can invest in primary care, and come into contact with people diagnosed with intellectual disability at this immediate level, in order to more effectively attend to clients during the acute stages of the change process (Muir, 2012).

HEALTH PROMOTION AND PREVENTION FOR INDIVIDUALS DIAGNOSED WITH INTELLECTUAL DISABILITY

According to AOTA (2013), occupational therapy's belief of engagement in meaningful occupations that support health is parallel to that of Healthy People 2020. Wilcock (2006) emphasized that an occupation-based health promotion intervention focuses on what the person can and wants to do as the primary concern, and that health is the outcome. It is through our occupations that we become healthy and have the potential to improve our health and well-being (Lamb & Metzler, 2014; Muir, 2012). The World Health Organization defines health promotion as "the process of enabling people to increase control over their health and its determinants, and thereby improve their health" (WHO, 2006).

It is established that access to health promotion and disease prevention activities are lower for individuals with intellectual disability than those in the general population, particularly for regular annual screenings, recommended physical activity, and oral health care (Oullette-Kuntz, 2005; Rimmer & Yamaki, 2006). Occupational therapy practitioners routinely promote healthy lifestyles through programs that address smoking cessation, obesity prevention, and other health promotion interventions (Donnelly et al., 2014; Lamb & Metzler, 2014). Individuals with intellectual disability are often at a higher risk for obesity, unhealthy lifestyles, and the negative secondary conditions associated with these same comorbidities. This creates opportunities for occupational therapy practitioners to provide individual treatment, self-management, self-determination strategies, counseling, and lifestyle planning in the primary care setting (Krahn, Hammond, & Turner, 2006; Koverman, Royeen, & Stoykov, 2017). Therefore, occupational therapy practitioners have an opportunity to create noticeable impacts, using the lens of occupations to prevent diseases and promote health for the people experiencing typical conditions associated with intellectual disability. Refer to Table 16-1 using a case example applied to a three tiered prevention model.

Table 16-1. Three Tiers of Prevention

Case Example Highlighting Occupational Therapy Practitioners' Contribution to Primary Care for Individuals With Intellectual Disability

A 60-year-old woman with intellectual and developmental disabilities presents for an annual health exam with her caregiver from her residential group home. Prior to making this appointment, the client's caregiver called to report that the client has not been sleeping well, has had increased behavioral and emotional outbursts during the day, frequent periods of difficulty recalling previous events, and was not taking her blood pressure medication consistently.

The client has a history of sleep apnea, type 2 diabetes, and recent diagnosis of congestive heart failure. At the time of her last exam, she was prescribed a new diuretic medication, instructed to weigh herself daily to monitor for any fluid weight gain, and to call the office if there were any questions. The client was given the automated after-visit summary sheet produced from her electronic health record with these instructions and advised to provide information to the staff at her group home.

For this current annual visit, the client arrives with her new caregiver. At the time of intake, the client reports she sustained a minor injury following a fall a few weeks ago and notices that she becomes easily tired when performing her basic activities of daily living. The client states that she does not like her continuous positive airway pressure (CPAP) machine and thinks she has been taking her medication regularly, but to mention that she does not like "a lot of pills" in her mouth. The caregiver who brought her to her annual visit states that there have been changes at the group home, including new people and different schedules. Upon her annual exam, it is noted she has some weight gain, and that her blood pressure and A1C levels are elevated. The nurse practitioner reviews the medications with the client, tells the client she needs to change her diet to a low sodium and diabetic diet, to weigh herself every day, and to schedule a follow up visit in 1 month.

(continued)

TABLE 16-1. THREE TIERS OF PREVENTION (CONTINUED)

TIERED PREVENTION CONSIDERATIONS*	EXAMPLES OF THE OCCUPATIONAL THERAPY PROCESSES IN PRIMARY CARE SERVICE DELIVERY* *(Performance of an occupational profile is inherently suggested here.)*	POTENTIAL ROLES OF OCCUPATIONAL THERAPY PRACTITIONERS IN PRIMARY CARE SETTING*	RESEARCH EVIDENCE AND RELATED RESOURCES GUIDING PRACTICE
Primary Prevention			
• Determine routines, roles, and habits that impact adherence to healthy habits, nutrition and physical activity • Identify barriers and supports to occupations that promote health • Review the client's primary care health risk screening site's items that address prevention	Evaluation options: • Assess self-efficacy for balance, stability, and fear of falling using Falls Efficacy Scale • Assess functional mobility for reaching items using Functional Reach Test/Modified Functional Reach Test • Assess client's occupational adaptation and readiness for change to support recommended health behaviors using the Occupational Circumstances Assessment Interview and Rating Scale (OCAIRS)	• Individual provider • Consultant	Evaluations: • Falls Efficacy Scale (Tinetti, Richman, & Powell, 1990) available at www.sralab. org/rehabilitation-measures/tinetti-falls-efficacy-scale • Functional Reach Test/Modified Functional Reach Test (Weiner, Duncan, Chandler, & Studenski, 1992) available at www.sralab.org/rehabilitation-measures/functional-reach-test-modified-functional-reach-test • OCAIRS Version 4.0, (Forsyth et al, 2005) available at www.moho.uic.edu/productDetails.aspx?aid=35

(continued)

TABLE 16-1. THREE TIERS OF PREVENTION (CONTINUED)

TIERED PREVENTION CONSIDERATIONS*	EXAMPLES OF THE OCCUPATIONAL THERAPY PROCESSES IN PRIMARY CARE SERVICE DELIVERY* (Performance of an occupational profile is inherently suggested here.)	POTENTIAL ROLES OF OCCUPATIONAL THERAPY PRACTITIONERS IN PRIMARY CARE SETTING*	RESEARCH EVIDENCE AND RELATED RESOURCES GUIDING PRACTICE
Primary Prevention	Intervention options: • Educate in techniques to utilize preferred occupations that promote healthy food choices and increase activity level • Provide motivational interviewing techniques to influence health behavior change using meaningful occupations and engage the client in specific action plans by asking permission, eliciting change, exploring importance with open-ended questions, and emotion-seeking skills • Address lifestyle modifications taking into consideration access to exercise facilities, transportation, cognitive abilities to use exercise equipment, meal preparation skills, and access to social/in-person supports		Interventions: • Motivational interviewing and occupational therapy (Corcoran, Baum, & Dunn, 2017; Miller & Rollnick, 2013) • Lifestyle Redesign program modified to individual level (Clark, Azen, et al., 1997; Clark, Blanchard, et al., 2015)

(continued)

TABLE 16-1. THREE TIERS OF PREVENTION (CONTINUED)

TIERED PREVENTION CONSIDERATIONS*	EXAMPLES OF THE OCCUPATIONAL THERAPY PROCESSES IN PRIMARY CARE SERVICE DELIVERY* *(Performance of an occupational profile is inherently suggested here.)*	POTENTIAL ROLES OF OCCUPATIONAL THERAPY PRACTITIONERS IN PRIMARY CARE SETTING*	RESEARCH EVIDENCE AND RELATED RESOURCES GUIDING PRACTICE
Primary Prevention			
	• Provide review of home safety measures identifying safety hazards via pictorial methods (e.g., pictures in the Home Safety Self-Assessment Tool [HSSAT])		• Fall Prevention in Primary Care (Mackenzie et al., 2013) • Home Safety Training (Horowitz, Almonk, & Vasil, 2016) • HSSAT (Tomita, Saharan, Rajendron, Schweitzer, & Nochajski, 2014)
Secondary Prevention			
• Sleep apnea • Sensory regulation • Cognitive changes • Caregiver/environmental supports and strains	Evaluation options: • Assess sensory needs using Sensory Integration Inventory–Revised for Individuals With Developmental Disabilities • Assess environmental supports for occupational performance related to medical management of chronic conditions using Residential Environment Impact Scale (REIS) • Screen for dementia behaviors using Dementia Screening Questionnaire for Individuals with Intellectual Disabilities (DSQIID)	• Individual provider • Care coordinator • Consultant	Evaluations: • Sensory Integration Inventory–Revised for Individuals With Developmental Disabilities (Hanschu & Reisman, 1992) • REIS Version 4.0 (Fisher et al., 2014) available at www.moho.uic.edu/productDetails.aspx?iid=5 • DSQIID (Deb, Hare, Prior, & Bhaumik, 2007) available at www.birmingham.ac.uk/documents/college-les/psych/ld/lddementiascreeningquestionnaire.pdf

(continued)

TABLE 16-1. THREE TIERS OF PREVENTION (CONTINUED)

TIERED PREVENTION CONSIDERATIONS*	EXAMPLES OF THE OCCUPATIONAL THERAPY PROCESSES IN PRIMARY CARE SERVICE DELIVERY* *(Performance of an occupational profile is inherently suggested here.)*	POTENTIAL ROLES OF OCCUPATIONAL THERAPY PRACTITIONERS IN PRIMARY CARE SETTING*	RESEARCH EVIDENCE AND RELATED RESOURCES GUIDING PRACTICE
Secondary Prevention			
	Intervention options: • Provide sensory regulation techniques to decrease arousal states and regulate behavior • Establish effective nighttime routines, habits, and environments • Link potential behavior difficulties to sleep disruption and/or dementia behaviors • Collaborate with caregiver/in-person supports and client on adaptive methods to implement occupations in context to client's surroundings/environment, routines, and habits that promote sensory regulation		Interventions: • Sensory Integration for Self-Injurious Behavior (Smith, Press, Koenig, & Kimnealy, 2005) • Sleep hygiene (Gutman et al, 2017; Leland et al, 2014)

(continued)

TABLE 16-1. THREE TIERS OF PREVENTION (CONTINUED)

TIERED PREVENTION CONSIDERATIONS*	EXAMPLES OF THE OCCUPATIONAL THERAPY PROCESSES IN PRIMARY CARE SERVICE DELIVERY* *(Performance of an occupational profile is inherently suggested here.)*	POTENTIAL ROLES OF OCCUPATIONAL THERAPY PRACTITIONERS IN PRIMARY CARE SETTING*	RESEARCH EVIDENCE AND RELATED RESOURCES GUIDING PRACTICE
Tertiary Prevention			
• Routines, roles, and habits that impact adherence to diet, medication, and weight monitoring for chronic conditions • Client's environmental barriers and supports to occupation	Evaluation options: • Assess problematic occupations and client prioritization and satisfaction using the Canadian Occupational Performance Measure (COPM) • Assess self-efficacy to perform self-management and behaviors using the Chronic Disease Self-Efficacy Scale (6-Item Short Form)	• Individual provider • Care coordinator • Group facilitator	Evaluations: • COPM (Law et al., 2014) available at http://www.thecopm.ca • Chronic Disease Self-Efficacy (6-Item Short Form; Lorig, Stewart, Ritter, Gonzalez, & Laurent, 1996) available at www.selfmanagementresource.com/docs/pdfs/English_-_self-efficacy_for_managing_chronic_disease_6-item.pdf

(continued)

Table 16-1. Three Tiers of Prevention (continued)

Tiered Prevention Considerations*	Examples of the Occupational Therapy Processes in Primary Care Service Delivery* *(Performance of an occupational profile is inherently suggested here.)*	Potential Roles of Occupational Therapy Practitioners in Primary Care Setting*	Research Evidence and Related Resources Guiding Practice
Tertiary Prevention	Intervention options: • Address medication management via use of routines, adapted visual reminders, talking glucometers, and adapted pill boxes • Provide peer group mentoring via Stanford Chronic Disease Self-Management Program • Consider oral defensiveness, oral health, and/or oral dysfunction and modification on medication administration • Instruct and provide strategies to successfully use a talking blood glucose monitor • Educate in techniques to utilize preferred occupations that promote healthy food choices and increase activity level		Interventions: • Self-management and multi-comorbidity management (Leland et al., 2017; Ory et al., 2013; Richardson et al., 2014) • Medication management (Murphy, Somerville, Keglovits, Hu, & Stark, 2017; Sanders & Van Oss, 2013; Schwartz & Smith, 2016)

*Note that areas of consideration listed in the table are not exclusive to only one level of prevention or occupational therapy process; these may be applicable/suitable at other levels with different processes

AOTA's (2013) position paper on promotion of health and well-being defines the three levels of prevention as (1) primary prevention through education or efforts to prevent onset or reduce incidence of medical conditions, injuries, or diseases, (2) secondary prevention through early detection via screenings after the onset of a medical condition to minimize or cease the presence of the condition, and (3) tertiary prevention through interventions that are intended to prevent the progression of a condition. The following provides brief examples of how tiered prevention objectives are applied to typical conditions associated with intellectual disability.

Primary Preventive Care

This level of prevention is geared to prevent onset or reduce incidence of medical conditions, injuries, or diseases. Examples of areas to focus on specific to individuals with intellectual disability are physical activity, sexual health, fall prevention, oral health, and visual screenings (Koverman et al., 2017; Mackenzie, Clemson, & Roberts, 2013; Muir, 2012). Prevention efforts that focus on education in these areas will avoid the development of diabetes due to obesity, falls related to reduced vision and lack of physical mobility/activity, oral cavities leading to poor nutrition and further difficulty with communication and intelligibility, and unhealthy or unsafe sexual health practices/relationships leading to sexually transmitted diseases or sexual abuse.

Secondary Preventive Care

Focus at this tier is on early detection via screenings after the onset of a medical condition typical to individuals with intellectual disability. Examples include sleep hygiene for obstructive sleep apnea (Gutman et al., 2017; Leland, Marcione, Schepens Niemec, & Kelkar Don Fogelberg, 2014), sensory regulation/modulation and environmental modifications for sensory sensitivities, proper postural support for congenital spinal abnormalities, and on-going management of behavioral and mental health needs.

Tertiary Preventive Care

At this level of prevention, the goal is to prevent disease progression, a situation that is inherently applicable to individuals with intellectual disability who have multiple comorbidities. Occupational therapy has been proven to assist in addressing chronic disability needs (Killian et al., 2015; Leland et al., 2017) and provides cost-effective services with savings (Metzler, Hartmann, & Lowenthal, 2012; Rexe et al., 2013). Frequently diagnosed chronic conditions seen in individuals with intellectual disability include diabetes, dementia, cardiovascular disease, and coronary artery disease. Self-management interventions, by adhering to medication regimens, lifestyle modifications, and assessing environmental barriers, are effective means to address chronic conditions.

OCCUPATIONAL THERAPY APPROACHES IN PRIMARY CARE

Although other primary care team members contribute to these prevention methods, occupational therapy focuses on identifying the occupations, the supports or barriers to health as determined by task performance, routines, habits, roles, and the context surrounding the client. All these factors are considered in how they promote engagement in positive, healthy occupations. The ability to effectively educate, collaborate, and coordinate the care required for individuals with intellectual disability and their supports is essential to the integration and successful delivery of occupational therapy services in the primary care setting.

Educate

Research states that training for primary care professionals is not adequate to support this population (Perry et al., 2014). Primary care physicians and practice nurses are aware they are not adequately addressing the health needs of people with intellectual disability but they do not know how to change this problem. Examples of evidence for needed training are that primary care physicians often speak only to the caretakers during conversations, instead of to the clients directly, illustrating unconscious biases that assume adults with intellectual disability are not capable of making health care decisions (Werner, Yalon-Chamovitz, Rinde, & Heymann, 2017). Occupational therapy practitioners could educate the primary care team on adaptive methods to converse and engage the client within the client's cognitive and communicative abilities. Additionally, educating the team on the role of occupational therapy within the primary care setting is often needed and essential to fostering trust amongst interprofessional teams (Donnelly et al., 2013; Koverman et al., 2017; McColl et al., 2009).

Communication and self-reporting are often challenges for those with intellectual disability, and can lead to difficulty interacting in the community as well as with primary care providers in a fast-paced clinic. Thus, communication problems can lead to great difficulty for primary care providers to respond to symptoms, address needs, and properly diagnose conditions. Another challenge to communication is that the direct support staff attending the visit with the client with intellectual disability may not have the medical history available to relay to the health care professional (Brown & Censullo, 2008; Lennox et al., 2004).

Communicating with people with intellectual disability and providing strategies for the home and community, as well as in the primary care office, can enhance overall function and improve health care services. For example, this may include teaching a client to use augmentative and alternative communications, designing a visual schedule to better communicate needs to caregivers (Muir, 2012) or assisting the client to use the "ask for it" health advocacy kit, which is a structured health diary (Lennox et al., 2004). The use of pictorials vs. written verbiage on assessment tools and questionnaires would reduce the health literacy disparity for this population. Communicating complicated disease processes and client factors, in the context of occupational performance, may be particularly helpful to people with intellectual disability to understand the impact on their daily life and thus aid in the collaboration between the physician, client, and family. Translating information on how to medically manage a condition, to daily life through occupations, also helps to fill in the gaps and match the health literacy level to the individual's abilities.

Collaborate

Interprofessional collaboration within the primary care setting is noted to influence client outcomes and is a key component to delivering efficacious and efficient care, particularly for clients with multiple chronic and complex conditions, such as individuals with intellectual disability (Epping-Jordan, Pruitt, Bengoa, & Wagner, 2004). Primary care physicians need to be aware that treating people with intellectual disability requires engaging multiple disciplines, including occupational therapy practitioners. Muir (2012) states that occupational therapy practitioners can assist the primary care physicians in lessening the impact of a disease process. Interprofessional primary team collaboration with occupational therapy practitioners during the assessment and intervention services (Donnelly et al., 2013), is beneficial and essential for individuals with intellectual disability who require numerous types of services from various professionals. Studies have demonstrated that occupational therapy practitioners assist primary care teams in achieving the triple aim of the ACA and reinforces the importance of interprofessional collaboration (Dahl-Popolizio et al., 2017). Interprofessional collaboration occurs effectively and efficiently with the use of today's electronic health records. The physical colocation of the occupational therapy practitioner within the primary care clinic also facilitates informal and formal communication with the primary care team.

Collaboration with the individual with intellectual disability and their family members or in-person supports is vital. The literature reveals the need for comprehensive health assessments in primary care that address not only the specific needs for these individuals, but also actively engage the supports within their environment for effective and comprehensive treatment of the client's health issues (Naaldenberg et al., 2015). Collaboration with the individual with intellectual disability, and/or their family members in the primary care clinic, is considered shared decision making and is a model of practice formally adopted by CMS (2016). In the primary care setting, Rubin (2006) highlights the need to treat, not only the needs of the client, but the needs of the caregivers, family, and community, as part of the client's environment, as well. The client's environment impacts occupational performance and co-occupations and is being recognized as more significant in the primary care setting.

Coordinate

An essential component to effective health care service delivery is ensuring the individual receives the appropriate level of care at the right place, the right time, and with the right provider. Individuals with intellectual disability attend routine, annual health examinations at a much lower rate than the general population (Ware & Lennox, 2016). Various studies (Krahn et al., 2006; Ware & Lennox, 2016) suggest that more frequent routine health checkups would benefit this population by targeting specific health issues. The occupational therapy practitioner would be able to effectively intervene to ensure these services are received due to the keen understanding of the client's occupational abilities and environmental supports or barriers, which would implicate the accessibility of such services. Coordinating these necessary services encompasses a level of advocacy, which in turn supports overall health and participation in occupation and promotes fairness and equality (AOTA, 2014a). It may be initiated in the form of the practitioner assisting the client to access community support services. Also, enabling the client's understanding and awareness of their own level of self-determination, and then progress toward empowering the client with intellectual disability to become their own change agent for their health care needs.

Roles of an Occupational Therapy Practitioner in Primary Care

Occupational therapy practitioners are able to provide the holistic approach by understanding the individual with intellectual disability's acute care needs, potential use of long-term services and supports, and needed follow up for transitional care upon discharge from hospital or post–acute care setting. Individuals with intellectual disability also require access to other ancillary services and supports within the community to assist in managing multiple chronic morbidities that affect basic activity of daily living and instrumental activity of daily living performance and dependency on others for transportation in the community. People with intellectual disability have many health care needs along the continuum of services they receive, due to their complex multiple comorbidities, numerous caregivers/in-person assistance, and typical group home residential facility locations (Brown & Censullo, 2008; Ervin et al., 2014).

The role of the occupational therapy practitioner in primary care should be as a generalist who focuses on function and engagement in daily activities using an efficient, targeted evaluation and succinct interventions (Dahl-Poplizio et al., 2016). Occupational therapists may be individual providers, consultants, case managers, and advocates within the primary care settings (AOTA, 2014b). The focus of intervention is to remediate, prevent, promote health, and establish healthy occupational routines (Muir, 2012). Health care reform is not only changing the clinic practices, which impacts the functions of primary care clinic, but it is also changing the processes and, thereby, developing new roles for the primary care team.

Role as Care Coordinator or Case Manager

As health care payment reforms are supporting the role of care coordination, positions within the primary care setting are being established, creating opportunities for occupational therapy practitioners to assume these roles (Robinson, Fisher, & Broussard, 2016). For instance, a PCMH or ACO is now responsible to coordinate the client's care using care coordinators who follow individuals with higher levels of risk, as determined by a health risk stratification tool. Occupational therapy practitioners who have a general skill set (i.e., they are familiar with various populations and conditions that are considered high risk groups) and who have had community-based experience, are particularly equipped to take on this type of care coordination role within a PCMH or ACO setting. Once a care coordinator is assigned to the individual client who has higher health risks factors, such as an individual diagnosed with intellectual disability, that potential occupational therapy care coordinator provides in-person and/or telephonic encounters to facilitate communication amongst team care providers, schedule appointments, and performs traditional, annual health risk assessments, which are augmented with occupational therapy processes.

Role as Consultant

The occupational therapy practitioner provides consulting services to the primary care team through different means, either conjointly with the primary care provider during the office encounter, or through interdisciplinary communication with the primary care team, who identifies a potential client that requires an occupational therapy consult. Benefits of providing consulting services at the time of the primary care office encounter with the provider offers an ideal opportunity to educate them on the value of occupational therapy. This is particularly helpful at the onset of initiating any occupational therapy services in the clinic, as it serves to generate awareness and subsequent consultation requests once a clear understanding of the profession's unique contribution is relayed.

Role as Single Provider

Depending on the internal operations of the primary care clinic, it may be best suited for occupational therapy services to be delivered as a separate individual encounter visit with the client and the practitioner following the primary care physician encounter. As an individual provider, the occupational therapy practitioner is able to allot greater time and perform follow-up sessions for individuals with intellectual disability who require more comprehensive services, such as management of chronic conditions, family or caregiver education, follow through on environmental modifications, and/or longer term behavioral/mental health services.

Role as Group Facilitator

The efficacy of peer mentor groups and those that focus on self-management for chronic conditions provide suitable roles for occupational therapy practitioners to engage as a group facilitator. The occupational therapy practitioner could oversee a group of individuals diagnosed with intellectual disability and encourage peer members to incorporate healthy habits. An occupation-based lens identifies appropriate routines and occupations that support desired healthy habits for individuals with intellectual disability, and could provide a more relevant and effective means of communicating real strategies to the individual on how to take control of their own health.

Conclusion

Williamson, Contreras, Rodriguez, Smith, and Perkins' (2017) scoping review on health care access for adults with intellectual disability stresses the importance of occupational therapy practitioners developing interventions that improve access within the health care environment. Individuals with intellectual disability who have access to preventative, primary health care services, promotes a greater likelihood of participation in occupations, which creates occupational choice and promotes occupational justice. Occupational therapy practitioners' presence in the primary care setting encourages individuals with intellectual disability to have more control over their services, identify occupations that support health, and the environmental surrounding that influence the client's ability to engage in those occupations. Occupational therapy practitioners' approach to interprofessional collaboration, coordination, and education contributes toward achieving the Triple Aim (Berwick, Nolan, & Whittington, 2008) for today's primary care setting.

Metzler et al. (2012) and Muir (2012) both suggest there are endless possibilities for occupational therapy practitioners in the primary care setting, and hope that occupational therapy will help transform this setting into one that truly encompasses the entire person, family, and community. The community of individuals who are diagnosed with intellectual disability and their family and support systems could benefit from these possibilities, which in turn manifests into endless possibilities for participation in meaningful occupations.

References

Altschuler, J., Margolius, D., Brodenheimer, T., & Grumbach, K. (2012). Estimating a reasonable patient panel size for primary care physicians with team-based task delegation. *Annals of Family Medicine, 10,* 396-400. doi: 10.1370/afm.1400

American Association of Intellectual and Developmental Disabilities. (2008). Self-determination. Retrieved from https://aaidd.org/news-policy/policy/position-statements/self-determination#.WS8VK2jyu70

American Occupational Therapy Association. (2013). Occupational therapy in the promotion of health and well-being. *American Journal of Occupational Therapy, 67,* S47-S59. doi: 10.5014/ajot.2013.67S47

American Occupational Therapy Association. (2014a). Occupational therapy practice framework: Domain and process, 3rd edition. *American Journal of Occupational Therapy, 68*(Suppl. 1), S1-S48.

American Occupational Therapy Association. (2014b). The role of occupational therapy in primary care. Retrieved from http://www.aota.org/-/mediaC226E3FF7DF84A6B 8/64394125D919B5E.ashx.

American Academy of Family Physicians. (2016). Primary care. Retrieved from http://www.aafp.org/about/policies/all/primary-care.html

Axmon, A., Karlsson, B., & Ahlstrom, G. (2016). Health care utilization among older persons with intellectual disability and dementia: A registry study. *Journal of Intellectual Disability Research, 60,* 1165-1177. doi: 10.1111/jir.12338

Berwick, D. M., Nolan, T. W., & Whittington, J. (2008). The Triple Aim: Care, health, and cost. *Health Affairs, 27*(3), 759-769. doi: 10.1377/hlthaff.27.3.759

Brown, M., & Censullo, M. (2008). Supporting safe transitions from home to health care settings for individuals with intellectual disabilities. *Topics in Geriatric Rehabilitation, 24,* 74-82.

Channon, A. (2014). Intellectual disability and activity engagement: Exploring the literature from an occupational perspective. *Journal of Occupational Science, 21,* 443-458. doi: 10.1080/14427591.2013.829398

Centers for Medicare & Medicaid Services. (2016). Beneficiary engagement and incentives models: Shared decision making model. Retrieved from https://www.cms.gov/Newsroom/MediaReleaseDatabase/Fact-sheets/2016-Fact-sheets-items/2016-12-08-2.html

Centers for Medicare & Medicaid Services. (2017). Comprehensive primary care plus. Retrieved from https://innovation.cms.gov/initiatives/comprehensive-primary-care-plus/

Clark, F., Azen, S.P., Zemke, R., Jackson, J., Carlson, M., Mandel, D., … Lipson, L. (1997). Occupational therapy for independent-living older adults: A randomized controlled trial. *Journal of American Medical Association, 278,* 1321-1326.

Clark, F. Blanchard, J., Sleight, A., Cogan, A., Floríndez, L., Gleason, S., … Vigen, C. (2015). *Lifestyle redesign: The intervention test in the USC well elderly studies* (2nd ed.). Bethesda, MD: AOTA Press.

Corcoran, M.A., Baum, C., & Dunn, W. (2017). Using naturalistic measurement methods to understand occupational performance. In M. Law, C. Baum, & W. Dunn (Eds.). *Measuring occupational performance: Supporting best practice in occupational therapy* (3rd ed., pp. 69-81). Thorofare, NJ: SLACK Incorporated.

Cutchin, M., & Dickie, V. (2012). Transactionalism: Occupational science and the pragmatic attitude. In G. E. Whiteford & C. Hocking (Eds.), *Occupational science: Society, inclusion and participation* (pp. 23-37). Sussex, United Kingdom: Wiley-Blackwell Publishing, Ltd.

Dahl-Popolizio, S., Manson, L., Muir, S., & Rogers, O. (2016). Enhancing the value of integrated primary care: The role of occupational therapy. *Families, Systems, & Health, 34*, 270-280. doi: 10.1037/fsh0000208

de las Heras, C. G., Geist, R., Kielhofner, G., Fisher, G., Forsyth, K., & Kerschbaum, J. (2005). *Volitional Questionnaire* (V. 4). Chicago, IL: MOHO Clearinghouse.

Deb S., Hare M., Prior L., & Bhaumik S. (2007). Dementia Screening Questionnaire for Individuals With Intellectual Disabilities (DSQIID). *British Journal of Psychiatry, 190*, 440-444.

Donnelly, C., Brenchley, C., Crawford, C., & Letts, L. (2014). The emerging role of occupational therapy in primary care. *Canadian Journal of Occupational Therapy, 81*(1), 51-61. doi: 10.1177/0008417414520683

Epping-Jordan, J., Pruitt, S., Bengoa, R., & Wagner, E. (2004). Improving the quality of health care for chronic conditions. *Quality and Safety in Health Care, 13*(4), 299-305. doi: 10.1136/qshc.2004.010744

Ervin, D., Hennen, B., Merrick, J. & Morad, M. (2014). Health care for persons with intellectual and developmental disability in the community. *Frontiers in Public Health, 2*, 1-8. doi: 10.3389/fpubh.2014.00083

Fisher, G., Forsyth, K., Harrison, M., Agarola, R., Kayhan, E., Noga, P., ... Irvine, L., (2014). *Residential Impact Scale (REIS)* (V. 4.). Chicago, IL: MOHO Clearinghouse.

Forsyth, K., Deshpande, S., Kielhofner, G., Henriksson, C., Haglund, L., Olson, L., ... Kulkarni, S. (2005). *User's manual for the Occupational Circumstances Assessment Interview and Rating Scale: OCAIRS* (V. 4.0). Chicago, IL: MOHO Clearinghouse.

Garvey, J., Connolly, D., Boland, F., & Smith, S. (2015). OPTIMAL, an occupational therapy led self-management support programme for people with multimorbidity in primary care: A randomized controlled trial. *BMC Family Practice, 16*, 1-11. doi: 10.1186/s12875-015-0267-0

Gutman, S. A., Gregory, K. A., Sadlier-Brown, M. M., Schliisel, M. A., Schubert, A., Westover, L. A., & Miller, R. C. (2017). Comparative effectiveness of three occupational therapy sleep intervention: A randomized controlled study. *Occupational Therapy Journal of Research, 37*, 5-13. doi: 10.1177/1539449216673045

Hanschu, B., & Reisman, J. E. (1992). *Sensory Integration Inventory Revised—For individuals with developmental disabilities.* Hugo, MN: PDP Press

Hermans, H., & Evenhuis, H. (2014). Multimorbidity in older adults with intellectual disabilities. *Research in Developmental Disabilities, 35*, 776-783. doi: 10.1016/j.ridd.2014.01.022

Horowitz, B., Almonte, T., & Vasil, A. (2016). Use of Home Safety Self-Assessment Tool (HSSAT) within community health education to improve home safety. *Occupational Therapy in Health Care, 30*, 356-372. doi: 10.1080/07380577.2016.1191695

Killian, C., Fisher, G., & Muir, S. (2015). Primary care: A new context for the scholarship of practice model. *Occupational Therapy in Health Care*, 1-14. doi: 10.3109/07380577.2015.1050713

Krahn, G., & Fox, M. (2014). Health disparities of adults with intellectual disabilities: What do we know? What do we do? *Journal of Applied Research in Intellectual Disabilities, 27*, 431-446. doi: 10.1111/jar.12067

Krahn, G. L., Hammond, L., & Turner, A. (2006). A cascade of disparities: Health and health care access for people with intellectual disabilities. *Mental Retardation and Developmental Disabilities Research Reviews, 12*(1), 70-82. doi: 10.1002/mrdd.20098

Koverman, B. Royeen, L., & Stoykov, M. (2017). Occupational therapy in primary care: Structures and processes that support integration. *The Open Journal of Occupational Therapy, 15*, 11. doi: 10.1543/2168-6408.1376

Lamb, A. J., & Metzler, C. A. (2014). Health policy perspectives—Defining the value of occupational therapy: A health policy lens on research and practice. *American Journal of Occupational Therapy, 68*, 9-14. doi: 10.5014/ajot.2014.681001

Lauer, E., & McCallion, P. (2015). Mortality of people with intellectual and developmental disabilities from select U.S. Stated disability service systems and medical claims data. *Journal of Applied Research in Intellectual Disabilities, 28*, 395-405.

Law, M., Baptiste, S., Carswell, A., McColl, M. A., Polatajko, H., & Pollock, N. (2014). *The Canadian Occupational Performance Measure* (5th ed.). Toronto, ON, Canada: CAOT Publications.

Leland, N., Marcione, N., Schepens Niemec, S. L., Kelkar, K., & Fogelberg, D. (2014). What is occupational therapy's role in addressing sleep problems among older adults? *Occupational Therapy Journal of Research: Occupation, Participation and Health, 34*, 141-149. doi: 10.3928/15394492-20140513-01

Leland, N. E., Fogelberg, D. J., Halle, A. D., & Mroz, T. M. (2017). Health policy perspectives—Occupational therapy and management of multiple chronic conditions in the context of health care reform. *American Journal of Occupational Therapy, 71*, 7101090010. doi: 10.5014/ajot.2017.711001

Lennox, N., Taylor, M., Rey-Conde, T., Bain, C., Boyle, F., & Purdie, D. (2004). Ask for it: Development of a health advocacy intervention for adults with intellectual disability and their general practitioners. *Health Promotion International, 19*, 167-175.

Lennox, N., Van Driel, M. L., & van Dooren, K. (2015). Supporting primary health care professionals to care for people with intellectual disability: Research agenda. *Journal of Applied Research in Intellectual Disabilities, 28*, 33-42

Lorig, K., Stewart, A., Ritter, P., Gonzalez, V., & Laurent, D. (1996). *Outcome measures for health education and other health care interventions.* Thousand Oaks, CA: Sage Publications.

Mackenzie, L., Clemson, L., & Roberts, C. (2013). Viewpoint occupational therapists partnering with general practitioners to prevent falls: Seizing opportunities in primary health care. *Australian Occupational Therapy Journal, 60*, 66-70. doi: 10.1111/1440-1630.12030

McColl, M. A., Shortt, S., Godwin, M., Smith, K., Rowe, K., O'Brien, P., & Donnelly, C. (2009). Models for integrating rehabilitation and primary care: A scoping study. *Archives of Physical Medicine and Rehabilitation, 90*, 1523-1531. doi: 10.1016/j.apmr.2009.03.017

Melville, C. A., Cooper, S., Morrison, J., Smiley, E., Allan, L., Jackson, A., … Mantry, D. (2008). The prevalence and incidence of mental ill—health in adults with autism and intellectual disabilities. *Journal of Autism and Developmental Disorders, 38*(9), 1676-1688. doi: 10.1007/s10803-008-0549-7

Merrick, J., Merrick, E., Lunsky, Y., & Kandel, I. (2006). A review of suicidality in persons with intellectual disability. *Israel Journal of Psychiatry and Related Sciences, 43*(4), 258-264.

Metzler, C. A., Hartmann, K. D., & Lowenthal, L. A. (2012). Health policy perspectives—Defining primary care: Envisioning the roles of occupational therapy. *American Journal of Occupational Therapy, 66*(3), 266-270.

Miller, W. R., & Rollnick, S. (2013). *Motivational interviewing: Helping people change* (3rd ed.). New York, NY: Guilford Press.

Muir, S. (2012). Occupational therapy in primary health care: We should be there. *American Journal of Occupational Therapy, 66*(5), 506-510.

Murphy, M. C., Somerville, E., Keglovits, M., Hu, Y.-L., & Stark, S. (2017). In-Home Medication Management Performance Evaluation (HOME–Rx): A validity study. *American Journal of Occupational Therapy, 71*, 7104190020. doi: 10.5014/ajot.2017.022756

Naaldenberg, J., Banks, R., Lennox, N., Ouellette-Kunz, H., Meijer, M., & van Schrojenstein Lantman-de Valk, H. (2015). Health inequity in people with intellectual disabilities: From evidence to action applying an appreciate inquiry approach. *Journal of Applied Research in Intellectual Disabilities, 28*, 3-11. doi: 10.1111/jar.12130

Oguni, H. (2013). Epilepsy and intellectual and developmental disabilities. *Journal of Policy and Practice in Intellectual Disabilities, 10*(2), 89-92.

Ory, M. G., Ahn, S., Jian, L., Smith, M. L., Ritter, P., Whitelaw, N., & Lorig, K. (2013). Successes on national study on the chronic disease self-management program: Meeting the Triple Aim of health care reform. *Medical Care, 51*, 992-998.

Ouelette-Kuntz, H. (2005). Understanding health disparities and inequities faced by individuals with intellectual disabilities. *Journal of Applied Research in Intellectual Disabilities, 18*, 113-121.

Patient-Centered Primary Care Collaborative. (2017). *The impact of primary care practice transformation on cost, quality, and utilization: A systematic review of research published in 2016.* Retrieved from https://www.pcpcc.org/resource/impact-primary-care-practice-transformation-cost-quality-and-utilization

Patient Protection and Affordable Care Act, Pub. L. 111-148, § 3502, 124 Stat. 119, 124 (2010).

Perry, J., Felce, D., Kerr, M., Bartley, S., Tomlinson, J., & Felce, J. (2014). Contact with primary care: The experience of people with intellectual disabilities. *Journal of Applied Research in Intellectual Disabilities, 27*(3), 200-211.

Rabin, R. (2014). 15-minute visit takes a toll on the doctor-patient relationship. Retrieved from http://www.kaiserhealthnews.org/stories/2014/april/21/15-minute-doctor-visits.aspx

Rexe, K., Lammi, B., & von Zweck, C. (2013). Occupational therapy: Cost-effective solutions for changing health system needs. *Healthcare Quarterly, 16*, 69-75.

Richardson, J., Loyola-Sanchez, A., Sinclair, S., Harris, J., Letts, L., MacIntyre, N. J., … Ginis, K. (2014). Self-management interventions for chronic disease: A systematic scoping review. *Clinical Rehabilitation.* Retrieved from http://cre.agepub.com/content/early/2014/04/29/0269215514532478

Roberts, P., Farmer, M. E., Lamb, A. J., Muir, S., & Siebert, C. (2014). The role of occupational therapy in primary care. *American Journal of Occupational Therapy, 68*(Suppl. 3), S25-S33.

Robinson, M., Fisher, T., & Broussard, K. (2016). Role of occupational therapy in case management and care coordination for clients with complex conditions. *American Journal of Occupational Therapy, 70*, 70020900010.

Rimmer, J. H., & Yamaki, K. (2006). Obesity and intellectual disability. *Mental Retardation and Developmental Disabilities Research Review, 12*, 22-27.

Rubin, L. I. (2006). Severe and profound disabilities. In L. I. Rubin. & A. C. Crocker. (Eds.), *Medical care for children and adults with developmental disabilities* (pp. 591-602). Baltimore, MD: Paul H. Brookes Publishing Co.

Sanders, M. J., & Van Oss, T. (2013). Using daily routines to promote medication adherence in older adults. *American Journal of Occupational Therapy, 67*, 91-99.

Schwartz, J. K., & Smith, R. O. (2016). Intervention promoting medication adherence: A randomized, Phase I, small-N study. *American Journal of Occupational Therapy, 70*, 7006240010.

Scott, H. M., & Havercamp, S. M. (2014). Mental health for people with intellectual disability: The impact of stress and social support. *American Journal on Intellectual and Developmental Disabilities, 119*(6), 552-564.

Smith, S. A., Press, B., Koenig, K. P., & Kinnealey, M. (2005). Effects of sensory integration intervention on self-stimulating and self-injurious behaviors. *American Journal of Occupational Therapy, 59*, 418-425.

Stanford Medicine. (2017). Chronic disease self-management program (Better Choices, Better Health Workshop). Retrieved from http://patienteducation.stanford.edu/programs/cdsmp.html

Sullivan, W., Berg, J. M., Bradley, E., Cheetham, T., Denton, R., Heng, J., ... McMillan, S. (2011). Primary care of adults with developmental disabilities. Canadian consensus guidelines. *Canadian Family Physician, 57,* 541-553

Surrey Place Centre. (2011). Primary care. Retrieved from http://www.surreyplace.on.ca/resources-publications/primary-care

Tinetti, M. E., Richman, D., & Powell, L. (1990). Falls efficacy as a measure of fear of falling. *Journal of Gerontology, 45*(6), 239-43.

Tomita, M., Saharan, S., Rajendron, S., Schweitzer, J., & Nochajski, S. (2014). Development of psychometrics and use of Home Safety Self-Assessment Tool (HSSAT). *American Journal of Occupational Therapy, 68*(6), 711-718.

Townsend E., & Wilcock, A. A. (2004) Occupational justice and client-centered practice: A dialogue in progress. *Canadian Journal of Occupational Therapy, 71,* 75-87. doi: 10.1177/000841740407100203

U.S. Department of Health and Human Services. (2010). *Multiple chronic conditions: A strategic framework: Optimal health and quality of life for individuals with multiple chronic conditions.* Washington, D.C.: Author.

Vanderbilt Kennedy Center. (2014). Healthcare for adults with intellectual and developmental disabilities. Retrieved from http://vkc.mc.vanderbilt.edu/etoolkit/

Ware, R., & Lennox, N. (2016). Characteristics influencing attendance at a primary care health check for people with intellectual disability: An individual participant data meta-analysis. *Research in Developmental Disabilities, 55,* 235-241. doi: 10.101016/j.ridd.2016.04.012

Weiner, D. K., Duncan, P. W., Chandler, J., & Studenski, S. A. (1992). Functional reach: A marker of physical frailty. *Journal of the American Geriatric Society, 40,* 203-207.

Weise, J., Pollack, A., Britt, H., & Trollor, J. N. (2016). Primary health care for people with an intellectual disability: An exploration of demographic characteristics and reasons for encounters from the BEACH program. *Journal of Intellectual Disability Research, 60,* 1119-1127. doi: 10.1111/jir.12301

Werner, S., Yalon-Chamovitz, M., Rinde, T., & Heymann, A. D. (2017). Principles of effective communication with patients who have intellectual disability among primary care physicians. *Patient Education and Counseling, 100*(7), 1314-1321. doi: 10.1016/j.pec.2017.01.022

Wilcock, A. (2006). *An occupational perspective of health.* Thorofare, NJ: SLACK Incorporated.

Willamson, H., Contreras, G., Rodriguez, E., Smith, J., & Perkins, E. (2017). Health care access for adults with intellectual and developmental disabilities: A scoping review. *Occupational Therapy Journal of Research: Occupation, Participation, and Health,* 1-10.

Woodbury-Smith, M. (2016). Improving the uptake of health screening among individuals with intellectual disability. *Developmental Medicine and Child Neurology, 58,* 1265-1272. doi: 10.1111/dcmn.13193

World Health Organization. (2015). Primary care evaluation tool. Retrieved from http://www.euro.who.int/en/health-topics/Health-systems/primary-health-care/country-work/primary-care-evaluation-tool

17

Older Adults With Intellectual Disability

E. Adel Herge, OTD, OTR/L, FAOTA

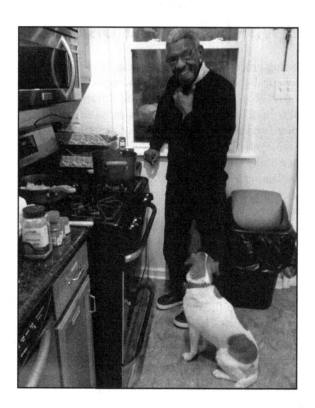

Key Words: aging process, intellectual disability, older adult

Bryze, K.
Occupational Therapy for Adults With Intellectual Disability (pp. 205-217).
© 2020 Taylor & Francis Group.

It was once believed that individuals with intellectual disability would have a shortened life expectancy (Alexander, Bullock, & Maring, 2008; Kim, El Hoyek, & Chau, 2011). Due to advances in medical care and better support service systems, individuals with intellectual disability are living longer, with the life expectancy of those with mild disabilities nearing that of the nondisabled, aging population (Perkins & Moran, 2010). There are an estimated 9.2 million individuals in the United States who are diagnosed with intellectual disability (Nochajski, 2000), with the number of these adults over the age of 60 projected to increase to 1.2 million by 2030 (Heller, Janicki, Marks, Hammel, & Factor, 2008). While this number represents only 2% of the overall U.S. population (Krahn, Hammond, & Turner, 2006), the majority of older adults with intellectual disability live, work, and receive services (including health care) in the community.

Adults with intellectual disability receive medical care in the same environments as nondisabled, older adults. This chapter will provide insight into the aging process for adults with intellectual disability, the underlying theories of aging with disabilities, and recommended practices for providing intervention and supports for these adults. Recommendations for the role of occupational therapy on interprofessional teams will be presented, as well as the ways practitioners can support older adults with intellectual disability and their caregivers in the future.

AGING PROCESS AND ADULTS WITH INTELLECTUAL DISABILITY

Evidence shows the aging process of adults with intellectual disability mirrors that of the nondisabled population. The physical changes, prevalence, and types of chronic conditions are similar to all individuals as they age (Gibbs, Brown, & Muir, 2008; Perkins & Moran, 2010). However, adults with intellectual disability may have a higher prevalence of medical conditions, with many conditions being unrecognized and undiagnosed or poorly managed (Havercamp, Scandlin, & Roth, 2004; Hemm, Dagnan, & Meyer, 2015; Krahn et al., 2006; Kim et al., 2011; Sullivan et al., 2006), and may demonstrate greater frailty and age-related changes earlier than the nondisabled population (Evenhuis, Hermans, Bastiaanse, & Echteld, 2012). Specific groups are at higher risk for impairment. For example, individuals with Down syndrome are reportedly at higher risk for hearing impairment (Haveman et al., 2011), heart conditions, and dementia (Bowers, Webber, & Bigby, 2014). Women with Down syndrome experience menopause at earlier ages (Coppus et al., 2010), which may increase their risk for breast cancer (Alexander et al., 2008; Wilkinson & Cerreto, 2008) and dementia (Coppus et al., 2010). Women with intellectual disability also experience osteoporosis at an accelerated rate, which may be due to genetics, sedentary lifestyle, and/or long-term use of medications (Alexander et al., 2008).

Researchers report differences in the number of preventable health conditions, which are often unrecognized by families or caregivers (Bowers et al., 2014), underdiagnosed, or diagnosed late by health care providers (Haveman et al., 2011; Sullivan et al., 2006). Lifestyle factors have been linked to poorer overall health status (Alexander et al., 2008; Haveman et al., 2011). While the evidence linking living situations with health status remains unclear (Janicki et al., 2002; Lewis & Stenfert-Kroese, 2010), sedentary lifestyles, decreased engagement in physical activity, and poor dietary habits have been linked to chronic conditions.

There is evidence of disparities in emotional and mental health issues, which are associated with living environments, social connections, and life events. In a study of adults with intellectual disability across 14 European countries, older adults were more likely to live in larger institutions and were more socially isolated than younger adults with intellectual disability (Haveman et al., 2011). Adults aging with intellectual disability experience higher incidences of anxiety and depression associated with changes in physical health, loss of mobility, and loss of leisure activities, and are less likely to have emotional support for their mental health problems (Havercamp et al., 2004; Hermans & Evenhuis, 2012).

Access to health care services can also be impacted due to issues with consent (Broughton & Thomson, 2000; Prevatt, 1998; Wilkinson & Cerreto, 2008), reimbursement (Bowers et al., 2014), and environmental barriers. Physical environmental barriers include inaccessible clinics and difficulty with positioning (i.e., for mammography or gynecological examinations). Social-environmental issues include difficulty communicating with the health care provider (Tracey, 2007), poorly trained health care providers (Gibbs et al., 2008; Michael & Richardson, 2008), negative attitudes by health care providers (Lewis & Stenfert-Kroese, 2010), lack of knowledge or skill sets to care for individuals with intellectual disability (Gibbs, Brown, & Muir, 2008; Sowney & Barr, 2006), and lack of appropriate guidelines for clinical screening and assessment (Mizen, Macfie, Findlay, Cooper, & Melville, 2012; Sullivan et al., 2006).

Dementia

Research indicates that adults aging with Down syndrome are at higher risk of developing dementia than the general population (Kim et al., 2011; Sheehan, Ali, & Hassiotis, 2014; Strydom, Hassiotis, King, & Livingston, 2009). The manifestation of dementia in adults with intellectual disability differs from that of the general population. For example, adults with Down syndrome often exhibit behaviors that resemble frontal lobe dysfunction before changes in language or memory present (Sheehan et al., 2014; Strydom et al., 2009). Changes in emotion, personality, and behavior (e.g., aggression, anxiety) or other maladaptive behaviors (e.g., restlessness, disturbances in sleep-wake cycles, social withdrawal, apathy, uncooperativeness, depressed mood) can often occur (Ball et al., 2006). Other manifestations can include difficulty with communicating, understanding directions, and completing self-care activities, as well as wandering behaviors, low mood, or tiring easily (Adams et al., 2008; Prasher & Filer, 1995).

Diagnoses of dementia in adults with intellectual disability is complicated, due to lack of baseline information, comorbidities (Llewellyn, 2011), lack of standardized criteria (Sheehan et al., 2014), and a limited number of assessments specifically designed for this population (Zeilinger, Stiehl, & Weber, 2013). Early and accurate diagnosis is critical to establishing a comprehensive plan of care to support the adult with intellectual disability and dementia. This includes addressing all the medical, physical, and social needs of the individual and educating and equipping family and staff caregivers in strategies to support the person in maintaining a high quality of life (Dicks, Jackson, Pasokhy, Catty, & Symes, 2015; Llewellyn, 2011; Wilkinson & Cerreto, 2008)

Environmental and Caregiver Considerations

Many adults who are aging with intellectual disability previously lived in large residential facilities and these institutions continue to exist in many states. The physical, social, and cultural environments of many institutions were based on congregate care for large groups of people who needed assistance with self-care and who exhibited maladaptive behaviors (Kim et al., 2011). Institutional environments are characterized by low stimuli, low staffing ratios, and limited occupational engagement (Wolfensberger, 1991). Currently, adults with intellectual disability, who have significant medical needs that require nursing care and substantial supports, reside in nursing homes, which suffer from the same challenges as residential institutions and carry with them similar challenges for occupational engagement.

Whether family member or paid staff, the essential person in the life of an adult aging with intellectual disability is the caregiver who provides direct support. This person provides the critical assistance needed to enable the adult to participate in all aspects of life, including assistance for basic self-care, community mobility, social participation, productivity, and leisure occupations. Parents caring for their adult child at home perhaps experience simultaneous challenges with aging, which further stresses the caregiving role. Wang (2012) revealed that care relationships between aging parents and their adult children can become reciprocal, with the adult child actually providing some level of care for his or her parent. While families find caring for their adult child emotionally rewarding, the need for future planning becomes more evident as the parent ages and the tasks associated with caregiving became more challenging (Dillenburger & McKerr, 2011).

Adults aging with intellectual disability may also live in residences in the community in which they receive support from paid caregiving staff. This support can be intermittent or continual depending on the needs of the adult with intellectual disability. Staff are vital to the quality of services and the daily life experience of adults with intellectual disability (Rose, Kent, & Rose, 2012; Vassos, Nankervis, Skerry, & Lante, 2013). As the extent and types of care change with aging individuals' needs, staff may experience increased levels of stress, especially if they lack the training and skills necessary to manage the complications of aging. Residential staff often fail to recognize pain in adults with intellectual disability, believing that aches and pains are part of normal aging (Buys, Aird, & Miller, 2012; Lewis & Stenfert-Kroese, 2010).

Staff play a primary role in supporting adults with intellectual disability with their increased medical and psychological needs (Buys et al., 2012). Increased number of physician appointments, more involved specialists (e.g., cardiologists, endocrinologists), changes in the environment or daily routine, greater use of adaptive equipment, increased need for physical assistance, and changing activity patterns are all components of staff responsibilities with adults with intellectual disability who are aging (Buys et al., 2012; Chng, Stancliffe, Wilson, & Anderson, 2013). Staff working directly with aging adults with intellectual disability also face the complex challenges associated with end of life care, dying, and death. Staff often participate in end of life care decisions and may even provide palliative care for individuals living at home. While staff report providing care at the end of life to be a positive experience, there exists a number of challenges to providing high quality, patient-centered end of life care (Flynn, Brown Salomons, Burns Salomons, & Keywood, 2009).

Perspectives on Aging

Aging adults with intellectual disability report experiencing changes in physical appearance, physical health, mobility, and activity patterns (e.g., transitioning from work to retirement) (Burke, Taylor, Urbano, & Hodapp, 2012; Strnadová, Cumming, Knox, Parmenter, & Lee, 2015). Illness and changes in physical health, fears about the future, loss of parents and family members, and fears about their own death are counterbalanced with seeing aging as a positive experience, with more time for social activities, gaining wisdom, increased opportunities for travel, and learning new skills (Burke et al., 2012; Strnadová et al., 2015). Overall, adults with intellectual disability appear to have the same concerns and priorities about aging as the nondisabled population. Environmental factors, such as living situations and the nature and degree of staff/caregiver support, were identified as significant supports or barriers to facilitating the adult's ability to make their own choices and participate in desired activities while aging (Dodevska & Vassos, 2013; Shaw, Cartwright, & Craig, 2011; Strnadová et al., 2015). Understanding and acknowledging the personal experience of aging will help occupational therapy practitioners design client-centered interventions that address the adult's priorities and concerns.

Transitions and Loss

Aging for any person is characterized by transitions; shifting from active work to retirement, lessening of skills and changes in routines, secondary to the physiological processes of aging, the loss of family, friends, and loved ones to death and illness, changes to living arrangements, and perhaps unfulfilled dreams. The adult aging with intellectual disability also experiences transition and loss. While many of these losses are the same as his or her typical age peers, variations may be due to life history, the environments in which they have lived or are living, and the nature and degree of cognitive impairment. Adults with intellectual disability may have experienced frequent changes in significant relationships, such as caregivers due to staff turnover or changes in job responsibility or schedules, but can include loss of family and friends or housemates due to relocation, illness, or death.

Adults aging with intellectual disability may experience personal losses associated with the loss of skills, such as mobility, valued leisure activities (Sinai, Bohnen, & Strydom, 2012), or independence in activities of daily living. As life events accumulate for the aging adult with intellectual disability, challenges to the places and sense of safety or security may ensue. The accumulation of challenging life events are experienced by the aging adult and correlated with higher rates of depression and anxiety symptoms, which may be due to individuals' lack of control over the events and limited coping skills associated with the cognitive impairment (Ballan & Sormanti, 2014; Hermans & Evenhuis, 2012).

Individuals with intellectual disability experience grief, although the cognitive impairment associated with intellectual disability may contribute to an individual's difficulty fully understanding a situation and why a loss has occurred (e.g., staff turnover, death of a family member, the permanency of death; Ballan & Sormanti, 2014; McEvoy, MacHale, & Tierney, 2012). Long standing relationships with family and caregivers, who provide assistance and support for the basic and intimate aspects of self-care, can lead to strong attachments. When caregivers are no longer a primary support, the individual may experience an overwhelming sense of loss and grief, regardless of the severity of the individual's level of cognitive disability (Hurst, 2009). Tables 17-1 and 17-2 describe best practices to support individuals with intellectual disability in grief and loss.

ROLE OF THE OCCUPATIONAL THERAPIST: BEST PRACTICES

Best practice in health care for aging adults with intellectual disability should mirror that of the nondisabled aging adult. A comprehensive, seamless, client-centered service delivered by a well-trained, fully functioning interprofessional team is the ideal; however, the experiences of providers and families belay this reality. Table 17-3 presents suggestions for occupational therapists working on interprofessional teams.

Working as a member of the interprofessional team, occupational therapy practitioners contribute their expertise to promoting health through engagement in occupation (American Occupational Therapy Association [AOTA], 2014). Depending on the need of the individual and his or her context, this can take many forms. Occupational therapists can advocate for adults aging with intellectual disability and their caregivers to receive the same quality of health care as any other patient. The occupational therapist can also work with health care providers to modify protocols to help facilitate physical examinations. Occupational therapy practitioners can provide education and training in the use of strategies to reduce anxiety, make recommendations for positioning for screening tests, or use adaptive strategies to help adults with intellectual disability communicate with their providers (Lennox et al., 2007; Lennox et al., 2013; Prater & Zylstra, 2006; Regnard et al., 2007).

Occupational therapists can advocate for, support, and implement interventions for adults with intellectual disability to be proactive and take responsibility for their own health through participation in health promotion programs (Heller, Fisher, Marks, & Hsieh, 2014). For example, lifestyle design programs can be established to help aging individuals with intellectual disability establish healthy occupational routines, whether adding physical activity into their day, establishing healthy eating patterns, engaging in social interaction, or participating in activities to promote relaxation and manage stress (Herge, 2008). In a scoping review of health promotion programs for adults with intellectual disability, Heller et al. (2014) found a variety of innovative community based programs that demonstrated significant benefits for participants. The researchers stated the need for adaptation of programs to include better utilization of adaptive equipment for persons with physical disabilities, integration of principles of self-determination, and greater consideration given to the preferences of aging adults with intellectual disability (Heller et al., 2014).

TABLE 17-1. BEST PRACTICES TO SUPPORT INDIVIDUALS WITH INTELLECTUAL DISABILITY THROUGH GRIEF AND LOSS
1. ALL SUPPORT SHOULD BE PROVIDED WITH THE APPROPRIATE CULTURAL CONTEXT
Occupational therapy practitioners are uniquely qualified to examine context and to develop appropriate interventions that respect and acknowledge the individual as the primary subject. Valuing and respecting the client's beliefs can help encourage active participation and guide interventions more efficiently (AOTA, 2014).
2. RECOGNIZE THE SYMPTOMS AND BEHAVIOR ASSOCIATED WITH GRIEVING
The process of grieving and the length of time moving through the process vary. Some individuals may learn how to integrate grief into their own lives and continue living (Stewart & Tolliver, 2015).
3. INCLUDE THE INDIVIDUAL WITH INTELLECTUAL DISABILITY IN CONVERSATION AND PARTICIPATION IN THE RITUALS
Families and caregivers often desire to protect the individual with intellectual disability from the extent of the loss (Morgan & McEvoy, 2014; Read & Elliott, 2007) or avoid sharing all the information. Researchers suggest the individual be brought into the conversation. Being direct and honest initiates the process of support and coping when the individual recognizes that something is wrong/different. Caregivers should take opportunities to teach/reinforce that death is part of life. Experts say that the individual is encouraged to actively participate in religious practices and rituals of their faith tradition (e.g., funerals, memorials services, other rituals that mark the passage) in order to facilitate the grieving process (Read & Elliott, 2007).
4. RECOGNIZE THAT ENGAGEMENT IN OCCUPATIONS MAY VARY
The individual may have limited interest in occupations he or she they previously enjoyed and may even show regression in his or her the ability to perform activities (Hurst, 2009). Participation in occupations that support memories (e.g., searching through photographs) or connecting the individual with the person or object of loss may replace occupations they previously enjoyed while the individual processes the loss. Meaningful occupations that provide support and comfort should be encouraged; this is not the time to teach new skills (Hurst, 2009).
5. PROVE SOCIAL SUPPORT
Support of caregivers, families, and support groups can mediate the effects of and facilitate the process of grieving; however, be mindful of the type and quality of support as some adults with intellectual disability may experience additional stress (McEvoy et al., 2012).
6. BE PATIENT
Grieving takes time and there is no magic solution to hurry the process. Experts recommend you "be with" the individual who is grieving, give them space and time to experience the journey of grief, and listen as they share his or her thoughts and feelings. Specific strategies are included in Table 17-2 (Stewart & Tolliver, 2015).

Occupational therapists can also help educate health care providers, families, and staff in evidence based, proven strategies to support aging individuals with intellectual disability toward successful aging. Occupational therapists can educate caregivers in activity modification and environmental adaptation to help individuals remain active and engaged as the physiological changes associated with aging occur. Most health care professionals do not receive pre-service training in the health care needs of aging adults with intellectual disability (Lennox et al., 2007). Occupational therapists can help providers understand the unique needs of the aging individual with intellectual disability and his or her caregivers to help alleviate misconceptions, be more comfortable interacting with, and providing care.

TABLE 17-2. STRATEGIES TO SUPPORT AN INDIVIDUAL WITH INTELLECTUAL DISABILITY IN GRIEF

- Give full eye contact and attention.
- Recognize their desire to tell the story repeatedly as this helps process the grief.
- Use verbal and nonverbal communication strategies to be "in tuned" with the person.
- Use open-ended phrases to illicit the conversation and encourage them to talk.
- Use active listening to paraphrase back to the speaker what you hear.
- Reflect their feelings even to the point of giving them words to use to describe their feelings.

TABLE 17-3. TIPS FOR OCCUPATIONAL THERAPISTS WORKING WITH THE INTERPROFESSIONAL TEAM

1. ASK THE QUESTION

Through the evaluation process of assembling the occupational profile and analyzing the individual's current occupational performance, the occupational therapist develops a hypothesis of what could be happening for the individual at the time. Share this hypothesis with the interprofessional (i.e., health care and caregiving) team and expand their perspective of all the aspects of the adult with intellectual disability who is aging. Is the change in individual's behavior due to a change in physiological status? Increase in pain? Change in sensory abilities (i.e., hearing or vision), mental or emotional health (e.g., onset of depression)? Communicate your ideas to the team and collaborate with them in exploring strategies to uncover the answer.

2. EMPOWER THE INDIVIDUAL AND HIS OR HER CAREGIVERS

Occupational therapists recognize that engagement in occupations is central to an individual's identity and sense of competence (AOTA, 2014). We recognize that continued engagement in occupations supports an individual's health and wellness. Direct support staff, caregivers, program specialists, and day/residential program supervisors and staff providing support to adults aging with intellectual disability are often seeking strategies to help adults with intellectual disability age successfully. They are often caught between helping a person adjust to the changes associated with aging and the loss of skills and assisting the person in remaining active in valued activities both in and outside the home. Empowering individuals and their caregivers to be active participants engaging in valued occupations brings meaning and value to the individual and the caregiver (Mahoney & Roberts, 2011). Occupational therapists design intervention plans that support the individual in being active in their own health promotion (i.e., setting personal health goals) and health care access (Haveman et al., 2011).

3. BUILD ON THE EVIDENCE

Occupational therapy is a science driven, evidence-based profession. The evidence for effective occupational therapy services in the aging adult with intellectual disability may be emerging at the current time but occupational therapy practitioners should not be discouraged. This creates the opportunity for occupational therapy to create the evidence. Occupational therapy practitioners should use the current evidence of best practice in health care and other professions as a basis for developing science driven, evidence-based programs. By adding the unique perspective of occupational therapy to these programs, we will create our own evidence of how occupational therapy services meet the occupational needs of this underserved population and their caregivers.

4. MEASURE OUTCOMES

Occupational therapy practitioners should always include outcome measurement as part of their intervention plan. Collecting solid outcome data in a systematic way is an ideal method of monitoring and evaluating the success of your intervention plan or the need for modification. In addition to showing if the individual is meeting the target goal, the data also informs the interprofessional team of the success of the plan and enhances the value of the program, as well as the benefits of occupational therapy services.

Ethical Considerations

Provider agencies, such as nursing homes or assisted living facilities, are turning to assistive technology and telecare as potential solutions to transform the delivery of health care (Perry, Beyer, & Holm, 2009). To increase autonomy, the individual must be aware that the technology has been put in place and be able to provide consent (Perry et al., 2009), yet these individuals must have the right to privacy, especially when actively engaged in the bathroom or bedroom. *Surveillance technology* is an example of one emerging source of telecare that raises ethical concerns for aging adults with intellectual disability. Surveillance technology is defined as "electronic equipment that allows the visual and acoustic monitoring of people or registers their activities" (Niemeijer, Frederiks, Depla, Eefsting, & Hertogh, 2013, p. 28). Researchers have shared various perspectives on the benefits and concerns of using this type of technology to help serve and protect individuals with disabilities. Many health professionals perceive using surveillance technology as an aid rather than a substitute for physical monitoring of clients, or combining the old routine of personal monitoring with electronic monitoring; however, several important aspects of technology need to be considered.

Alarm fatigue occurs when motion in the environment leads to overuse or excessive repetition of auditory/acoustic alarms. Not only does this disturbance upset the individual for whom the monitoring was implemented but the other clients and staff in the surrounding environment as well. To apply to the principle of beneficence, when an individual appears restless but is not necessarily being harmed, it may be feasible for staff to turn off the alarm for a short period of time while remaining within close proximity to the individual for safety (Niemeijer et al., 2013). When he or she becomes settled, staff can turn the alarm back on and resume rounds. Health professionals who utilize this strategy must have adequate knowledge of adults aging with intellectual disability and, more importantly, knowledge of the individuals directly involved in the conflict. Motion sensors may allow these clients to have more freedom; however, there is always room for error with technology. To apply the principle of non-maleficence, one client, who may not be allowed outdoors, may accidentally slip through an automatic door. If his or her personal monitor/GPS is not working, more troubling events may occur (Niemeijer et al., 2013).

There are concerns that the use of surveillance technology might distract organizations from the need to provide more staff and better training (Niemeijer et al., 2013), thus, acts of justice come into play. Perry, Firth, Puppa, Wilson, and Felce (2012) discuss levels of support provided by staff in conjunction with telecare and assistive technology devices. The levels of support included how much support would be required if it was always delivered by the most experienced team members; how much additional support would be required for arranged and spontaneous events (e.g., social trips, support with personal care, behavioral issues); and how telecare could help to change the delivery of staff support (Perry et al., 2012). To increase autonomy for aging adults with intellectual disability, support may be reduced at particular times rather than being completely withdrawn (Perry et al., 2012). The ability for staff to develop close relationships with the individual may also enhance the skills provided. A closer relationship would allow for a calmer environment, more focused care, and increased support in personal skill development; whereas, a more distant relationship with more general skills, would be required to serve those who present with the greatest needs (Perry et al., 2012).

CONCLUSION

The occupational therapist brings a specialized perspective to the interprofessional, health care team. The increase of longevity for adults with intellectual disability brings great challenges, but also great opportunities, for occupational therapists. New and innovative models of service delivery will be needed to support aging adults with intellectual disability in maintaining a high quality of life. These will include programs that support healthy aging of adults with intellectual disability; integrate technology and environmental adaptations to help the adults with intellectual disability "age in place"; maintain engagement in valued activities; and educate, support, and train family and staff caregivers in best practices for aging, dementia care, and end of life care. Inclusive, participatory research, which includes adults with intellectual disability as co-researchers (Bigby, Frawley, & Ramcharan, 2014; O'Brien, McConkey, & García-Iriarte, 2014), will increase our understanding of the experience of aging and the factors that support or hinder this process. This type of investigative inquiry will provide opportunities for aging adults with intellectual disability to be active in determining their own destiny and will inform our programs to be truly client centered. With expertise in evaluation and analysis of the person, task, and environment, (AOTA, 2014) occupational therapists are uniquely qualified to support aging adults with intellectual disability to maintain occupational engagement in their environment. The occupational therapy practitioner brings his or her understanding of the value of occupational engagement and participation in supporting the health and well-being of the aging adult with intellectual disability. Occupational therapy practitioners can work with members of the interprofessional, health care team to address the barriers to healthy aging and develop client-centered programs that specifically address client needs and interests.

REFERENCES

Adams, D., Oliver, C., Kalsy, S., Peters, S., Broquard, M., Basra, T., … McQuillan, S. (2008). Behavioural characteristics associated with dementia assessment referrals in adults with Down syndrome. *Journal of Intellectual Disability Research, 52*(4), 358-368.

Alexander, L. M., Bullock, K., & Maring, J. R. (2008). Challenges in the recognition and management of age-related conditions in older adults with developmental disabilities. Topics in geriatric rehabilitation. *Aging with a Developmental Disability, 24*(1), 12-25. doi: 10.1097/01.TGR.0000311403.16802.f8

American Occupational Therapy Association. (2014). Occupational therapy practice framework: Domain and process, 3rd edition. *American Journal of Occupational Therapy, 68*(Suppl. 1), S1-S48.

Ball, S. L., Holland, A. J., Hon, J., Huppert, F. A., Treppner, P., & Watson, P. C. (2006). Personality and behavior changes mark the early stages of Alzheimer's disease in adults with Down's syndrome: Findings from a prospective population-based study. *International Journal of Geriatric Psychiatry, 21*, 661-673. doi: 10.1002/gps.1545

Ballan, M. S., & Sormanti, M. (2014). Trauma, grief and the social model: Practice guidelines for working with adults with intellectual disabilities in the wake of disasters. *Review of Disability Studies*. Retrieved from https://www.rdsjournal.org/index.php/journal/article/view/339

Bigby, C., Frawley, P., & Ramcharan, P. (2014). A collaborative group method of inclusive research. *Journal of Applied Research in Intellectual Disabilities, 27*(1), 54-64.

Bowers, B., Webber, R., & Bigby, C. (2014). Health issues of older people with intellectual disability in group homes. *Journal of Intellectual & Developmental Disability, 39*(3), 261-269. doi: 10.3109/13668250.2014.936083

Broughton, S., & Thomson, K. (2000). Women with learning disabilities: Risk behaviours and experiences of the cervical smear test. *Journal of Advanced Nursing, 32*(4), 905-912.

Burke, M. M., Taylor, J. L., Urbano, R., & Hodapp, R. M. (2012). Predictors of future caregiving by adult siblings of individuals with intellectual and developmental disabilities. *American Journal on Intellectual and Developmental Disabilities, 117*(1), 33-47.

Buys, L., Aird, R., & Miller, E. (2012). Service providers' perceptions of active ageing among older adults with lifelong intellectual disabilities. *Journal of Intellectual Disability Research, 56*(12), 1133-1147. doi: 10.1111/j.1365-2788.2011.01500

Chng, J., Stancliffe, R., Wilson, N., & Anderson, K. (2013). Engagement in retirement: An evaluation of the effect of active mentoring on engagement of older adults with intellectual disability in mainstream community groups. *Journal of Intellectual Disability Research, 57*(12), 1130-1142.

Coppus, A. M., Evenhuis, H. M., Verberne, G., Visser, F. E., Eikelenboom, P., van Gool, W. A., … van Duijn, C. M. (2010). Early age at menopause is associated with increased risk of dementia and mortality in women with Down syndrome. *Journal of Alzheimer's Disease, 19*(2), 545-550.

Dicks, S., Jackson, S., Pasokhy, A., Catty, N., & Symes, M. (2015). Training for staff who care for clients with dementia: Stacey Dicks and colleagues explore the benefits of training for carers of people with learning disabilities whose clients are more likely than the rest of the population to develop Alzheimer's. *Learning Disability Practice, 18*(9), 28-32.

Dillenburger, K., & McKerr, L. (2011). 'How long are we able to go on?' Issues faced by older family caregivers of adults with disabilities. *British Journal of Learning Disabilities, 39*(1), 29-38.

Dodevska, G. A., & Vassos, M. V. (2013). What qualities are valued in residential direct care workers from the perspective of people with an intellectual disability and managers of accommodation services? *Journal of Intellectual Disability Research, 57*(7) 601-615.

Evenhuis, H. M., Hermans, H. M., Bastiaanse, L. P., & Echteld, M. A. (2012). Frailty and disability in older adults with intellectual disabilities: Results from the healthy ageing and intellectual disability study. *Journal of the American Geriatrics Society, 60*(5), 934-938. doi: 10.1111/j.1532-5415.2012.03925

Flynn, M., Brown Salomons, H., Burns Salomons, S., & Keywood, K. (2009). The palliative care experiences of adults with learning disabilities/intellectual disability: The implications for ethical decision making. *International Journal on Disability and Human Development, 8*(1), 25-32.

Gibbs, S., Brown, M., & Muir, W. (2008). The experiences of adults with intellectual disabilities and their carers in general hospitals: A focus group study. *Journal of Intellectual Disability Research, 52*(12), 1061-1077.

Haveman, M., Perry, J., Salvador-Carulla, L., Walsh, P., Noonan, Kerr, M., … Weber, G. (2011). Ageing and health status in adults with intellectual disabilities: Results of the European POMONA II study. *Journal of Intellectual & Developmental Disability, 36*(1), 49-60. doi: 10.3109/13668250.2010.549464

Havercamp, S. M., Scandlin, D., & Roth, M. (2004). Health disparities among adults with developmental disabilities, adults with other disabilities, and adults not reporting disability in North Carolina. *Public Health Reports, 119*(4), 418-426. doi: 10.1016/j.phr.2004.05.006

Heller, T., Fisher, D., Marks, B., & Hsieh, K. (2014). Interventions to promote health: Crossing networks of intellectual and developmental disabilities and aging. *Disability and Health Journal, 7*(1), S24-S32.

Heller, T., Janicki, M. P., Marks, B., Hammel, J., & Factor, A. (2008). Brief report: State of the science symposium on aging and developmental disabilities. *Journal of Policy and Practice in Intellectual Disabilities, 5*(4), 286-288.

Hemm, C., Dagnan, D., & Meyer, T. D. (2015). Identifying training needs for mainstream health care professionals, to prepare them for working with individuals with intellectual disabilities: A systematic review. *Journal of Applied Research in Intellectual Disabilities, 28*(2), 98-110.

Herge, E. A. (2008) A web based intervention to empower adults with intellectual disabilities (ID) to take charge of their health. Unpublished evidence-based capstone project

Hermans, H., & Evenhuis, H. M. (2012). Life events and their associations with depression and anxiety in older people with intellectual disabilities: Results of the HA-ID study. *Journal of Affective Disorders, 138*(1), 79-85.

Hurst, R. A. J. (2009). What might we learn from heartache? Loss, loneliness, and pedagogy. *Feminist Teacher, 20*(1), 31-41.

Janicki, M. P., Davidson, P., Henderson, C., McCallion, P., Taets, J., Force, L., … Ladrigan, P. (2002). Health characteristics and health services utilization in older adults with intellectual disability living in community residences. *Journal of Intellectual Disability Research, 46*(4), 287-298.

Kim, N., El Hoyek, G., & Chau, D. (2011). Long-term care of the aging population with intellectual and developmental disabilities. *Clinics in Geriatric Medicine, 27*(2), 291-300.

Krahn, G. L., Hammond, L., & Turner, A. (2006). A cascade of disparities: Health and health care access for people with intellectual disabilities. *Mental Retardation and Developmental Disabilities Research Reviews, 12*(1), 70-82.

Lennox, N., Bain, C., Rey-Conde, T., Purdie, D., Bush, R., & Pandeya, N. (2007). Effects of a comprehensive health assessment programme for Australian adults with intellectual disability: A cluster randomized trial. *International Journal of Epidemiology, 36*(1), 139-146. doi: dyl254

Lennox, N., Brolan, C., Dean, J., Ware, R., Boyle, F., Taylor Gomez, M., … Bain, C. (2013). General practitioners' views on perceived and actual gains, benefits and barriers associated with the implementation of an Australian health assessment for people with intellectual disability. *Journal of Intellectual Disability Research, 57*(10), 913-922.

Lewis, S., & Stenfert-Kroese, B. (2010). An investigation of nursing staff attitudes and emotional reactions towards patients with intellectual disability in a general hospital setting. *Journal of Applied Research in Intellectual Disabilities, 23*(4), 355-365.

Llewellyn, P. (2011). The needs of people with learning disabilities who develop dementia: A literature review. *Dementia, 10*(2), 235-247. doi: 10.1177/1471301211403457

Mahoney, W., & Roberts, E. (2011). Co-occupation in a day program for adults with developmental disabilities. *Journal of Occupation Science, 16*(3), 170-179. doi: 10.1080/14427591.2009.9686659

McEvoy, J., MacHale, R., & Tierney, E. (2012). Concept of death and perceptions of bereavement in adults with intellectual disabilities. *Journal of Intellectual Disability Research, 56*(2), 191-203. doi: 10.1111/j.1365-2788.2011.01456

Michael, J., & Richardson, A. (2008). Health care for all: The independent inquiry into access to health care for people with learning disabilities. *Tizard Learning Disability Review, 13*(4), 28-34.

Mizen, L. A., Macfie, M. L., Findlay, L., Cooper, S. A., & Melville, C. A. (2012). Clinical guidelines contribute to the health inequities experienced by individuals with intellectual disabilities. *Implementation Science, 7,* 42-5908-7-42. doi: 10.1186/1748-5908-7-42

Morgan, N., & McEvoy, J. (2014). Exploring the bereavement experiences of older women with intellectual disabilities in long-term residential care: A staff perspective. *OMEGA: Journal of Death and Dying, 69*(2), 117-135. doi: 10.2190/OM.69.2

Niemeijer, A., Frederiks, B., Depla, M., Eefsting, J., & Hertogh, C. (2013). The place of surveillance technology in residential care for people with intellectual disabilities: Is there an ideal model of application? *Journal of Intellectual Disability Research, 57*(3), 201-215. doi: 10.1111/j.1365-2788.2011.01526

Nochajski, S. M. (2000). The impact of age-related changes on the functioning of older adults with developmental disabilities. *Physical & Occupational Therapy in Geriatrics, 18*(1), 5-21.

O'Brien, P., McConkey, R., & García-Iriarte, E. (2014). Co-researching with people who have intellectual disabilities: Insights from a national survey. *Journal of Applied Research in Intellectual Disabilities, 27*(1), 65-75.

Perkins, E. A., & Moran, J. A. (2010). Aging adults with intellectual disabilities. *Journal of the American Medical Association, 304*(1), 91-92. doi: 10.1001/jama.2010.906

Perry, J., Beyer, S., & Holm, S. (2009). Assistive technology, telecare, and people with intellectual disabilities: Ethical considerations. *Journal of Medical Ethics, 35*(2), 81-86. doi: 10.1136/jme.2008.024588

Perry, J., Firth, C., Puppa, M., Wilson, R., & Felce, D. (2012). Targeted support and telecare in staffed housing for people with intellectual disabilities: Impact on staffing levels and objective lifestyle indicators. *Journal of Applied Research in Intellectual Disabilities, 25*(1), 60-70.

Prasher, V. P., & Filer, A., (1995). Behavioural disturbance in people with Down's syndrome and dementia. *Journal of Intellectual Disability Research, 39*(5), 432-436.

Prater, C. D., & Zylstra, R. G. (2006). Medical care of adults with mental retardation. *American Family Physician, 73*(12), 2175-2183.

Prevatt, B. (1998). Gynecologic care for women with mental retardation. *Journal of Obstetric, Gynecologic, & Neonatal Nursing, 27*(3), 251-256.

Read, S., & Elliott, D. (2007). Exploring a continuum of support for bereaved people with intellectual disabilities: A strategic approach. *Journal of Intellectual Disabilities, 11*(2), 167-181.

Regnard, C., Reynolds, J., Watson, B., Matthews, D., Gibson, L., & Clarke, C. (2007). Understanding distress in people with severe communication difficulties: Developing and assessing the Disability Distress Assessment Tool (DisDAT). *Journal of Intellectual Disability Research, 51*(4), 277-292.

Rose, N., Kent, S., & Rose, J. (2012). Health professionals' attitudes and emotions towards working with adults with intellectual disability (ID) and mental ill health. *Journal of Intellectual Disability Research, 56*(9), 854-864. doi: 10.1111/j.1365-2788.2011.01476

Shaw, K., Cartwright, C., & Craig, J. (2011). The housing and support needs of people with an intellectual disability into older age. *Journal of Intellectual Disability Research, 55*(9), 895-903.

Sheehan, R., Ali, A., & Hassiotis, A. (2014). Dementia in intellectual disability. *Current Opinion in Psychiatry, 27*(2), 143-148. doi: 10.1097/YCO.0000000000000032

Sinai, A., Bohnen, I., & Strydom, A. (2012). Older adults with intellectual disability. *Current Opinion in Psychiatry, 25*(5), 359-364. doi :10.1097/YCO.0b013e328355ab26

Sowney, M., & Barr, O. G. (2006). Caring for adults with intellectual disabilities: Perceived challenges for nurses in accident and emergency units. *Journal of Advanced Nursing, 55*(1), 36-45.

Stewart, B. W., & Tolliver, M. A. (2015).

"Being with" people with I/DD experiencing grief and loss. The Arc. Retrieved from https://futureplanning.thearc.org/pages/learn/where-to-start/webinars/archived-webinars

Strnadová, I., Cumming, T. M., Knox, M., Parmenter, T. R., & Lee, H. M. (2015). Perspectives on life, wellbeing, and ageing by older women with intellectual disability. *Journal of Intellectual and Developmental Disability, 40*(3), 275-285.

Strydom, A., Hassiotis, A., King, M., & Livingston, G. (2009). The relationship of dementia prevalence in older adults with intellectual disability (ID) to age and severity of ID. *Psychological Medicine, 39*(01), 13-21.

Sullivan, W. F., Heng, J., Cameron, D., Lunsky, Y., Cheetham, T., Hennen, B., ... Swift, I. (2006). Consensus guidelines for primary health care of adults with developmental disabilities. *Canadian Family Physician, 52*(11), 1410-1418.

Tracey, M. (2007). Key points in caring for older adults with intellectual/developmental disabilities. *Geriatric Nursing, 28*(1), 43-44.

Vassos, M., Nankervis, K., Skerry, T., & Lante, K. (2013). Work engagement and job burnout within the disability support worker population. *Research in Developmental Disabilities, 34*(11), 3884-3895.

Wang, K. Y. (2012). The care burden of families with members having intellectual and developmental disorder: A review of the recent literature. *Current Opinion in Psychiatry, 25*(5), 348-352. doi: 10.1097/YCO.0b013e3283564248

Wilkinson, J. E., & Cerreto, M. C. (2008). Primary care for women with intellectual disabilities. *Journal of the American Board of Family Medicine, 21*(3), 215-222. doi: 10.3122/jabfm.2008.03.070197

Wolfensberger, W. (1991). Reflections on a lifetime in human services and mental retardation. *American Journal of Mental Retardation, 29*(1), 1-15.

Zeilinger, E. L., Stiehl, K. A., & Weber, G. (2013). A systematic review on assessment instruments for dementia in persons with intellectual disabilities. *Research in Developmental Disabilities, 34*(11), 3962-3977.

ADDITIONAL RESOURCES

National Task Group on Intellectual Disabilities and Dementia Practices | http://aadmd.org/ntg

The Arc | www.thearc.org

Vanderbilt Kennedy Center for Excellence in Developmental Disabilities

    Toolkit for Primary Care Providers | http://vkc.mc.vanderbilt.edu/etoolkit

    Tips and Resources | https://vkc.mc.vanderbilt.edu/assets/files/tipsheets/copinglosstips.pdf

U.S. Department of Health and Human Services Administration for Community Living | www.acl.gov/Programs/index.aspx#Disabilities

Eastern Pennsylvania–Delaware Geriatric Education Center

    Older Adults and Technology Toolkit | http://epadgec.jefferson.edu/pdfs/seniortechtoolkit.pdf

    Education Toolkit | http://epadgec.jefferson.edu/education8.cfm

Finger Lakes Geriatric Education Center | https://www.urmc.rochester.edu/medicine/geriatrics/flgec/intellectual-and-developmental-disabilities.aspx

University of Wyoming Geriatric Education Center | http://www.uwyo.edu/wycoa/index.html

Geriatric Education Center of Greater Philadelphia | http://www.med.upenn.edu/gec/Educational-Materials.shtml

18

Consultation, Collaboration, and Coaching
The Role of Occupational Therapy

Kimberly Bryze, PhD, OTR/L

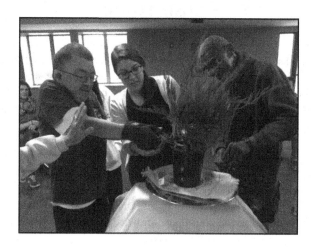

Key Words: coaching, collaboration, collaborative style, consultation

Bryze, K.
Occupational Therapy for Adults With Intellectual Disability (pp. 219-227).
© 2020 Taylor & Francis Group.

Occupational therapy practitioners may work with adults with intellectual disability in various settings and contexts through direct or indirect means. Occupational therapy for this population is often provided on a part-time or as-needed basis, using a consultative approach, given that organizations are often dependent upon the state budget or other limited funding sources for therapy services. However, skillful consultation requires both science and art. Utilizing occupational therapy knowledge and skills, the practitioner will utilize both science and art in the provision of consultation services. The practitioner must also demonstrate thoughtfulness and an other-centered approach for consultation to be effective for the other professionals, direct service staff, and clients with whom consultation takes place.

This chapter will present the similarities and differences between traditional (often referred to as *expert*) consultation, collaboration, and coaching. Each of these approaches evolves from certain assumptions the practitioner holds about the persons with whom the practitioner works and is based on ways in which one values interactive processes. Slightly different skill sets are required for each approach. The attitudes and values of each approach are congruent with those professed by occupational therapy, yet the benefits of collaborative approaches are highlighted. Application to occupational therapy, through presentation of a case example with an adult with intellectual disability will also be included.

CONSULTATION

Consultation is the act of exchanging information and opinions in order to solve a problem, reach a better understanding of something, or to make a decision. The consultant has more knowledge of, skill in, or familiarity with the challenge or problem that initiates the consultative work. Consultation may occur within a professional or health care setting, such as when an occupational therapist consults with a physician or when a consultant is specifically brought into a setting (e.g., a residential home) to help shed light on a particular problem in that context.

In occupational therapy practice, the practitioner is perceived as the expert in the role of consultant, while the consultee, typically a staff member, is perceived as the effector or implementer of the strategies recommended or prescribed by the occupational therapy consultant. Such consultation is most often directed toward enhancing the skills of the person with whom the consultant works (i.e., the consultee), to improve the targeted performance of the adult with intellectual disability. The consultation may focus on enhancing the consultee's knowledge, training in certain skills for working with the persons with intellectual disability, or may focus on designing and implementing a specific program for an individual. Such expert consultation may involve training other professionals or direct care staff in specific solutions to problems, or developing programs to meet particular needs within an agency, or consulting with case managers or qualified intellectual disability professionals regarding home or work environments, and how they impact particular persons with intellectual disability. Consultation may also address specific strategies for managing performance limitations of an individual with intellectual disability given body function limitations and may involve modifying tasks or adapting the environment in some way.

Consultation commonly implies a dynamic between the consultant and consultee, wherein, the consultant is in the position of expert. With the consultant's charge to help solve problems, educate others, train particular strategies or skills, design and establish approaches for managing the problem, implement systems for documentation of the various strategies, and many more tasks, the consultant's style may inadvertently resort to an authoritative, or *expert consultant*, role. As this consultant enters the situation, identifies the problems, initiates solutions, delegates tasks, then leaves until the next consulting time, the consultees are left with the responsibility to carry out the plans. The success or failure of the strategies implemented often rest on the consultees. In the worst case, the failure of a plan may be perceived to be due to some limitation of the persons with intellectual disability for whom the consultation process was initiated. Of course, consultation does not have to be such a grim experience. However, the attitudes and beliefs that guide an occupational therapy consultant must be thoughtfully examined and resultant behaviors and interactions must be consistent with the values that guide the consultancy.

COLLABORATIVE CONSULTATION

Consultation, as a general category of service delivery, may also reflect a more dynamic, interactional process of interpersonal collaboration, or a unique style of interacting with another professional. Collaborative consultation has several qualities or interactive characteristics, based on the consultant's beliefs and values, which differentiate it from an expert consultative model. In the special education literature, different authors (Bundy, 1991, 1995; Friend, 2000; Friend & Cook, 1990, 1991, 1992, 2010) have written extensively and articulated clearly the characteristics of collaborative consultation. They elaborate on the circumstances under which collaboration is actualized, in terms of the voluntary participation on the part of the partners, parity between or among the partners, and the partners' shared goals for collaboration, participation, accountability, and resources (Friend & Cook, 1990). The term *collaboration* simply means working together. Collaborative consultation has been defined in the special education literature as:

> [A]n interactive process that enables teams of people with diverse expertise to generate creative solutions to mutually defined problems. The outcome is enhanced, altered, and produces solutions that are different from those that the individual team member would produce independently. The major outcome of collaborative consultation is to provide comprehensive and effective programs for students with special needs within the most appropriate context. (Idol, Paolucci-Whitcomb, & Nevin, 2001, p. 1)

Collaboration is, therefore, conceptualized as a dynamic framework for efforts that endorse interdependent and coequal styles of interaction between the partners, working jointly to achieve common goals in a decision-making process. Collaboration is a broad, overarching process in which problems and successes, resources and solutions are shared between partners (Coben, Thomas, Sattler, & Morsink, 1997).

With a clear definition of collaboration, the occupational therapy practitioner must also understand the components of collaboration. Boshoff and Stewart (2013) emphasize the difference between teamwork, which is considered the action, and collaboration, which is considered the knowledge or underlying attitude. Collaboration requires open communication, knowledge and competence within one's discipline, problem-solving skills, conflict resolution skills, shared values and goals, established ground rules, defined team roles and responsibilities, an established formal meeting schedule, administrative support, and an equal exchange of ideas (Barnett & O'Shaughnessy, 2015; Bose & Hinojosa, 2008; Boshoff & Stewart, 2013). All of these components support the idea that professional partners must be comfortable giving up their real or perceived title as expert and must be willing to approach the relationship with open communication and mutual respect. Clearly, collaboration is a more complex form of interaction than most realize, to be used as a mindset rather than an end-goal (Kennedy & Stewart, 2011).

Effective collaborative consultation is supported by several critical elements: (1) voluntary participation in the team; (2) coequal status; (3) engagement in shared decision making; (4) communicating and informing each other of their unique impressions and areas of professional expertise; (5) work toward a common goal; and (6) shared accountability for the success of the adults with intellectual disability. As such, collaborative partners (i.e., consultant and consultee) work together voluntarily and willingly enter the collaborative, working relationship. Each partner has coequal status, and shares responsibility for the decision making and design of strategies directed toward meeting a common goal. Moreover, the goal is identified and agreed upon by all partners. Further, the partners communicate often and inform each other of progress, challenges, and their reasoning.

Each partner brings his or her unique impressions and areas of professional expertise and both share the commitment to and responsibility for the outcomes.

Collaborative consultation emerges from a culture of collaboration (Caron & McLaughlin, 2002), or a framework or set of possibilities from which to choose, and through which action steps are filtered or checked as the shared work progresses. Culture is considered to be an amalgam of shared meanings and values and the characteristics of culture are important to communication. The occupational therapy consultant and the consultees must create or develop their culture of collaboration to effectively share knowledge and support a common vision of improving the quality of life or performance of the persons with intellectual disability whom they serve.

Collaborative partners jointly identify the problems, work together to prioritize goals, establish action steps and suggest recommendations, share the work across time, and each have a stake in the benefits, as well as the problems, encountered along the way. Collaborative consultation involves individuals with differing expertise working cooperatively to solve a problem involving the persons with intellectual disability. Collaborative relationships must extend beyond the emphasis on problem solving to collectively direct the energies and abilities of all members toward the creation of a system that supports and nurtures each client served (Johnston & Brinamen, 2012).

Collaboration may also stand on its own, as a style of interacting and working with others, without the risk of stepping into an assumed role or responsibility for instructing or telling another professional what needs to be done, as is more common with consultation. Therefore, collaboration may also be described as a style for direct interaction between the collaborative partners, as they work toward a common goal. As a style, collaboration becomes authentic when it is linked effectively to another process or activity, such as consulting or problem-solving (Cook & Friend, 2010). More often, collaboration is a process used by individuals, teams, or schools (Giangreco, 1995) for the planning, development, and monitoring of interdisciplinary interventions (Barnes & Turner, 2001). It is a dynamic process that requires constant growth from those who practice it. Within teams, it involves the active processes of developing goals and objectives, initiating strategies, collaboratively monitoring these strategies, and reviewing the collective efforts related to specific outcomes.

Whether a style or a process, collaboration requires an ethical stance to be made by the professionals in their work together (Friend & Cook, 1990). One's ethical stance endorses a set of actions or behaviors, which are based on one's beliefs, values, and roles (Friend & Cook, 1992). A stance for collaboration presumes that one's beliefs and values reflect attitudes that shape how participants act in collaborative interactions. Collaboration is based on beliefs held regarding the collaborative partner, persons served, and process of consultation itself. An essential characteristic of the collaborative process is trust in one's colleagues, and the commitment of time and energy to the collaboration facilitates increased trust, and genuine respect for the other participants (Dreiling & Bundy, 2003; Friend & Cook, 1990).

The collaborative consultation relationship has been examined with particular traits identified within examples of effective, collaborative consultants (Johnston & Brinamen, 2012). The authors' recommendations are for consultants to adopt a style, use inquiry instead of inquisition, avoid acting as an outside authority, appreciate subjective experience, convey authentic caring and genuine compassion, and share vulnerability. Each of these components fosters the spirit of collaboration, which must be created and supported. Collaboration is much more of a "relational process of reflective facilitation" than a problem-solving endeavor (Johnston & Brinamen, 2012, p. 230).

As mentioned earlier, trust in one's colleagues and the commitment of time and energy to collaboration, facilitates genuine respect for the other team members (Dreiling & Bundy, 2003; Friend & Cook, 1990). The individuals' shared commitment and vision for their work together can guide them into their collective future. Occupational therapy consultants must be prepared to become change agents and aim to implement more collaborative models of service delivery in the home, vocational, and leisure settings where adults with intellectual disability live, work, and recreate.

Supports and Barriers to Collaboration

There are both supports and barriers to the occupational therapy practitioner's ability to collaborate within the various settings that serve adults with intellectual disability. The collaborative process is facilitated when the consultant uses language that is understandable to the consultees, providing all partners with the equal opportunity to have a voice and discuss the interventions or strategies (Phelan & Ng, 2015). Having positive and open communication between the occupational therapy practitioner and staff members while discussing interventions and progress also supports the collaboration process (Asher & Nichols, 2016). It is helpful to arrange set meeting times for consultation and to provide training or in-service opportunities for specific strategies, approaches, and formative methods in order to monitor progress and handle challenges that arise in the process.

As there is often a lack of adequate funding and resources to support the time and effort needed for collaborative efforts, some professionals may be led to default to problem-focused, expert consultation. At face value, such problem-based consultation appears to be more time efficient, although it may not be as effective for the persons served. Further, the benefits of face-to-face meetings are substantial, but the use of technology and virtual meetings should not be eliminated. Skype (Microsoft), Zoom, or other virtual meetings using computer technology may be a viable method for maintaining collaborative relationships, especially when time or distance is a barrier for collaborative approaches (e.g., rural areas, large urban areas where traffic impacts time management).

Occupational therapy practitioners can provide in-services, resources, and support interprofessional education efforts. The consulting practitioner will be most effective if one is willing to meet the consultees' working style and interpersonal characteristics in a flexible manner. If administrative support, whether financial or the allocation of time for meeting together, can be provided, collaborative efforts may be further strengthened.

Collaborative efforts are fostered when recommended interventions are embedded within authentic environments, and the occupational therapy practitioner works alongside a staff member to assess dynamically whether the recommended intervention or process will be beneficial for a particular client or situation. Willingness to "get one's hands dirty" often goes a long way toward building trust and communication with challenging situations or clients who demonstrate their frustration or fear in aggressive ways (Silverman, Hong, & Trepanier-Street, 2010). Gaining this insider's perspective on the problems in real time will help solidify the collaborative partnership for deriving appropriate recommendations and implementing effective solutions. There are many different methods of approaches that can be utilized, not all of them appropriate for each situation, but the willingness on the part of the consultant to engage, participate, and work with the consultee indicates a respect and value for the other partner in the collaborative relationship.

COACHING

Coaching is becoming more evident in occupational therapy literature and offers a strength-based approach to help others problem solve and overcome challenges. Coaching is described as:

> An asset-based appreciative approach highly congruent with enabling lasting occupational change.... The emphasis is to coach people to take responsibility for self-direction in naming priorities and goals, which are most meaningful to them. Coaching involves collaboratively identifying challenges, setting goals and working towards the goals set. The coach may offer feedback on occupational performance in order to support and enhance occupational development. (Townsend & Polatajko, 2007, p. 119)

The aim of coaching is to create a supportive environment within the context of relationship and interaction to enable client readiness and motivation for change. Coaching is client centered and draws on the strengths and abilities of the consultee. As a method, coaching is inherently problem oriented, but such a problem-focused stance may inadvertently accentuate the perceived power of the occupational therapy consultant. A specific form of coaching, solution-focused coaching, offers a way for the coach to assume a stance of trust in the client and employs efforts toward the client generating solutions for themselves. Solution-focused coaching intends to not direct the client in any particular way but draw from the client's creativity and expertise in the situation.

Solution-focused coaching was used with teams of staff who served adults with intellectual disability in the Netherlands (Roeden, Maaskant, Bannink, & Curfs, 2012), to examine whether this approach helped the teams attain their goals of solving client-related problems. A protocol was used by the coaches in this intervention study, with consistent steps taken during each session designed to facilitate positive solutions, attainment of goals, and enhance the quality of relationships with clients. Thirteen teams of staff participated in the study. The coach utilized the steps of exploring each team's self-identified problem with the participants, setting a specific goal related to the problem, asking specific questions during each of the coaching sessions (e.g., monitoring their progress toward meeting their goals on a 1 to 10 scale, exploring the competence and confidence of the team members, asking open-ended questions), then providing feedback. Results indicated that the teams experienced positive changes in goal attainment, proactive thinking, and the quality of relationships. It was determined that solution-focused coaching can be a useful approach to build relationships, facilitate self-efficacy, and foster working together as caregivers for individuals with intellectual disability (Roeden et al., 2012).

Solution-focused coaching requires the coaches to remain open to collaborative shaping of interventions, remain intentionally respectful, and demonstrate trust in the consultee's capacity for seeking and implementing creative solutions to the problems they identify and set as goals (Baldwin et al., 2013). Such an approach requires skill in reframing problems and challenges, using key questions with an open, curious mind, and strong skills in the therapeutic use of self, in order to connect and relate to the client. Strength-based coaching may be effective in supporting staff members to deal proactively with problems involved with their care (Roeden, Maaskant, & Curfs, 2014). "Therapists' ability to maintain a strengths-based, client-driven process that facilitates client engagement and empowerment is critical" when using solution-focused coaching (Baldwin et al., 2013, p. 478).

Occupational therapy practitioners using coaching should proceed with caution and monitor outcomes carefully. Further research is needed to determine the utility for coaching applications within occupational therapy practice, especially with different populations and across various settings (Kessler & Graham, 2015). However, the underlying beliefs and value for the partners in such a coaching approach is consistent with the collaborative process and style presented earlier in this chapter. Occupational therapy practitioners should examine their attitudes and interpersonal style considering specific consultancy opportunities, to determine whether expert consultation, collaborative consultation, or solution-focused coaching methods might be most appropriate and consistent with one's therapeutic approach. Perhaps an example of one collaborative consultative experience would be helpful.

CASE EXAMPLE

Margie's Work Dance

I (the author) was asked to consult with an agency's day program/workshop, as one of their clients was just returning to work after a medical leave of absence. I had consulted with this agency in the past and had had interactions with the client. Margie was 39 years old, diagnosed with Down syndrome, and had experienced a cervical neck injury (cervical spondylolisthesis) that resulted from a car accident. Cervical fusion and 2 months of rehabilitation in a subacute care center were accomplished, and Margie returned to her group home and to work. The rehabilitation center therapists sent Margie home with a list of exercises to do several times each day but Margie was not motivated and refused (loudly) to do them. Margie was primarily left-handed, but the injury left her with residual right arm weakness, and she rarely used it to hold or support objects during work tasks and had difficulty managing her lunch containers. She reportedly used both arms during dressing and personal, self-care tasks, but staff reported that she seemed to "forget" her right arm when doing tasks at a table, such as during meals, working at her workstation, or working on her puzzles after dinner. Her primary work supervisor, Karen, stated their main concerns were two-fold: (1) that Margie "would not use both hands to work," and (2) staff's fears that she would move too fast and fall, potentially hurting herself on the concrete floors or tables, chairs, and people in the workshop setting. Even after her recent medical leave of absence, Margie was quite energetic, preferring to walk quickly and change directions abruptly when someone or something interesting caught her eye. Margie was curious, highly social, and "clumsy." In the week prior to my consulting appointment, she had fallen recently when hurrying across the room to talk to a peer, but she was unable to use both arms to protect herself as she fell forward, possibly due to the weaker right arm.

After learning from Karen the concerns and staff's desire to "keep Margie safe" and "get her to use both hands," I wanted to spend time observing Margie as she worked at her workstation. When Karen led me to the workstation, Margie promptly stood and hugged me tightly in greeting. Her hug was firmer with her left arm than her right. I hugged her back, firmly, indirectly indicating that she could hug me tighter. The right-side weakness was obvious to me. After explaining that I was glad to see her back at work and that I'd like to see what she was working on that day, she sat down and resumed her work. Her task that day was to fill small plastic bags with 10 nuts and 10 bolts, then place each filled bag into a box located toward the right side of the table. She had a bin with sections for the nuts and for the bolts situated toward her left side on the table. I noted that the plastic bags had been opened and the edges folded over to keep them open. A wooden jig (template) with 2 rows of 10 indentations for each of the nuts and bolts, was positioned on the table at her midline. The bin to hold the filled plastic bags was positioned on the table to her right.

Margie sat in an armchair at the table and used her left hand to take nuts and bolts from the bin on her left and place them into the wooden jig indentations. She then attempted to place the nuts and bolts, one or two at a time, into a pre-opened plastic bag using only her left hand. Her right arm remained in her lap, and she made no attempt to bring it up to the table to help her left hand (although she had readily raised both arms at the shoulder to hug me). She struggled for several minutes but placed all 20 items into the plastic bag and placed the filled bag into the bin on her right side. As she moved her left arm in the horizontal plane, she shifted her trunk position by elevating her shoulder and abducting her left elbow as she grasped the items, placed them in the bag, and reached for items on the table. Karen prompted Margie verbally to use her right hand. Margie raised her right arm and placed her forearm onto the table close to the wooden jig but did not attempt to hold the jig or plastic bag. Her forearm soon slipped back onto her lap and she used her left hand.

I said that it seemed hard for her to keep her right arm up on the table. Margie agreed but then explained and demonstrated that she could open, close, and pinch with her right hand. I asked her if she would like to use both hands, to which she replied, "I used to." As her chair was positioned approximately 10 inches from the table, I asked her permission to help push her chair in a bit more. As I pushed her a few inches closer to the table, I angled the chair so her right elbow and forearm could rest more comfortably on the table while still being able to easily reach with her left arm. She attempted to reach her right hand toward an opened plastic bag but compensated with shoulder elevation and squishing the bag closed. I asked her how we could make holding the plastic bags easier for her. She told me that her hand "needs to stay open" so the bag wouldn't squish closed. Karen asked, "Would a cup in her hand help?" She walked to her desk and brought back a 3-inch in diameter metal pencil cup. Margie held the cup in her right hand and I suggested that she place the plastic bag into the cup, which she did using her left hand. With the support of the table, the cup in her right hand, and a slightly angled position, she was able to complete her work tasks with greater speed and accuracy. "This is much better," Margie said.

Leaving Margie to her work, Karen and I discussed the exercises that were intended to help improve the range of motion and strength in Margie's right arm. Karen had worked with the house staff to encourage Margie to do the exercises with her peers after lunch, during break times, or while others were watching a movie or playing table games with each other. Karen told me that she tried to exercise with Margie on Friday afternoon when work was slow, and the other clients were watching a movie or playing table games with each other. Margie was not one to sit and watch a movie, and table games were not enjoyable to her, so Karen thought that this might be another opportunity to try to follow through on the exercises but Margie continued to refuse. I asked what Margie does like besides socializing with others during break times. She and several other clients had a consistent Ladies Group at lunch and break times, always sitting together at one table, socializing and enjoying each other's company. Karen happened to mention that the Ladies Group had loved watching Richard Simmons exercise tapes one week when there was no work, which led to a conversation about "Sweating to the Oldies" as one of his workout tapes recommended. Karen stated that she would be willing to try these tapes and perhaps the Ladies Group would workout as a special session once per week to begin.

I returned to the agency 2 weeks later and Karen and Margie had adjusted the seating position at the workspace for different work tasks (e.g., folding letters for stuffing envelopes, affixing stickers onto plastic buckets of animal food). I learned that the workout tapes and sessions were successful and going to be done 3 times that week and beyond. Margie told me that she called the workout sessions "dancing" and explained that she saw on television what appeared to be a creative, exotic dance with ribbons, with several dancers in colorful costumes. I asked Margie if she had ever danced with ribbons before (remembering back to old gym classes with "dances" in the curriculum). She told me no but that she wanted to do that. Karen went to find something ribbon-like from the activity closet and returned with chiffon scarves. Margie gathered her ladies and they enacted a spontaneous ribbon (scarf) dance to music from an iPod (Apple). As she danced, Margie used both her arms, watched her friends' movements to imitate them, and expelled quite a bit of energy during this break time—all without "exercising."

Karen and Margie continued to find creative movement experiences over the next couple of months. While Margie's right arm strength never returned to pre-injury, she spontaneously used both arms in leisure, work, and self-care tasks that required bilateral movement. She demonstrated greater stability, and staff were no longer fearful that she would fall, as they observed what appeared to be better coordination. Margie also demonstrated renewed enthusiasm for learning new work tasks. Moreover, the Ladies Group won first place in the talent show at the agency's winter holiday party.

CONCLUSION

This chapter presented issues and strategies pertinent to occupational therapy consultation, collaboration, and coaching. Occupational therapy practitioners often serve as consultants to adults with intellectual disability given the constraints of funding that preclude monies for ongoing, direct interventions. Consultative approaches are often more common and can be extremely powerful in services delivered to adults with intellectual disability, agencies, or communities. An important focus of these consultative approaches is the underlying attitude or value for working with, supporting, and developing partnerships with the other professionals, staff, and family members who are the recipients of our consultation efforts. Further, collaborative consultation, if done well, can be a powerful intervention approach for occupational therapy for adults with intellectual disability.

REFERENCES

Asher, A., & Nichols, J. D. (2016). Collaboration around facilitating emergent literacy: Role of occupational therapy. *Journal of Occupational Therapy, Schools, & Early Intervention, 9*, 51-73.

Baldwin, P., King, G., Evans, J., McDougall, S., Tucker, M. A., & Servais, M. (2013). Solution-focused coaching in pediatric rehabilitation: An integrated model for practice. *Physical & Occupational Therapy in Pediatrics, 33*, 467-483.

Barnes, K. J., & Turner, K. D. (2001). Team collaborative practices between teachers and occupational therapists. *American Journal of Occupational Therapy, 55*, 83-89.

Barnett, J. E. H., & O'Shaughnessy, K. (2015). Enhancing collaboration between occupational therapists and early childhood educators working with children on the autism spectrum. *Early Childhood Education Journal, 43*(6), 467-472.

Bose, P., & Hinojosa, J. (2008). Reported experiences from occupational therapists interacting with teachers in inclusive early childhood classrooms. *American Journal of Occupational Therapy, 62*, 289-297.

Boshoff, K., & Stewart, H. (2013). Key principles for confronting the challenges of collaboration in educational settings. *Australian Occupational Therapy Journal, 60*, 144-147.

Bundy, A. C. (Ed.). (1991). *Making a difference: OTs and PTs in public schools.* Chicago, IL: University of Illinois at Chicago.

Bundy, A. C. (1995). Assessment and intervention in school-based practice: Answering questions and minimizing discrepancies. *Physical & Occupational Therapy in Pediatrics, 15*, 69-88.

Caron, E. A., & McLaughlin, M. J. (2002). Indicators of beacons of excellence schools: What do they tell us about collaborative practices? *Journal of Educational and Psychological Consultation, 13*, 285-313.

Coben, S. S., Thomas, C. C., Sattler, R. O., & Morsink, C. V. (1997). Meeting the challenge of consultation and collaboration: Developing interactive teams. *Journal of Learning Disabilities, 30*, 427-432.

Cook, L., & Friend, M. (2010). The state of the art of collaboration on behalf of students with disabilities. *Journal of Educational and Psychological Consultation, 20*, 1-8.

Dreiling, C. S., & Bundy, A. C. (2003). A comparison of consultative model and direct—indirect intervention with preschoolers. *American Journal of Occupational Therapy, 57*, 566-569.

Friend, M. (2000). Perspective: Myths and misunderstandings about professional collaboration. *Remedial and Special Education, 21*, 130-132.

Friend, M., & Cook, L. (1990). Collaboration as a predictor for success in school reform. *Journal of Educational and Psychological Consultation, 1*, 69-86.

Friend, M., & Cook, L. (1991). Principles for the practice of collaboration. *Preventing School Failure, 35*(4), 6.

Friend, M., & Cook, L. (1992). The ethics of collaboration. *Journal of Educational and Psychological Consultation, 3*(2), 181-184.

Friend, M., & Cook, L. (2010). *Interactions: Collaboration skills for school professionals* (6th ed.). Upper Saddle River, NJ: Pearson/Merrill.

Giangreco, M. F. (1995). Related service decision-making: A foundational component of effective education for students with disabilities. *Physical & Occupational Therapy in Pediatrics, 15*, 47-67.

Idol, L., Paolucci-Whitcomb, P., & Nevin, A. (2001). *Collaborative consultation.* Austin, TX: Pro-Ed.

Johnston, K., & Brinamen, C. F. (2012). The consultation relationship—From transactional to transformative: Hypothesizing about the nature of change. *Infant Mental Health Journal, 33*, 226-233.

Kennedy, S., & Stewart, H. (2011). Collaboration between occupational therapists and teachers: Definitions, implementation and efficacy. *Australian Occupational Therapy Journal, 58*, 209-214.

Kessler, D., & Graham, F. (2015). The use of coaching in occupational therapy: An integrative review. *Australian Occupational Therapy Journal, 62*, 160-176.

Phelan, S. K., & Ng, S. L. (2015). A case review: Reframing school-based practices using a critical perspective. *Physical & Occupational Therapy in Pediatrics, 35*, 396-411.

Roeden, J. M., Maaskant, M. A., Bannink, F. P., & Curfs, F. M. G. (2012). Solution-focused coaching of staff of people with severe and moderate intellectual disabilities: A case series. *Journal of Policy and Practice in Intellectual Disabilities, 9*, 185-194.

Roeden, J. M., Maaskant, M. A., & Curfs, L. M. (2014). Processes and effects of solution-focused brief therapy in people with intellectual disabilities: A controlled study. *Journal of Intellectual Disability Research, 58*, 307-320.

Silverman, K., Hong, S., & Trepanier-Street, M. (2010). Collaboration of teacher education and child disability health care: Transdisciplinary approach to inclusive practice for early childhood pre-service teachers. *Early Childhood Education Journal, 37*(6), 461-468.

Townsend, E. A., & Polatajko, H. J. (2007). *Enabling occupation II: Advancing an occupational therapy vision for health, well-being and justice through occupation.* Ottawa, ON, Canada: CAOT Publications.

19

Visions for the Future

Ricardo C. Carrasco, PhD, OTR/L, FAOTA and
Kelsea Rose A. Grampp, OTD, OTR/L

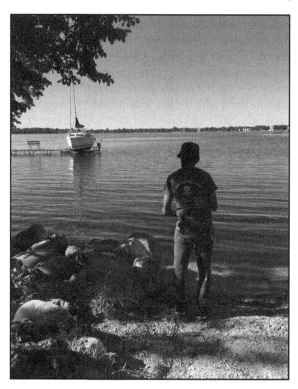

Key Words: advocacy, levels of occupational science research,
occupational alienation, occupational injustice, occupational science

Bryze, K.
Occupational Therapy for Adults With Intellectual Disability (pp. 229-241).
© 2020 Taylor & Francis Group.

The American Occupational Therapy Association's (AOTA's) (2007) Centennial Vision identifies that occupational therapy as a profession strives to become a "powerful, widely recognized, science-driven, and evidence-based profession with a globally connected and diverse workforce meeting society's occupational needs." In 2017, this vision expanded to include specific action steps that occupational therapy will take to remain a key stakeholder in a dynamic and changing health care system through Vision 2025 (AOTA, 2016). Therefore, AOTA's Centennial Vision and Vision 2025 demand that occupational therapy practitioners not only identify barriers of occupational participation and performance for adults with intellectual disability, but also develop a science-driven, evidence-based practice to improve this population's quality of life through occupational engagement. This chapter aims to distinguish a vision of occupational therapy practice for adults for intellectual disability by (1) identifying current issues surrounding this population, (2) discussing funding and services available to adults with intellectual disability, (3) calculating the need for advocacy and legislation, (4) summarizing the promotion of occupational justice, and (5) to relating research guided by occupational science.

CURRENT ISSUES

As discussed in previous chapters, in regard to their diagnosis, adults with intellectual disability present with a unique set of client factors that often lead to a lower quality of life compared to adults without disabilities (Simões & Santos, 2016). For instance, Cooper, Smiley, Morrison, Williamson, and Allan (2007) estimated that 40% of adults with intellectual disability also have mental illness. These conditions commonly include psychotic disorders, affective disorders, anxiety disorders, obsessive-compulsive behavior, and sleep disorders (Cooper et al., 2007). It becomes important to understand the implication of a mental health illness because these conditions and disorders are often negatively correlated to the quality of life, health, and wellness of the individual with intellectual disability (Cooper et al., 2007) and his or her family (McIntyre et al., 2002). A young adult with intellectual disability's mental health and perceived negative behaviors are strongly correlated to a family's decision to seek an out-of-home placement or institutionalization for that individual (McIntyre, Blacher, & Baker, 2002). Placing an individual with intellectual disability in an out-of-home placement becomes of concern when considering the context and environment provided by an institution. Caregivers providing care for adults with intellectual disability in out-of-home placements often do not have adequate support, structure, and education to provide the highest level of care for their residents (McVilly, Stancliffe, Parmenter, & Burton-Smith, 2006). The challenges of housing individuals with intellectual disability in out-of-home placements or institutions include higher rates of loneliness and lower quality of life compared to adults with intellectual disability who live at home with their families (McVilly et al., 2006).

Aging is a major concern of the general population, but the implications of aging are of greater concern for the adult with intellectual disability population and their families. Later in life, adults with intellectual disability have increased multimorbidity compared to the overall population (Hermans & Evenhuis, 2014). These adults have higher rates of mental health illness and perceived negative behaviors when compared to the general population. In turn, these increased health concerns lead to more unmet needs compared to the overall population (Krahn, Hammond, & Turner, 2006). Unmet needs often include supported employment, housing, day programs, access to health care services, and leisure activities (Burke & Heller, 2017). To further evaluate the severity of the unmet needs of this population, adults with intellectual disability who are nonverbal or from minority backgrounds and have health concerns, are exponentially more likely to have a greater number of unmet needs (Burke & Heller, 2017). Unmet needs lead to more chronic conditions, ailments, and lack of preventative care, further increasing the marginalization of this population.

In addition to the higher rate of unmet needs, if an individual with intellectual disability is competitively employed, as only an estimated 18% of adults with intellectual disability are (Dean & Burke, 2017), they are also unlikely to have health insurance or a pay scale above the national minimum wage (Heyman, Stokes, & Siperstein, 2016). The lack of health insurance and minimum wage pay scale continue to be contributors to their needs being unmet, as they will likely have severe financial struggles when there are any health issues. Adults with intellectual disability fall victim to the health care system, as they do not have adequate access to health care services with appropriate attention to care needs and education on the importance of health prevention (Krahn et al., 2006).

Today and historically, there are persistent societal views that young adults with intellectual disability are incapable of benefiting from a post-secondary education, and thus, are not prepared for the hidden curriculum of post-secondary education during high school (Arnold & Rybski, 2010; Garrison-Wade, 2012; Oertle & Bragg, 2014). The hidden curriculum identified in the post-secondary education of adults with intellectual disability is disability awareness and disclosure, adult-based navigation, and persisting challenges with adaptive behaviors (Berg, Jirikowic, Haerling, & MacDonald, 2017). If adults with intellectual disability are not given the opportunity to explore and successfully study post-secondary education from a societal and institutional standpoint, their lives are then further marginalized due to lack of education and exposure.

The context and environment of today's society does not support community involvement of adults with intellectual disability, and thus, creates strong barriers in their community participation (Umeda et al., 2017). Despite the definite community barriers to these individuals, this population has a strong desire to participate in their community (Hall, 2016). Accepting, identifying, and then responding to the existing barriers for adults with intellectual disability through support services in the community will provide for a better quality of life than institutionalization (Felce, 2017). Although community services are not always included in today's funded programs, costs would be dependent upon the funding structure and planned investment prior to deinstitutionalization (Felce, 2017). Community inclusion would be greatly improved through assessing current issues that adults with intellectual disability face, allowing occupational therapy practitioners to better advocate and create evidence-based treatment interventions to promote occupational participation and performance for this population (Francisco & Carlson, 2002).

FUNDING AND SERVICES

There are numerous funding sources and services available for adults with intellectual disability, but there is still a significant portion of these adults with unmet needs. The challenge becomes one of discerning which programs and funding sources are available to each individual and then the individual and their family accessing those resources (Centers for Parent Information & Resources, 2017). Public websites, such as Centers for Parent Information & Resources (2017), provide parents and families with a detailed list of resources available, organized by employment, post-secondary education, recreation, independent living, assistive technology, and disability living. In terms of employment, the Department of Vocational Rehabilitation is a national, federal-state program that provides services to adults with intellectual disability in order for them to gain employment, with each state having a central vocational rehabilitation agency (Centers for Parent Information & Resources, 2017). The Job Accommodation Network is a free resource for guidance on accommodations for individuals with disabilities with a toll-free hotline (Centers for Parent Information & Resources, 2017). Another invaluable resource made available to this community is the ADA [Americans with Disabilities Act] National Network, funded through the U.S. Department of Health and Human Services, which provides a list of resources available on their website (ADA National Network, 2017). The ADA National Network website offers state-specific networks, ADA fact sheets and publications, and specific topics to different populations (ADA National Network, 2017). Goodwill Industries International is a private organization that offers training and support to individuals with intellectual disability (Goodwill Industries International, 2017).

In addition to employment, post-secondary education is often a main concern for adults with intellectual disability and their families, so the individual can obtain better employment to support their future. Although there are multiple organizations that seek to provide resources to support adults with intellectual disability receiving a post-secondary education, there are far less services and resources available compared to organizations and resources made available to gain employment (Centers for Parent Information & Resources, 2017). The Association on Higher Education and Disability (2017) is a multidisciplinary, professional organization for professionals to gain an understanding of the supports in place for adults with intellectual disability to pursue a higher education. The National Center for College Students with Disabilities (NCCSD; 2017) is a federally funded, national association for college students with any disability, their families, and college faculty, who are in need of assistance or guidance, through post-secondary education. In addition to the individuals who work with the student with intellectual disability, the NCCSD also provides support to faculty members with any disabilities (NCCSD, 2017).

In terms of recreation programs and supports, there are far more opportunities for support for individuals with physical disabilities compared to individuals with cognitive impairments (Centers for Parent Information & Resources, 2017). The United States Adaptive Recreation Center (USARC) works with public centers, including hospitals, schools, and park and recreation centers, to assist individuals with physical and cognitive impairments to support their participation. Additionally, USARC also offers seasonal recreational programing for children and adults with physical and cognitive impairments (USARC, 2017). On the USARC website, there is a list of city specific, adaptive programs (USARC, 2017). Recreation programs and supports can be overlooked, as they are not an immediate need, but they do positively impact community involvement.

In addition to federal programs, there are multiple privately-run organizations that assist individuals with intellectual disability (Benefits.gov, 2017). The University of Kansas sponsors the Research and Training Center on Independent Living, which is outlined on their website, and features resources and products available for adults (University of Kansas, 2017). Although the Research and Training Center on Independent Living does not focus exclusively on helping adults with intellectual disability, they do offer a wide array of project-specific, center-wide training programs (University of Kansas, 2017). The training programs vary greatly from purpose to context and are available for the individual with disability and the health care professional (University of Kansas, 2017). Smaller private organizations, such as the Research and Training Center on Independent Living, in addition to the Social Security Administration (SSA), maximize the resources adults with intellectual disability can receive and all available options should be considered these individuals and their families.

Assistive technology has the ability to transform people's lives through simplification, to promote occupational participation and performance. Specifically, for adults with intellectual disability, assistive technology has the ability to remind people of their schedules and transform the way they participate in their chosen occupations. The Center of Technology and Disability (CTD; 2017) provides free resources on assistive technology to state and local leaders, teachers, families, and service providers. The CTD (2017) website includes a wealth of resources for transition including the following subcategories: assistive technology planning, independent living, post-secondary, technology tools, and transition to employment/workforce. It is important for occupational therapy practitioners to become aware of assistive technology that may be beneficial for adults with intellectual disability in order to increase their occupational participation.

The federal program for funding of Medicaid Managed Care fluctuates greatly depending upon the political landscape of the country (Chatterjee & Sommers, 2017). Conservative policy makers have declared their intention to repeal the Patient Protection and Affordable Care Act and diminish Medicaid funding and, in 2016, proposed a funding cut of Medicaid by approximately 50% (Chatterjee & Sommers, 2017). Proposed funding cuts will lead to an increase of individuals, both with and without disabilities, with unmet needs and higher state taxes (Chatterjee & Sommers, 2017). In light of policy changes, there is a current trend of Medicaid state programs to transition to a model often called *managed long-term services and supports*, with the rationale behind the transition being to decrease funding costs (Williamson, Perkins, et al., 2017). Although this overall change in policy is still being implemented across the United States, occupational therapy must position itself well to inform stakeholders about the best practices and needs of their clients (Williamson, Contreras, et al., 2017). To further consider changes in the Medicaid funding program, as it is both federal and state policy, the state of Florida will be considered. The Florida Senate proposed Senate Bill 916, which further cuts funding for Statewide Medicaid Managed Care, requiring prepaid plans for network providers and decreasing availability for consumers (Chatterjee & Sommers, 2017; The Florida Senate, 2017). On the other end of the spectrum is the state of California, which is a larger state than Florida and tends to be more liberal in its funding for Medicaid Managed Care (Kaiser Family Foundation, 2017). Under the current Medicaid Managed Care program in California, 12.3 million Americans are provided with health care and long-term care coverage. The American Health Care Act, proposed in 2017, would redesign the current Medicaid Managed Care program and eliminate the guarantee of services provided under the plan to millions of Americans (Kaiser Family Foundation, 2017). In today's ever-changing political climate, it becomes increasingly important for occupational therapy practitioners to understand legislation in the state where they are licensed to practice.

Despite the proposed changes in the American Health Care Act of 2017, the United States federal government has developed a screening instrument through a website to help identify resources available to an individual (Benefits.gov, 2017). One of the resources available is the SSA, which provides cash benefits to individuals with disabilities who are unable to work for 1 year or more, or who have terminal disabilities affecting their ability to work (SSA, 2017). The State Technology Act Projects is provided through the Rehabilitation Services Act and is a state-funded program to assist individuals with disabilities in using assistive technology (National Public Website on Assistive Technology, 2017). It is important for occupational therapy practitioners to have an understanding of the political atmosphere in order to provide the best services to their clients and advocate for their needs.

In looking to the future, one must dissect the present and past. Opportunities for occupational therapy practitioners working in the previously discussed agencies is unprecedented. Occupational therapy practitioners have a unique skill set, in which they are more than qualified to work in agencies and help individuals with intellectual disability learn how to find the resources for which they qualify for themselves. When occupational therapy re-examines its current job trends and expands its boundaries more client-centered treatment options become available. It is possible that through occupational therapy practitioners working in more diversified work settings (e.g., government agencies) they are better able to assist adults with intellectual disability in ways that have not been previously explored.

ADVOCACY AND LEGISLATION

The Occupational Therapy Practice Framework: Domain and Process, Third Edition (AOTA, 2014) states that occupational therapy services can be provided directly to an individual client, or a group of individuals, or through advocacy or consultation, and thus, advocacy is an important function of an occupational therapy practitioner (Stover, 2016; Yerxa, 1990). *Advocacy*, as defined by the AOTA (2014), is the empowerment of clients to seek resources and efforts in reaching full occupational participation and performance and promoting occupational justice. Advocacy is showing up for a client in ways that are not always billable but are rather the right thing to do, as in writing letters, attending hearings, advocating for policy change, and educating clients on the importance of self-advocating (Stover, 2016).

It is easy to understand the implications of being an occupational therapy practitioner, and the responsibility of advocating for clients, but it becomes more difficult to create an action plan to become an advocate. Stover (2016) suggests the first step to becoming an advocate is to become aware and educate oneself on specific policies. In addition to becoming aware of policies and legislation that specifically affects clients, it is important to understand the full scope of occupational therapy practice, and to advocate to stakeholders on the medical necessity of occupational therapy services for all clients (Stover, 2016).

It is suspected that the definitions of certain terms will become a point of contention within the changing health care arena in the United States (Stover, 2016). For instance, the qualifying process will be re-examined to determine if an individual has a disability, which will impact his or her eligibility for benefits. Another term under deep inspection will be *medical necessity*, as it is defined as "key term in insurance companies' coverage decisions that usually refers to the medical appropriateness of a particular intervention in a particular case" (Hill, 2012, p. 449). The term medical necessity has variations of its definition, which allows for different stakeholders to interpret its impact on funding differently (Stover, 2016). Knowledge and understanding of key terms will remain a crucial concern of health care stake holders, as legislation is based on definitions to determine eligibility of specific groups of people.

Advocacy can be related through the following different system levels: occupational therapy programs; local, state, and national policy and government; and state and national occupational therapy associations. Occupational therapy programs, including their curricula, faculty members, and fieldwork educators, produce the future practitioners of the profession. Occupational therapy programs can facilitate students to become advocates who are more aware of their civic duties in their future careers through implementing community-based service learning experiences (Maloney, Myers, & Bazyk, 2014). This chapter's second author attests to community-based learning experiences, promoting the value of advocating for individuals with intellectual disability when enrolled at the entry-level, Doctor of Occupational Therapy program at Nova Southeastern University in Fort Lauderdale, Florida. Experiences afforded to occupational therapy students promote a deep-seated responsibility for advocating for underserved people in the community, such as adults with intellectual disability. To advocate for adults with intellectual disability on a local, state, and, even national, level involves becoming an active participant in the conversation of health care policy.

An occupational therapy practitioner is an expert at task analysis and providing the tools for a community program to provide engaging and meaningful activities for adults with intellectual disability for increased participation. On a state level, it is possible to contact and write to state representatives to voice concern over the changes in Medicaid Managed Care, and to better educate on the value of occupational therapy to the adult with intellectual disability population. To advocate on a national level can be somewhat more time consuming, but it is possible. Other than joining the politic arena as a state representative, one is able to participate in his or her state organization for occupational therapy and the AOTA.

PROGRAM IMPLEMENTATION AND POLICY CHANGES

As occupational therapy practitioners, we must be mindful of the policy changes in health care and continue to adapt and grow as a profession to provide the most client-centered, evidence-based services to our clients (Leland, Fogelberg, Halle, & Mroz, 2017). Underserved and at-risk populations, including adults with intellectual disability, face an increased risk of occupational injustice in addition to lack of health care services. Occupational therapy has a place in primary care to provide more comprehensive treatments for adults with intellectual disability (Murphy, Griffith, Mroz, & Jirikowic, 2017). Occupational therapy provides a valid skill set to primary care through implementation of activity analysis and recommendation of compensatory strategies (Roberts et al., 2014). Occupational therapy services in primary care would be able to provide the appropriate recommendations for adults with intellectual disability at the most convenient time, when they are already receiving health care services. The inclusion of occupational therapy in primary care would allow practitioners to provide the timeliest services to their clients, when their occupational performance is likely already being hindered due to a medical condition or lack of preventive care.

A recommended way to serve their clients in a changing health care arena is to provide organization-level consults. Rather than providing treatment interventions to an individual, an occupational therapy practitioner would apply the same recommendations to an organization, and thus provide organization-level consultation (Umeda et al., 2017). Umeda et al. (2017) presents a case study of occupational therapy students providing consultation and collaboration within a science center museum. The students were able to provide a sensory guide, adventure planner, visual schedule, tip sheet for parents, and staff development and training. Parents and museum staff members reported that children and adults with intellectual and developmental disabilities were better able to participate and enjoy the experiences provided by the science center museum (Umeda et al., 2017).

Through changes in policy, adults with intellectual disability are transitioning from living in institutional residential settings to community-based living. An important area for consideration for program implementation and policy change is supported community inclusion, due to the impact on occupational participation and performance, as discussed in this chapter. Identified areas of improvement to support community inclusion, are transportation, post-secondary education, and social supports in group environments (Hall, 2016). Through organization level consultation, occupational therapy is able to create and improve upon transportation, post-secondary education, and social support programs and organizations (King et al., 2017).

In addition to adults with intellectual disability requiring support for inclusion in the community, their families, caregivers, and friends also will benefit from occupational therapy consultation. Families, caregivers, and friends often have difficulties grading activities for the individual with intellectual disability in their lives. Caregivers report that they tend to do the entire activity for their loved one, and are unsure of what they are actually able to complete and with what level of support and supervision. This lack of awareness leads to a feeling of caregiver burnout. Through occupational therapy consultation, caregivers would be able to learn how to provide the "just right challenge" (Ayres, 1979) and create a network of caregivers to provide support (AOTA, 2014).

As mentioned, young adults with intellectual disability are frequently not taught the necessary skills required for successful participation in post-secondary education (Berg et al., 2017). Through occupational therapy school consultation, teachers, staff, and the individuals with intellectual disability would be able to better prepare for the transition from secondary to post-secondary school. This facilitated transition would allow adults with intellectual disability to gain better supported and competitive employment with potentially higher earning salaries and benefits.

An occupation-based employment program is effective for promoting employment for adults with intellectual disability (Dean & Burke, 2017). Case-Smith, Cleary, and Persch (2015) identify that job matching is a collaborative process, with occupational therapy being a key stakeholder when current job matching outcomes are poorly defined. Occupational therapy practitioners need to identify effective outcome measurements for job matching for adults with intellectual disability.

Occupational therapy practitioners may also consult with day programs for adults with intellectual disability in order to provide supports to the staff and in turn provide better occupational experiences for the clients (Mahoney, Roberts, Bryze, & Parker Kent, 2016). Additionally, there is a need for federally funded programs, where adults with intellectual disability can be provided with cost effective housing and supported employment to help cover their living costs (Johnson, Bagatell, & Devault, 2017).

PROMOTING OCCUPATIONAL JUSTICE AND PARTICIPATION

When people are not adequately involved in their chosen meaningful occupations, they can experience feelings of disconnectedness, isolation, and loss of power (Mahoney et al., 2016). These feelings of hopelessness, cultivated through lack of occupational participation, directly impact occupational participation and performance. An *occupational gap*, described by Connor, Wolf, Foster, Hildebrand, and Baum (2014), is when there is a difference between what an individual desires and what the individual actually does for participation. The potential client factors of adults with intellectual disability, the current context, and an environment that frequently affects them (AOTA, 2014) create the possibility for these adults to be at risk for occupational injustices and occupational alienation (Mahoney et al., 2016). Adults in day programs who are not given the proper support or meaningful choices to participate in chosen occupations are at risk of occupational alienation (Townsend & Wilcock, 2004). Occupational justice identifies that "humans are occupational beings," and that participation in meaningful occupations determines the health and quality of life of a person (Stadnyk, Townsend, & Wilcock, 2010, p. 330). When individuals are not able to achieve occupational participation in meaningful occupations, they experience occupational injustice, and their health and quality of life decreases (Stadnyk et al., 2010). Complications of intellectual disability further increase their risk for occupational injustice and alienation.

The Intersection of Occupational Science and Occupational Therapy

Earlier scholarly debate identified a need for separation between the science and the practice of occupation and vice versa, and, later, to articulate the value of occupational science for the practice of occupational therapy (Clark et al., 1993; Mosey, 1993; Yerxa, 2009). It is imperative to continue these healthy discussions; however, conversations need to progress toward building more productive interactions, which lead to collaborations and expanding the scope of occupational science scholarship. Conversations about the evolution of the relatively young science of occupation has spread beyond the United States, especially with its emergence in other countries. South America, for example, highlights that non-English speakers are at a disadvantage, and hindered during global conversations, collaboration, and information sharing in occupational science (Magalhães, Farias, Rivas-Quarneti, Alvarez, & Serrata Malfitano, 2018). Occupational therapy and occupational science have the potential to support domestic and global collaborations that address occupational disparities (e.g., occupational injustice, disruption, deprivation) and including the decolonization of theoretical frameworks (Laliberte Rudman, 2018). Likewise, occupational scientists can draw from educational reformers, such as Philip Magnus, John Dewey, Octavia Hill, Maria Montessori, Eduard Lindeman, and Thomas Kidner, when articulating social and economic justice with occupational engagement and participation (Townsend & Friedland, 2016).

Challenge for Scholarship to Benefit Individuals With Intellectual Disability

During her Ruth Zemke Lecture in Occupational Science, Pierce (2012) posited the promise of occupational science and described occupational science research in four levels that can be applied to study different aspects of occupation (Pierce, 2014). Occupation is a "transactional experience" where people experience interactions among themselves, their environment, and other people, communities, and organizations, as they participate in their chosen occupations (Dickie, Cutchin, & Humphry, 2006). As such, this allows for conceptualization of an individual's participation and engagement in occupations, environment, and context. Understanding occupation as a transactional experience, and furthering research in occupational science, allows occupational therapy practitioners to advocate for adults with intellectual disability through the identification of the supports needed for community involvement and for more independent living (Lamb & Metzler, 2014). The concepts and levels of research provided by occupational science allows occupational therapy practitioners to describe the varied occupations of adults with intellectual disability and draw from related disciplines, such as psychology and anthropology. Then, to further explain the occupations of adults with intellectual disability, predict their occupations across time, and apply this information to foster changes to current and future occupational therapy practice, designed to reduce occupational injustices for this population.

Deciding to contribute to best practice is an intentional choice. Clinicians and committed researchers can select to read and/or conduct occupational therapy and/or occupational science research in one or more of four levels. Descriptive in nature, the first level of research aims to describe occupation and serves as the basis for all other levels (Pierce, 2014). An example of a study at this level describes the experiences of loneliness and the daily occupations of adults with intellectual disability (McVilly et al., 2006). The second level, or relational research, combines research from other disciplines with the construct of occupation (Pierce, 2014). This fosters collaboration with other professions, such as anthropology, sociology, and psychology. For example, Simões and Santos (2016) examined the quality of life of individuals with and without intellectual disability by describing their daily occupations. The least developed of the four levels is the third level, or predictive research. It attempts to identify patterns of occupation across groups of individuals (Pierce, 2014). This level of research is closely connected to descriptive research and expands upon descriptive theories. This level is important to occupational therapy practice; however, it cannot be developed further until level one research more fully describes occupation (Pierce, 2014).

The level of occupational science research that is most related to occupational therapy practice is the fourth level, or prescriptive research. This level involves the application of occupational science to occupational therapy practice (Pierce, 2014), and further research at this level can provide scholarly work with systematic studies for the practice of occupational therapy (Howick, 2009). An example of prescriptive research is an exploratory study of 10 occupational therapy practitioners and their practice in community settings (Ramsey, 2011).

CONCLUSION

Adults with intellectual disability have greater unmet needs compared to the general population. Guided by Vision 2025 from the AOTA, occupational therapists and scientists have many opportunities to benefit individuals with intellectual disability. Introduced in 2016, the vision states "As an inclusive profession, occupational therapy maximizes health, well-being, and quality of life for all people, populations, and communities through effective solutions that facilitate participation in everyday living" (AOTA, 2016). The literature provides exemplars of scholarly work of interest regarding the intellectual disability population. Some of them were mentioned in the earlier sections of this chapter and additional inspirations follow.

A recent scoping review that explored health care access by adults with intellectual and/or developmental disabilities revealed opportunities for occupational therapy to address health care access by engaging in research and developing interventions, which can lead to improved occupational participation and changes in the health care environment. There is a need to remove barriers to employment for individuals with intellectual disability. This will open opportunities beyond unskilled or low-skill employment. Future interventions aimed at vocational training need to include social and other experiences, which leads to better programming that leads to qualifications for higher level employment (McDaniels, 2016). Likewise, Haines, Wright, and Comerasamy (2018) suggested initiating a cultural shift in how occupational therapists and other professionals work with direct support workers. Appropriate collaboration can lead to improved education and training to open possibilities for improved quality of life for people with intellectual disability. Channon (2014) also expressed the need to address occupational barriers that impede the ability of individuals with intellectual disability to engage in meaningful activities. The barriers result in a lived experience of social injustice, highlighting the need to address participation factors in physical, social, political, and economic areas.

Comparing intervention strategies provides the opportunity for guidance toward best practice. Selanikyo, Yalon-Chamovitz, and Weintraub (2017) investigated school participation by students with intellectual and developmental disabilities by comparing results from two intervention models, providing a combination of in-service and collaborative consultation, which involved an interprofessional team, including an occupational therapist, and another model that provided an in-service program to teachers. Both groups had teacher participants. Subjects were school children from 8 to 20 years of age. The intervention aimed to improve three participation skills: communication, making choices, and initiation. The results showed that children in the collaborative consultation group improved in all areas, while the in-service group declined.

When compared to typical adults, individuals with intellectual disability are prone to diminished active occupational participation in using time and space. By providing educational and consultative services, occupational therapy can promote ways to diversify participation for individuals with intellectual disability to reduce dependency, increase mobility, and facilitate appropriate occupational choices (Crowe, Salazar, Kertcher, & LaSalle, 2015). Increasingly, students with intellectual and/or developmental disabilities are pursuing college education. Beyond academic preparation, individuals with intellectual and/or developmental disabilities have to learn social and other prerequisites that are not necessarily part of an explicit curriculum, which include employment, social support, and use of public transportation (Berg et al., 2017). Service providers can promote the development of these skills through a hidden curriculum, which are not necessarily outside the scope of occupational therapy

Gil-Llario, Morell-Mengual, Ballester-Arnal, and Díaz-Rodríguez (2018) considered the high level of sexual activity among individuals with intellectual disability, and studied a sample of equally distributed 180 men and 180 women. They proposed that educational programming is imperative to address gender specific content, abuse prevention, and use of effective prophylactics. Representation of individuals with intellectual disability in movies potentially affects access to meaningful and appropriate participation and achievement of occupational potential (Renwick, Fudge Schormans, & Shore, 2013). Most commonly, portrayal of individuals with intellectual and/or developmental disabilities project child-like or simplified participation in otherwise complex occupations, such as cognitively challenging jobs. This portrayal may influence the perception of movie consumers, who may have films as their only source of contact with these individuals.

This final chapter identified current issues surrounding individuals with intellectual disability, discussed funding and services available to adults with intellectual disability, calculated the need for advocacy and legislation, discussed the promotion of occupational justice, and related research guided by occupational science. Hopefully, this chapter painted a realistic vision and provided information that opened the door for the student or practitioner in their journey of occupational therapy and science, which can only benefit individuals with special needs, especially those with intellectual disability.

REFERENCES

American Disabilities Act National Network. (2017). Learn about the national network. Retrieved from https://adata.org/national-network

American Occupational Therapy Association. (2007). AOTA's centennial vision and executive summary. *American Journal of Occupational Therapy, 61*, 613-614. doi: 10.5014/ajot.61.6.613

American Occupational Therapy Association. (2014). Occupational therapy practice framework: Domain and process, 3rd edition. *American Journal of Occupational Therapy, 68*(Suppl. 1), S1-S48.

American Occupational Therapy Association. (2016). AOTA unveils Vision 2025. Retrieved from https://www.aota.org/AboutAOTA/vision-2025.aspx

Arnold, M. J., & Rybski, D. (2010). Occupational justice. In M. E. Scaffa, S. M. Reitz, & M. A. Pizzi (Eds.), *Occupational therapy in the promotion of health and wellness* (pp. 135-156). Philadelphia, PA: F. A. Davis.

Association on Higher Education and Disability. (2017). About AHEAD. Retrieved from https://www.ahead.org/about

Ayres, A. J. (1979). *Sensory integration and the child.* Torrance, CA: Western Psychological Services.

Benefits.gov (2017). Looking for benefits? Retrieved from https://www.benefits.gov

Berg, L. A., Jirikowic, T., Haerling, K., & MacDonald, G. (2017). Centennial topics: Navigating the hidden curriculum of higher education for postsecondary students with intellectual disabilities. *American Journal of Occupational Therapy, 71*, 7103100020. doi: 10.5014.ajot.2017.024703

Burke, M. M., & Heller, T. (2017). Disparities in unmet services needs among adults with intellectual and other developmental disabilities. *Journal of Applied Research in Intellectual Disabilities, 30*, 898-910. doi: 10.1111/jar.12282

Case-Smith, J., Cleary, D., & Persch, A. (2015). Current practices in job matching for individuals with intellectual and developmental disabilities. *American Journal of Occupational Therapy, 69*, 6911500099. doi: 10.5014/ajot.2015.69S1-PO4089

Center on Technology and Disability. (2017). Retrieved from www.ctdinstitute.org

Centers for Parent Information & Resources. (2017). Services for adults with disabilities. Retrieved from www.parentcenterhub.org/foradults

Channon, A. (2014) Intellectual disability and activity engagement: Exploring the literature from an occupational perspective, *Journal of Occupational Science, 21*(4), 443-458. doi: 10.1080/14427591.2013.829398

Chatterjee, P., & Sommers, B. D. (2017). The economics of Medicaid reform and block grants. *Journal of the American Medical Association, 317*(10), 1007-1008. doi: 10.1001/jama.2017.0901

Clark, F., Zemke, R., Frank, G., Parham, D., Neville-Jan, A., Hedricks, C., … Abreu, B. (1993). Dangers inherent in the partition of occupational therapy and occupational science. *American Journal of Occupational Therapy, 47*(1), 184-186. doi: 10.5014/ajot.47.2.184

Connor, L. T., Wolf, T. J., Foster, E. R., Hildebrand, M. W., & Baum, C. M. (2014). Participation and engagement in occupation in adults with disabilities. In D. Pierce (Ed.), *Occupational science for occupational therapists* (pp. 107-120). Thorofare, NJ: SLACK Incorporated.

Cooper, S., Smiley, E., Morrison, J., Williamson, A., & Allan, L. (2007). Mental ill-health in adults with intellectual disabilities: Prevalence and associated factors. *British Journal of Psychiatry, 190*, 27-35. doi: 10.1192/pjp.bp.106.022483

Crowe, T. K., Salazar, S., J., Kertcher, E. F., & LaSalle, J. (2015). Time and space use of adults with intellectual disabilities. *The Open Journal of Occupational Therapy 3*(2), 2. doi: 10.15453/2168-6408.1124

Dean, E., & Burke, K. (2017). Career development for adults with intellectual disability: Pilot outcomes from a community-based employment program. *American Journal of Occupational Therapy, 71*. doi: 10.5014/ajot.2017.71S1-RP401C

Dickie, V., Cutchin, M. P., & Humphry, R. (2006). Occupation as a transactional experience: A critique of individualism in occupational science. *Journal of Occupational Science, 13*(1), 83-93. doi: 10.1080/14427591.2006.9686573

Felce, D. (2017). Community living for adults with intellectual disabilities: Unravelling the cost effectiveness discourse. *Journal of Policy and Practice in Intellectual Disabilities, 14*(3), 187-197. doi: 10.1111/jppi.12180

The Florida Senate. (2017). CS/SB 916: Statewide Medicaid managed care program. Retrieved from www.flsenate.gov/Session/Bill/2017/00916/?Tab=BillHistory

Francisco, I., & Carlson, G. (2002). Occupational therapy and people with intellectual disability from culturally diverse backgrounds. *Australian Occupational Therapy Journal. 49*, 200-211.

Garrison-Wade, D. F. (2012). Listening to their voices: Factors that inhibit or enhance postsecondary outcomes for students with disabilities. *International Journal of Special Education, 27*, 113-125.

Gil-Llario, M. D., Morell-Mengual, V., Ballester-Arnal, R., & Díaz-Rodríguez, I. (2018). The experience of sexuality in adults with intellectual disability. *Journal of Intellectual Disability Research, 62*(1), 72-80. doi: 10.1111/jir.12455

Goodwill Industries International. (2017). Careers at Goodwill. Retrieved from http://www.goodwill.org/find-jobs-and-services/careers-at-goodwill

Haines, D., Wright, J., & Comerasamy, H. (2018). Occupational therapy empowering support workers to change how they support people with profound intellectual and multiple disabilities to engage in activity. *Journal of Policy and Practice in Intellectual Disabilities, 15*, 295-306. doi:10.1111/jppi.12257

Hall, S. A. (2016). Community involvement of young adults with intellectual disabilities: Their experiences and perspectives on inclusion. *Journal of Applied Research in Intellectual Disabilities, 30*, 859-871. doi: 10.1111/jar.12276

Hermans, H., & Evenhuis, H. M. (2014). Multimorbidity in older adults with intellectual disabilities. *Research in Developmental Disabilities, 35*(4), 776-783. doi: 10.1016/j.ridd.2014.01.022

Heyman, M., Stokes, J. E., & Siperstein, G. N. (2016). Not all jobs are the same: Predictors of job quality for adults with intellectual disabilities. *Journal of Vocational Rehabilitation, 44*, 299-306. doi: 10.3233/JVR-160800

Hill, J. B. (2012). What is the meaning of health? Constitutional implications of defining "medical necessity" and "essential health benefits under the Affordable Care Act. *Faculty Publications.* Retrieved from http://scholarlycommons.law.case.edu/faculty_publications/81

Howick, J. (2009). Oxford Centre for Evidence-based Medicine—Levels of evidence. Retrieved from www.cebm.net/oxford-centre-evidence-based-medicine-levels-evidence-march-2009

Johnson, K., Bagatell, N., & Devault, M. (2017). Beyond custodial care: Mediating the possibilities for meaningful participation in an institutional setting. *American Journal of Occupational Therapy, 17*, 7111510192p1. doi: 10.5014/ajot.2017.71S1-PO4059

Kaiser Family Foundation. (2017). Medicaid in California. Retrieved from http://files.kff.org/attachment/fact-sheet-medicaid-state-CA

King, E., Okodogbe, T., Burke, E., McCarron, M., McCallion, P., & O'Donovan, M. A. (2017). Activities of daily living and transition to community living for adults with intellectual disabilities. *Scandinavian Journal of Occupational Therapy, 24*(5), 357-365. doi: 10.1080/11038128.2016.1227369

Krahn, G. L., Hammond, L., & Turner, A. (2006). A cascade of disparities: Health and health care access for people with intellectual disabilities. *Developmental Disabilities Research Reviews, 12*(1), 70-82. doi: 10.1002/mrdd.20098

Laliberte Rudman, D. (2018). Occupational therapy and occupational science: Building critical and transformative alliances. *Brazilian Journal of Occupational Therapy, 26*(1), 241-249. doi: 10.4322/2526-8910.ctoEN1246

Lamb, A. J., & Metzler, C. A. (2014). Health policy perspectives—Defining the value of occupational therapy: A health policy lens on research and practice. *American Journal of Occupational, 68*, 9-14. doi: 10.5014/ajot.2014.681001

Leland, N. E., Fogelberg, D. J., Halle, A. D., & Mroz, T. M. (2017). Health policy perspectives—Occupational therapy and management of multiple chronic conditions in the context of health care reform. *American Journal of Occupational Therapy, 71*, 7101090010. doi: 10.5014/ajot.2017.711001

Magalhães, L., Farias, L., Rivas-Quarneti. N., Alvarez, L., & Serrata Malfitano, A. P. (2018). The development of occupational science outside the Anglophone sphere: Enacting global collaboration. *Journal of Occupational Science, 26*(2), 181-192. doi: 10.1080/14427591.2018.1530133

Mahoney, W. J., Roberts, E., Bryze, K., & Parker Kent, J. A. (2016). Brief report—Occupational engagement with adults with intellectual disabilities. *American Journal of Occupational Therapy, 70*, 7001350030. doi: 10.5014/ajot2016.016576

Maloney, S. M., Myers, C., & Bazyk, J. (2014). The influence of a community-based service-learning experience on the development of occupational therapy students' feelings of civic responsibility. *Occupational Therapy in Mental Health, 30*(2), 144-161. doi: 10.1080/0164212X.2014.91060

McDaniels, B. (2016). Disproportionate opportunities: Fostering vocational choice for individuals with intellectual disabilities. *Journal of Vocational Rehabilitation, 45*, 19-25. doi: 10.3233/JVR-160807

McIntyre, L. L., Blacher, J., & Baker, B. L. (2002). Behaviour/mental health problems in young adults with intellectual disability: The impact on families. *Journal of Intellectual Disability Research, 46*(3), 239-249. doi:10.1046/j.1365-2788.2002.00371.x

McVilly, K. R., Stancliffe, R. J., Parmenter, T. R., & Burton-Smith, R. M. (2006). 'I get by with a little help from my friends': Adults with intellectual disability discuss loneliness. *Journal of Applied Research in Intellectual Disabilities, 19*(2), 191-203.

Mosey. A. (1993). Partition of occupational science and occupational therapy. *American Journal of Occupational Therapy, 40*(9), 851-853.

Murphy, A. D., Griffith, V. M., Mroz, T. M., & Jirikowic, T. L. (2017). Health policy perspectives—Primary care for underserved populations: Navigating policy to incorporate occupational therapy into federally qualified health centers. *American Journal of Occupational Therapy, 71*, 7102090010. doi: 10.5014/ajot.2017.712001

National Center for College Students with Disabilities. (2017). Retrieved from http://www.nccsdonline.org

National Public Website on Assistive Technology. (2017). *State Tech ACT Projects*. Retrieved from http://assistivetech.net/webresources/stateTechActProjects.php

Oertle, K. M., & Bragg, D. D. (2014). Transitioning students with disabilities: Community college policies and practices. *Journal of Disability Policy Studies, 25*, 59-67. doi: 10.1177/1044207314526435

Pierce, D. (2012) Promise. *Journal of Occupational Science. 19*(4), 298-311, doi: 10.1080/14427591.2012.667778

Pierce, D. (2014). *Occupational science for occupational therapy*. Thorofare, NJ: SLACK, Incorporated.

Ramsey, R. (2011). Voices of community-practicing occupational therapists: An exploratory study. *Occupational Therapy in Health Care, 25*(2/3), 140-149. doi: 10.3109/07380577.2011.569856

Renwick, R., Fudge Schormans, A., & Shore, D. (2013). Hollywood takes on intellectual/developmental disability: Cinematic representation of occupational participation. *Occupation, Participation and Health, 34*(1), 20-31. doi: 10.3928/15394492-20131118-01

Roberts, P., Amini, D., Farmer, M., Lamb, A., Muir, S., & Siebert, C. (2014). Occupational therapy in primary care. American Occupational Therapy Association. Retrieved from http://www.aota.org/-/medical/Corporate/Files/Publications/Primary-Care-Position-Paper.PDF

Selanikyo, E., Yalon-Chamovitz, S., & Weintraub. N. (2017). Enhancing classroom participation of students with intellectual and developmental disabilities. *Canadian Journal of Occupational Therapy, 84*(2), 76-86. doi: 10.1177/0008417416661346

Simões, C., & Santos, S. (2016). Comparing the quality of life of adults with and without intellectual disability. *Journal of Intellectual Disability Research, 60*(4), 378-388. doi: 10.1111/jir.12256

Social Security Administration. (2017). Benefits for people with disabilities. Retrieved from https://www.ssa.gov/disability

Stadnyk, R. L., Townsend, E. A., & Wilcock, A. A., (2010) Occupational justice. In C. H. Christiansen, & E. A. Townsend (Eds.) *Introduction to occupation: The art and science of living* (2nd ed., pp. 329-358). Upper Saddle River, NJ: Pearson Education Inc.

Stover, A. D. (2016). Health policy perspectives—Client-centered advocacy. Every occupational therapy practitioner's responsibility to understand medical necessity. *American Journal of Occupational Therapy, 70,* 7005090010. doi: 10.5014/ajot.2016.705003

Townsend, E., & Friedland, J. (2016). Teaching occupation: 19th & 20th century educational reforms arising in Europe, the United Kingdom, and the Americas: Inspiration for occupational science? *Journal of Occupational Science, 23*(4), 488-495. doi: 10.1080/14427591.2016.1232184

Townsend, E., & Wilcock, A. A. (2004). Occupational justice and client-centered practice: A dialogue in progress. *Canadian Journal of Occupational Therapy, 71,* 75-87. doi: 10.1177/000841740407100203

Umeda, C. J., Fogelberg, D. J., Jirikowic, T., Pitonyak, J. S., Mroz, T. M., & Ideishi, R. I. (2017). Expanding the implementation of Americans with Disabilities Act for populations with intellectual and developmental disabilities: The role of organization-level occupational therapy consultation. *American Journal of Occupational Therapy, 71,* 7104090010. doi: 10.5014/ajot.2017.714001

United States Adaptive Recreation Center. (2017). Retrieved from http://usarc.org

University of Kansas. (2017). Research & training center on independent living. Retrieved from http://rtcil.org/training/overview

Williamson, H. J., Contreras, G. M., Rodriguez, E. S., Smith, J. M., & Perkins, E. A. (2017). Health care access for adults with intellectual and developmental disabilities: A scoping review. *Occupation, Participation and Health, 37*(4), 227-236. doi: 10:1177/1539449217714148

Williamson, H., Perkins, E., Lulinski, A., Armstrong, M., Baldwin, J., Levin, B., & Massey, O. (2017). Medicaid managed care and adults with intellectual or developmental disabilities and their family caregivers. *American Journal of Occupational Therapy, 71,* 7111510167p1. doi: 10.5014/ajot.2017.71S1-RP401A

Yerxa, E. J. (1990). An introduction to occupational science, a foundation for occupational therapy in the 21st century. *Occupational Therapy in Health Care, 6*(4), 1-17.

Yerxa, E. J. (2009). The infinite distance between the I and the it. *American Journal of Occupational Therapy, 63*(4), 490-497.

Financial Disclosures

Dr. Meghan G. Blaskowitz has no financial or proprietary interest in the materials presented herein.

Dr. Kimberly Bryze has no financial or proprietary interest in the materials presented herein.

Dr. Susan M. Cahill has no financial or proprietary interest in the materials presented herein.

Dr. Ricardo C. Carrasco has no financial or proprietary interest in the materials presented herein.

Katie Coakley has no financial or proprietary interest in the materials presented herein.

Dr. Mariana D'Amico has no financial or proprietary interest in the materials presented herein.

Dr. Evan E. Dean has no financial or proprietary interest in the materials presented herein.

Dr. Kelsea Rose A. Grampp has no financial or proprietary interest in the materials presented herein.

Dr. Joy Hammel has no financial or proprietary interest in the materials presented herein

Dr. Jenna Heffron has no financial or proprietary interest in the materials presented herein.

Dr. E. Adel Herge has no financial or proprietary interest in the materials presented herein.

Joy Hyzny has no financial or proprietary interest in the materials presented herein.

Dr. Anne F. Kiraly-Alvarez has no financial or proprietary interest in the materials presented herein.

Dr. Lisa Mahaffey has no financial or proprietary interest in the materials presented herein.

Dr. Wanda J. Mahoney has no financial or proprietary interest in the materials presented herein.

Dr. Monika Robinson has no financial or proprietary interest in the materials presented herein.

Dr. Alisa Jordan Sheth has no financial or proprietary interest in the materials presented herein.

Daniel Stumpf has no financial or proprietary interest in the materials presented herein.

Dr. Minetta Wallingford has no financial or proprietary interest in the materials presented herein.

Index

bathing, assistive devices for, 152
becoming, 139-142
behavior
    attention seeking, 35-36
    sensory contributions to, 80-81
being, 139-142
beliefs
    importance of, 141
    shaping occupational therapy approach, 42
    spiritual, 144
belonging, 139-142
Best Buddies Program, 65
best practice, 149, 209-212, 237-238
Boardmaker software, 78
boundaries, social skills and, 65-66
brain
    injury to, 2
    neural networks in, 30-31

Canadian Occupational Performance Measure
    (COPM), 126
care coordinator, 200
caregivers, 207-208
    family as, 62-63
    occupational therapy interventions with, 93
    support from, 101
case manager, 200
causal agency theory, 52-53
Centers for Medicare & Medicaid payment
    reforms, 185, 186
Centers for Parent Information & Resources,
    231
Certificate in Contemporary Living, 164
Checklist of Adaptive Living Skills (CALS), 79
choice making, 52, 54, 56, 57
Circle of Friends Program, 65
civil rights, impacting intellectual disability
    policy, 13-14
client, value of, 42-43
coaching, 220, 223-224, 226
    definition of, 223
    solution-focused, 223-224
    to support leisure participation, 130-131
Cognitive Orientation to daily Occupational
    Performance (CO-OP), 56
collaboration, 220, 221-222, 226
    in primary care setting, 198-199
    supports and barriers to, 223
collaborative partners, 222
collaborative style, 222
communication, assistive devices for, 154
community-based living, transitioning to, 20,
    235
Community First Choice option, 19
community housing options, 18
community integration movement, 111

community life
    barriers in, 231
    daily adaptations to, 46-47
    inclusion in, 235
    occupational therapy in, 6
community mobility devices, 154
competence/competency, 45
    essential elements of, 46
    individual, 45-46
competency-based model, 45-47
competitive employment, 113
Comprehensive Primary Care Plus Model, 185,
    186
computer technology, 156
conceptual models, 42, 43-49
Consolation House, 110
consultant role, 200
consultation, 220-221
    case example of, 224-226
    collaborative, 221-222
        supports and barriers to, 223
context
    with daily routine, 58
    participation in, 52-58
co-occupation, 103-104
coordination of health care services, 199
culture, collaborative, 222

daily routine, 58
dating, 65
day centers, 132-133
day program consultation, 235
decision making, 56
    supported, 176
deep touch pressure, 37
deinstitutionalization, 231
dementia, 207
depression, 65
developmental centers, 13
Developmental Disability Act Amendment, 111
developmental models, 43-44
diagnostic overshadowing, 30
dignity, 43, 47-48
disability
    as mismatch between abilities and
        environment, 55
    qualifying process for, 234
disability rights movements, 17
doing, 139-142
Down syndrome, 2
    dementia and, 207
dressing, assistive devices for, 152
Dunton, William Rush, 110
dynamic assessment, 77-78

Printed in the United States
by Baker & Taylor Publisher Services